Atlas of
HEART DISEASES

HEART DISEASE IN THE PRESENCE OF DISORDERS OF OTHER ORGAN SYSTEMS

Volume VI

Atlas of
HEART DISEASES

HEART DISEASE IN THE PRESENCE OF DISORDERS OF OTHER ORGAN SYSTEMS

Volume VI

VOLUME EDITOR

Michael H. Crawford, MD

Robert S. Flinn Professor
Chief, Division of Cardiology
The University of New Mexico School of Medicine
Albuquerque, New Mexico

SERIES EDITOR

Eugene Braunwald, MD, MD (Hon), ScD (Hon)

Hersey Professor of the Theory and Practice of Medicine
Harvard Medical School
Chairman, Department of Medicine
Brigham and Women's Hospital
Boston, Massachusetts

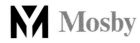

St. Louis Baltimore Boston Carlsbad Chicago Naples New York Philadelphia Portland
London Madrid Mexico City Singapore Sydney Tokyo Toronto Wiesbaden

Developed by Current Medicine Inc., Philadelphia

CURRENT MEDICINE

400 MARKET STREET, SUITE 700 • PHILADELPHIA, PA 19106

Development Editors .... *Diane Q. Forti,*
Maureen McNally

Designer .... *Lisa Caro*

Illustrators .... *Birck Cox, Wendy Jackelow,*
Liz Kazanecki,
Lisa Antonucci Messina

Art Director .... *Paul Fennessy*

Illustration Director .... *Ann Saydlowski*

Production .... *David Myers,*
Lori Holland

Indexing .... *Alexandra Nickerson*

Distribution rights for North America
and territories not listed below:
MOSBY-YEAR BOOK, INC.
11830 Westline Industrial Drive
St. Louis, MO 63146

In Canada: TIMES MIRROR
PROFESSIONAL PUBLISHING LTD.
130 Flaska Drive • Markham, Ontario
Canada L6G 1B8

Distribution rights for Central and
South America: NUEVA EDITORIAL
INTERAMERICANA, SA DE CV.

Distribution rights for Japan:
NANKODO CO LTD.

Distribution rights for Indian Subcontinent
and South East Asia (except Japan):
TIMES MIRROR INTERNATIONAL
PUBLISHERS, LTD.

Heart disease in the presence of disorders of other organ systems/volume editor,
Michael H. Crawford.
p. cm. – (Atlas of heart diseases; v. 6)
Includes bibliographical references and index.
ISBN 1-878132-28-8 (hardcover)
1. Cardiological manifestations of general diseases—Atlases. I.
Crawford, Michael H., 1943-. II. Series.
[DNLM: 1. Heart Diseases—etiology—atlases. WG 17 A8816 1996 v.6]
RC682.A818 1996 vol. 6
[RC682]
616.1'2 s—dc20
[616.1'2071]
DNLM/DLC   95-24438
for Library of Congress   CIP

Library of Congress Cataloging-in-Publication Data
ISBN 1-878132-28-8

Printed in Singapore by Imago Productions (FE) Ltd.

10   9   8   7   6   5   4   3   2   1

SERIES PREFACE

Disorders of the cardiovascular system are the most common causes of death and serious morbidity in the industrialized world. In 1991, more than 40% of all deaths in the United States were attributed to cardiac and vascular diseases. These conditions accounted for almost 5 million years of potential life lost.

Despite these sobering statistics, progress in cardiovascular medicine has been immense, and is, in fact, accelerating. Our understanding of the pathobiology of most forms of heart disease has advanced steadily and there have been enormous advances in the diagnosis, treatment, and prevention of cardiovascular disorders. For example, during just one decade, from 1981 to 1991, the overall death rates from cardiovascular disease declined by 26% and death rates from acute myocardial infarction and stroke declined by 32%. Similar progress has been made in other major cardiovascular disorders, including hypertension, valvular and congenital heart disease, congestive heart failure, and the arrhythmias.

The physician responsible for the care of patients with cardiovascular disease now has a number of vehicles available for obtaining up-to-date information, including excellent journals and textbooks of every conceivable size, scope, and depth. In developing new strategies for transmitting information about these conditions, it is important to consider that cardiovascular medicine is the most "visual" of medical specialties. Cardiovascular diagnosis is based on the recognition and understanding of a variety of graphic waveforms, images, decision trees, and microscopic sections. Treatment increasingly involves the intelligent use of algorithms, which are most effectively portrayed visually. Likewise, mechanical correction of cardiovascular disorders, whether catheter-based or surgical, can best be described pictorially. This *Atlas of Heart Diseases* has been designed to provide a detailed and comprehensive visual exposition of all aspects of cardiovascular medicine. Several thousand images, accompanied by detailed captions, have been carefully selected by expert authors and reviewed by the 12 distinguished Volume Editors. These images are now available separately in print and slide form and also will soon be formatted for CD-ROM use.

Many people deserve credit for the successful completion of this ambitious effort. The expertise and hard work of the authors and the devoted efforts of the Volume Editors naturally form the foundation of the *Atlas of Heart Diseases*. Great credit is also due to Abe Krieger, President of Current Medicine, who conceived the *Atlas* series; to Maureen McNally, the extremely effective Development Editor; and to Kathryn Saxon, who coordinated the efforts in my office.

All of us who have been engaged in this project hope that each individual volume, and the entire *Atlas*, will be useful to physicians of all specialties who are responsible for the care of patients with cardiovascular disorders, to investigators and teachers of cardiovascular medicine, and ultimately to the millions of patients worldwide with disorders of the heart and circulation.

Eugene Braunwald, MD

PREFACE

In the current cardiology practice arena, the ability to be a complete consultant in cardiovascular diseases is more important than ever. Now and in the near future, cardiologists will likely survive by either performing very highly specialized procedures or by being indispensable, broad-based consultants and caregivers in all aspects of cardiovascular disease. It is the latter role with which this part of the *Atlas of Heart Diseases* is concerned.

The 10 chapters in this part of the volume cover a wide spectrum of conditions that affect the cardiovascular system. Connective tissue diseases frequently involve the heart, often in clinically subtle ways; however, among patients with systemic lupus erythematosus, heart disease is the third most common cause of death. Most endocrine disorders have adverse effects on the heart. The best known is diabetes, which is a risk factor for atherosclerosis, but thyroid, adrenal, and growth hormone problems also cause cardiac disease. Hematologic diseases can have profound effects on the cardiovascular system. In addition to the circulatory effects of anemia, certain types of anemia can lead to organ infarction, hemochromatosis, and cardiac arrhythmias. Also, hematologic malignancies can directly invade or compress the heart. Abnormal blood coagulation frequently causes or exacerbates cardiac disease, and the various agents used to modify blood coagulation have become almost universal in the treatment of heart disease. Finally, many neuromuscular diseases adversely affect the heart, often leading to cardiomyopathy.

Pregnancy, which is not usually injurious to the heart, can aggravate other pre-existing heart conditions. A thorough knowledge of the hemodynamic changes that take place during normal pregnancy is important for managing the pregnant patient with heart disease. Nutritional and metabolic disorders may have profound effects on heart function, the most prominent of which is excessive alcohol intake, although other drugs and toxins frequently cause cardiac disorders. Cocaine use is a major problem, and has been the cause of death in prominent athletes. Usually, athletic activity strengthens the heart, but it can be risky in the person with pre-existing heart disease or in the presence of certain toxins. It is also important to be able to distinguish heart disease from changes in the heart that occur in response to athletic training. Finally, environmental conditions can affect the heart, such as high altitude, diving, and cold exposure. With the increased emphasis on physical fitness and recreational activities, environmentally related cardiac problems are being seen more frequently.

The major visual presentations of cardiovascular involvement in all of these conditions are presented throughout the chapters, along with considerable explanatory text. Pertinent diagnostic facts and forms of treatment are presented in tabular form. The information provided in the *Atlas* is an excellent brief review of clinical problems for the experienced physician, and an excellent visually oriented starting point for the novice. Thus, students, trainees, and physicians at all levels of expertise should find this volume of value in the current practice of cardiology.

Michael H. Crawford, MD

CONTRIBUTORS

JAMES D. ANHOLM, MD
Assistant Professor of Medicine
Loma Linda School of Medicine
Medical Director, Pulmonary
  Function Laboratory
Pulmonary Section
Jerry L. Pettis Veterans' Affairs Medical Center
Loma Linda, California

C. GUNNAR BLOMQVIST, MD
Professor of Internal Medicine
  and Physiology
Southwestern Medical School
Division of Cardiology
The University of Texas
  Southwestern Medical Center
Dallas, Texas

JAY C. BUCKEY, MD
Adjunct Assistant Professor of Medicine
Southwestern Medical School
Department of Internal Medicine
The University of Texas
  Southwestern Medical Center
Dallas, Texas

P. ANTHONY N. CHANDRARATNA, MD
Bauer and Bauer Rawlins Professor
  of Cardiology
Professor of Medicine
University of Southern California
Associate Chief of Cardiology
Director, Echocardiography/
  Graphics Laboratory
LAC/USC Medical Center
Los Angeles, California

DAVID R. FERRY, MD
Associate Professor of Medicine
Loma Linda University School of Medicine
Chief, Cardiology Section
Jerry L. Pettis Veterans' Affairs Medical Center
Loma Linda, California

MIHAI GHEORGHIADE, MD
Professor of Medicine
Northwestern University
  Medical School
Associate Chief of Cardiology
Chief, Cardiology Clinical Service
Northwestern Memorial Hospital
Chicago, Illinois

L. DAVID HILLIS, MD
James M. Wooten Chair in Cardiology
Professor of Internal Medicine
Associate Director, Division
  of Cardiology
The University of Texas
  Southwestern Medical Center
Co-director, Cardiac Catheterization
  Laboratory
Parkland Memorial Hospital
Dallas, Texas

J. LAWRENCE HUTCHISON, MD
Associate Professor of Medicine
  and Oncology
Senior Physician, Montreal General
  Hospital
McGill University
Montreal, Canada

STUART J. HUTCHISON, MD
Postdoctoral Fellow
Cardiology Division, Moffitt Hospital
University of California, San Francisco
San Francisco, California

LYNDA D. LANE, MS, RN
Senior Research Scientist
Division of Cardiology
The University of Texas
  Southwestern Medical Center
Dallas, Texas

RICHARD A. LANGE, MD

Jonsson-Rogers Chair in Cardiology
The University of Texas
  Southwestern Medical Center
Co-director, Cardiac Catheterization
  Laboratory
Parkland Memorial Hospital
Dallas, Texas

BENJAMIN D. LEVINE, MD

Assistant Professor of Medicine
Division of Cardiology
The University of Texas
  Southwestern Medical Center
Institute for Exercise
  and Environmental Medicine
Presbyterian Hospital
Dallas, Texas

JONATHAN R. LINDNER, MD

Clinical and Research Fellow
Cardiovascular Division
University of Virginia
  Health Sciences Center
Charlottesville, Virginia

BARRY J. MARON, MD

Director, Cardiovascular Research
  Division
Minneapolis Heart Institute Foundation
Minneapolis, Minnesota

ILEANA L. PIÑA, MD

Associate Professor of Medicine
Director, Cardiomyopathy
Director, Cardiac Rehabilitation
Temple University Hospital
Cardiomyopathy and
  Transplant Center
Philadelphia, Pennsylvania

CARLOS A. ROLDAN, MD

Assistant Professor of Medicine
Division of Cardiology
University of New Mexico Hospital
Albuquerque, New Mexico

B. SYLVIA VELA, MD

Assistant Professor
Department of Medicine
University of New Mexico
  School of Medicine
Staff Physician, Endocrinology Section
VA Medical Center
Albuquerque, New Mexico

**CHRIS WACHHOLZ,
RN, MBA**

Divers Alert Network (DAN)
Duke University Medical Center
Durham, North Carolina

CAROLE A. WARNES, MD

Associate Professor
Mayo Medical School
Consultant in Cardiovascular Diseases,
  Internal Medicine, and Pediatric Cardiology
Mayo Clinic
Rochester, Minnesota

STEPHEN M. ZAACKS, MD

Department of Internal Medicine
Northwestern University
  Medical School
Northwestern Memorial Hospital
Chicago, Illinois

ROSS R. ZIMMER, MD

Instructor
Department of Medicine
Division of Cardiology
Temple University Hospital
Philadelphia, Pennsylvania

CONTENTS

CHAPTER 4

ANTICOAGULANT, ANTITHROMBOTIC, AND THROMBOLYTIC THERAPY
Stephen M. Zaacks and Mihai Gheorghiade

CHAPTER 5

PREGNANCY AND THE HEART
Carole A. Warnes

CHAPTER 6

HEART DISEASE IN THE PRESENCE OF NEUROLOGIC DISEASE
Ileana L. Piña and Ross R. Zimmer

CHAPTER 7

ALCOHOL AND HEART DISEASE
Jonathan R. Lindner

RHEUMATIC AND CONNECTIVE TISSUE DISEASES AND THE HEART

CHAPTER

Carlos A. Roldan

Connective tissue diseases (CTDs) are of two types: *immune-mediated inflammatory* and *heritable*, or *noninflammatory*. The more common are the inflammatory type, which includes systemic lupus erythematosus (SLE), rheumatoid arthritis, scleroderma, ankylosing spondylitis (AS), and polymyositis-dermatomyositis (PM-DM). With the exception of AS, they affect mostly young women. The pericardium, myocardium, valve leaflets, conduction system, and great vessels may all be affected but with different rates of prevalence and degrees of severity. Of importance, these cardiac diseases are recognized clinically less often than is reflected by findings on echocardiographic and postmortem studies. The pathogenesis, natural history, and effects of therapy are still unclear.

The *SLE-associated cardiovascular diseases* are the best studied of the inflammatory CTDs. They are the third most common cause of death in patients with SLE after infectious and renal diseases. Valvular heart disease, pericarditis, and myocarditis or cardiomyopathy are the most common and most important of this group. Less common are coronary artery disease (CAD), arrhythmias or conduction disturbances, and pulmonary hypertension. Libman-Sacks vegetations, with their unique echocardiographic characteristics, are pathognomonic of SLE-related valvular heart disease.

Three possible pathogenic mechanisms may be responsible for SLE-related myocarditis: a primary acute, recurrent, or chronic immune-mediated myocarditis, which is the most common; epicardial or intramyocardial coronary arteritis, accelerated coronary atherosclerosis, coronary thrombosis, or coronary embolism, leading to ischemic dysfunction; and finally, severe valvular regurgitation. Dilated cardiomyopathy rarely ensues as a result of one or more of these mechanisms. Pulmonary hypertension in SLE patients has two etiologies: recurrent pulmonary embolism (the more common) and pulmonary vasculitis. Severe or recurrent pulmonary embolism or vasculitis can lead to severe pulmonary hypertension and cor pulmonale. In patients with SLE, the presence of up to 41% antiphospholipid antibodies in the form of anticardiolipin antibodies, the presence of lupus anticoagulant, or a false-positive VDRL test have been associated with arterial and venous thrombotic events. The true prevalence of SLE-associated pulmonary hypertension is not known.

The cardiovascular diseases associated with *rheumatoid arthritis* are produced by one or more of three mechanisms: nonspecific immune inflammation; vasculitis; and granulomatous deposition on the pericardium, myocardium, heart valves, coronary arteries, aorta, or conduction system. Consequently, pericarditis, myocarditis, valvular heart disease, conduction disturbances, coronary arteritis, aortitis, and cor pulmonale can occur. The prevalence of heart disease associated with rheumatoid arthritis is higher in patients who have had the disease a long time and who also have extra-articular and nodular disease, systemic vasculitis, or high rheumatoid factor levels. Although pericardial and myocardial diseases are the most frequent and clinically important, rheumatoid valvular disease is easily recognized because of its distinctive characteristics [6–9].

Cardiovascular diseases associated with *scleroderma* manifest predominantly as CAD, myocarditis, pericarditis, and less commonly valvular heart disease. Scleroderma-associated cardiovascular disease is the third most common cause of death after pulmonary and renal diseases, with death most often attributable to ischemic heart disease, heart failure, sudden cardiac death, and pericarditis [10–13].

The most important cardiovascular diseases associated with *ankylosing spondylitis* are aortitis with or without aortic regurgitation, conduction disturbances, mitral regurgitation, myocardial dysfunction, and pericarditis. Specific structural abnormalities can be seen in the aortic root and aortic and mitral valves. The cardiovascular diseases generally follow the arthritic syndrome by 10 to 20 years and are more common in patients who have had the disease for more than 20 years, those over age 50, and those with peripheral articular disease [14–16].

Cardiovascular diseases associated with *polymyositis-dermatomyositis* manifest predominantly as arrhythmias or conduction disturbances, myocarditis, and pericarditis. Dilated cardiomyopathy, mitral valve prolapse, coronary vasculitis, and cor pulmonale can also occur. Clinically overt heart disease is more common in PM than in DM. Men and women are similarly affected, and the presence of cardiovascular disease does not correlate with the activity, severity, or duration of PM-DM [17–20].

Marfan syndrome, Ehlers-Danlos syndrome, osteogenesis imperfecta, and *pseudoxanthoma elasticum* are the most important heritable or noninflammatory CTDs. They are characterized by an abnormal synthesis and composition of the collagen fibrils and therefore of the connective tissue. Marfan syndrome, Ehlers-Danlos syndrome, and osteogenesis imperfecta predominantly manifest as aortic root dilatation or aortic and mitral valve prolapse with regurgitation. In contrast, pseudoxanthoma elasticum manifests primarily as peripheral vascular disease and CAD [20–25].

Valvular, pericardial, myocardial, and great vessel abnormalities are the predominant manifestations of the cardiovascular diseases associated with both inflammatory and noninflammatory CTDs. Color Doppler transthoracic echocardiography is the most commonly used technique in the diagnosis, management, and follow-up of patients with these diseases because of its high sensitivity, specificity, and accuracy, as well as its availability, safety, and cost-effectiveness. Lately, with the advent of transesophageal echocardiography and its high-resolution images, the valvular and aortic root abnormalities associated with SLE, ankylosing spondylitis, and Marfan syndrome have been better characterized. Therefore, the principal features of the cardiovascular diseases associated with the two major classes of CTDs are illustrated in this chapter predominantly with transthoracic and transesophageal echocardiographic images.

GENERAL CONSIDERATIONS

GENERAL CONSIDERATIONS IN INFLAMMATORY CTDs

	PREVALENCE AND INCIDENCE	FEMALE/MALE RATIO	PREDOMINANT AGE, Y	MORTALITY
SLE	1.8–7.6/100,000/y	5–10:1	15–64	20% at 10 y
RA	0.5%–2.0% 0.2–0.4/100,000/y	2–4:1	20–60	30%–50% at 10 y
Scleroderma	0.4–2.0/100,000/y	3:1	30–50	27%–66% at 5 y
AS	0.10%–0.23% 6.6/100,000/y	1:4–10	35–64	5% at 10 y
PM-DM	0.2/100,000/y	3:1	10–14 and 45–64	28%–47% at 6–7 y

FIGURE 1-1. The immune-mediated inflammatory connective tissue diseases (CTDs) have a low prevalence and incidence, predominate in females (with the exception of ankylosing spondylitis [AS]), and are most prevalent between the second and fifth decades of life. Overall mortality is 5% to 50% at 5 to 10 years after onset of disease. PM-DM—polymyositis-dermatomyositis; RA—rheumatoid arthritis; SLE—systemic lupus erythematosus.

PREVALENCE OF CARDIOVASCULAR DISEASES ASSOCIATED WITH INFLAMMATORY CTDs BY TYPE OF EXAMINATION

	CLINICAL STUDIES, %	ECHOCARDIOGRAPHIC STUDIES, %	POSTMORTEM STUDIES, %
Systemic lupus			
Valve disease	Unknown	0–79	13–100
Pericarditis	12–52	4–54	43–100
Myocarditis	1–20	4–64	8–81
Ankylosing spondylitis			
Valve disease	0–5	17–38	20–30
Pericarditis	Unknown	0–14	Unknown
Myocarditis	<1	18–53	Unknown
Rheumatoid arthritis			
Valve disease	Unknown	0–30	23–75
Pericarditis	1–10	3–50	11–54
Myocarditis	<1	0–18	3–30
Scleroderma			
Valve disease*	Unknown	8–32	Up to 18
Pericarditis	5–15	21–41	33–42
Myocarditis	10–21	18–42	12–89
Polymyositis-dermatomyositis			
Valve disease*	Unknown	0–65	6–30
Pericarditis	17–23	5–54	Unknown
Myocarditis	3–44	5–25	50

FIGURE 1-2. The true prevalence of cardiovascular abnormalities associated with inflammatory connective tissue diseases (CTDs) is unclear. Their prevalence based on clinical, echocardiographic, and postmortem series varies widely. Variability in prevalence according to type of examination is related to several factors, such as differences in test sensitivity, the inclusion of asymptomatic patients from the clinical studies in contrast to those with the most severe forms of disease from the postmortem studies, and the fact that not all tests are applied to the same patient populations. *Asterisks* indicate that mitral valve prolapse is the most frequent disorder in these diseases.

GENERAL CONSIDERATIONS IN HERITABLE CTDs

	MARFAN SYNDROME	EHLERS-DANLOS SYNDROME	OSTEOGENESIS IMPERFECTA	PSEUDOXANTHOMA ELASTICUM
Inheritance	Autosomal-dominant	Autosomal-dominant (type IV) (90%)	Autosomal-dominant (60%), recessive (15%–20%), and sporadic (25%)	Predominantly autosomal-recessive, less often autosomal-dominant
Prevalence	4–6/100,000 births	—	1/60,000 births	—
Pathogenesis	Abnormal synthesis of collagen fibrils and elastin → loose medial elastic tissue → increased mucopolysaccharide deposits	Abnormal synthesis of procollagen → collagen fibrils → thin and irregular collagen fibrils	Abnormal synthesis of procollagen → collagen fibrils → irregular collagen fibrils	Fragmentation and calcification of elastic fibrils → elastic tissue disruption → fibrous proliferation and luminal narrowing
Organ systems affected	Eye: myopia, ectopia lentis, retinal detachment Musculoskeletal: loose joints, arachnodactyly, scoliosis and kyphosis, pectus excavatum Cardiovascular: aortic root and valve disease, mitral and tricuspid valve disease	Musculoskeletal: loose joints Cardiovascular: disease of large and medium-size arteries, aortic root and valve disease, mitral valve disease	Ears: deafness Teeth: dentinogenesis imperfecta Eyes: blue sclerae Musculoskeletal: fragile bones, loose joints, scoliosis and kyphosis Cardiovascular: aortic root and valve disease, mitral valve disease	Skin: Pseudoxanthomas Eyes: Angioid streaks Gastrointestinal: bleeding Cardiovascular: coronary artery disease, peripheral vascular disease, hypertension, mitral valve prolapse, endocardial fibroelastosis

FIGURE 1-3. The prevalence of the heritable connective tissue diseases (CTDs) is low. Their pathogenesis relates to the synthesis of abnormal collagen and elastic fibrils. In general, the distinction among Marfan syndrome, Ehlers-Danlos syndrome, and osteogenesis imperfecta is based on clinical features other than cardiovascular manifestations. Pseudoxanthoma elasticum, in contrast, is characterized by a high prevalence of coronary and peripheral vascular disease and sparing of the aortic root.

CHARACTERISTICS AND TREATMENT OF THE CARDIOVASCULAR DISEASES ASSOCIATED WITH HERITABLE CTDs

MARFAN SYNDROME

Prevalence up to 70%

Aortic root disease
  Dilatation of sinus of Valsalva, annulus, and root
  Aortic aneurysm
  Aortic dissection
    Type I DeBakey (most common)
    Type II (10%)
    Pregnancy increases risk
  Aortic valve prolapse and regurgitation
  Most common cause of premature death

Mitral valve disease
  Annular dilatation
  Elongated and thin leaflets
  Myxomatous degeneration and chordal rupture
  Mitral valve prolapse and regurgitation

Treatment
  β-blockers for root dilatation
  Aortic root homograft
  Valve replacement
  Infective endocarditis prophylaxis

EHLERS-DANLOS SYNDROME

Disease of large and medium-size arteries (most important)
  Spontaneous rupture of abdominal aorta, arch vessels, and limb arteries
  False aneurysms and fistulas
  Pregnancy increases risk for rupture

Mitral valve prolapse is frequent

Aortic root dilatation, dissection, rupture, and regurgitation are uncommon

Conduction disturbances are rare

Treatment
  β-blockers for root dilatation
  Aortic root homograft
  Valve replacement

OSTEOGENESIS IMPERFECTA

Aortic root and valve disease
  Sinus of Valsalva dilatation and aneurysms
  Aortic annular and root dilatation
  Aortic dissection
  Fenestration and prolapse of aortic cusps
  Aortic regurgitation

Mitral valve disease
  Fenestration of mitral valve leaflets
  Mitral valve prolapse
  Chordal rupture
  Mitral regurgitation

Treatment
  β-blockers for root dilatation
  Aortic root homograft
  Valve replacement
  Infective endocarditis prophylaxis

PSEUDOXANTHOMA ELASTICUM

Coronary artery disease
  Most important clinically
  Most common cause of premature death

Endocardial fibroelastosis, mainly of atria

Restrictive cardiomyopathy is rare

Increased prevalence of mitral valve prolapse, peripheral vascular disease, and hypertension

Treatment
  No specific therapy is available

FIGURE 1-4. Abnormal root dilatation, aortic aneurysm, aortic dissection, and aortic and mitral valve prolapse with regurgitation are the most common and characteristic cardiovascular manifestations of Marfan syndrome, Ehlers-Danlos syndrome, and osteogenesis imperfecta. In contrast, in pseudoxanthoma elasticum, premature coronary disease and peripheral vascular disease are the most prevalent features and the most common causes of death. CTDs—connective tissue diseases.

Immune-Mediated Inflammatory Connective Tissue Diseases

SYSTEMIC LUPUS ERYTHEMATOSUS

CHARACTERISTICS OF CARDIOVASCULAR DISEASES ASSOCIATED WITH SLE

VALVE DISEASE	PERICARDITIS	MYOCARDITIS	CORONARY ARTERY DISEASE

Categories
  Valve masses
  Valve thickening
  Valve regurgitation
  Valve stenosis
	Generally acute	Rarely detected clinically	Atherosclerotic and inflammatory diseases (arteritis) are uncommon (8%)

Libman-Sacks vegetations are pathognomonic of SLE	Most common during flares of SLE	May present as systolic or diastolic failure	Intramural CAD most common

Generally asymptomatic	Complications
	  Cardiac tamponade in up to 13%
	  Constrictive pericarditis in <1%
		Dilated cardiomyopathy is rare	Duration of SLE (>12 y) and of steroid therapy (>14 y) are important risk factors

Complications
  Congestive heart failure
  Infective endocarditis
  Cardioembolism
  Need for valve replacement
	Positive antinuclear antibodies in pericardial fluid is pathognomonic	Endomyocardial biopsy is diagnostic but not specific	Rarely due to embolism of Libman-Sacks vegetation coronary embolism

Effect of anti-inflammatory therapy not clear	NSAIDs and steroids are beneficial	Steroid therapy is beneficial	Steroids are beneficial for coronary arteritis

FIGURE 1-5. Cardiovascular diseases are the third most common cause of death after infectious and renal diseases in patients with systemic lupus erythematosus (SLE). Clinically, valvular heart disease characterized by the presence of Libman-Sacks vegetations is the most important of the cardiovascular manifestations associated with SLE. SLE-associated pericarditis is the most frequent cardiovascular disorder detected clinically because it often causes symptoms. Although myocarditis and coronary artery disease (CAD) are the least prevalent, they are associated with significant mortality and morbidity. Limited data are also available about the natural history of the cardiovascular diseases associated with SLE. NSAIDs—nonsteroidal anti-inflammatory drugs.

ECHOCARDIOGRAPHIC CHARACTERISTICS OF SLE-ASSOCIATED VALVE DISEASE

LIBMAN-SACKS MASSES	VALVE THICKENING	VALVE REGURGITATION
0%–31% prevalence	12%–50% prevalence	0%–79% prevalence
Pathognomonic of SLE	Generally diffuse	Mitral and aortic most important
Affect mitral and aortic valves most commonly	Can be localized to any leaflet portion	Most frequently mild in severity
Located most often on basal portions of leaflet	Predominantly of mitral and aortic valves	7%–41% prevalence of moderate-to-severe lesions
Located on atrial side of mitral valve and vessel side of aortic valve	Frequently associated with valve regurgitation (73%)	Frequently associated with valve thickening
Variable in size (0.2–0.85 cm^2) and shape, heterogeneous echodensity, and leaflet-dependent motion	Frequently associated with valve masses (50%)	Complications Heart failure Infective endocarditis Need for valve replacement
Frequently associated with valve thickening or regurgitation	Rarely involves mitral subvalvular apparatus	Rarely associated with valve stenosis (<3%)

FIGURE 1-6. Valve thickening and frequently associated valve regurgitation are the most common valve abnormalities associated with systemic lupus erythematosus (SLE). Nevertheless, Libman-Sacks vegetations and their unique echocardiographic features are considered pathognomonic of SLE-associated valve disease. Valve thickening and regurgitation or stenosis can be assessed by transthoracic echocardiography, but transesophageal echocardiography may be required to detect Libman-Sacks vegetations in patients with SLE in whom cardioembolism is suspected.

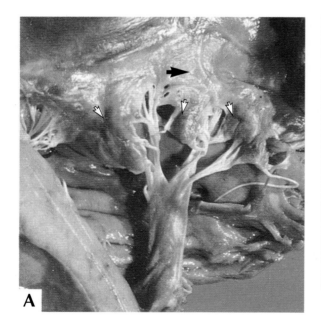 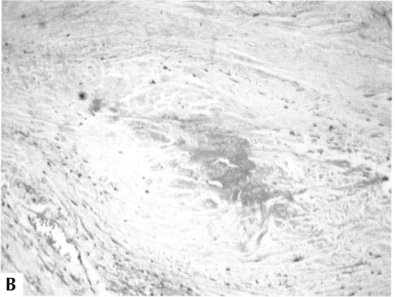

A **B**

FIGURE 1-7. Libman-Sacks vegetations on the mitral valve of a patient with SLE. **A,** Red, flat, multiple spreading lesions variable in size are present on the free margins or line of closure of the mitral leaflet (*large arrow*), consistent with Libman-Sacks vegetations (*small arrows*). **B,** The characteristic histology of Libman-Sacks vegetations consists of deep, eosinophilic areas of fibrinoid degeneration associated with minimal mononuclear infiltrate and some fibroblastic proliferation. Fibrinoid degeneration is visible at the edge of a mitral valve (×220). (*Adapted from* Farrer-Brown [26]; with permission.)

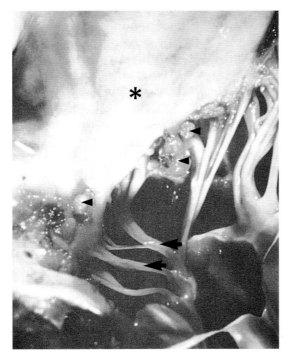

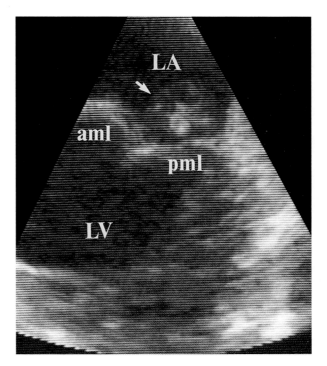

FIGURE 1-8. Multiple, small Libman-Sacks vegetations (*arrowheads*) with irregular borders and a warty appearance on the line of closure of the mitral leaflet (*asterisk*) in a patient with systemic lupus erythematosus (SLE). These valve masses are generally located on surfaces exposed to the forward flow of blood. The chordae tendineae are marked by *arrows*. (*Adapted from* Robbins [27]; with permission.)

FIGURE 1-9. Libman-Sacks vegetation and mitral valve thickening in a patient with systemic lupus erythematosus (SLE). Transesophageal semitangential echocardiographic view of the mitral valve revealing a large mass (*arrow*) with heterogeneous echodensity on the atrial side of the basal posterior mitral leaflet (pml). Associated diffuse thickening of the mitral leaflets can be seen. In addition, mild mitral regurgitation was noted. aml—anterior mitral leaflet; LA—left atrium; LV—left ventricle. (*Adapted from* Roldan and coworkers [1]; with permission from the American College of Cardiology.)

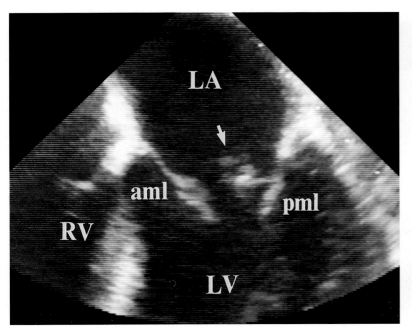

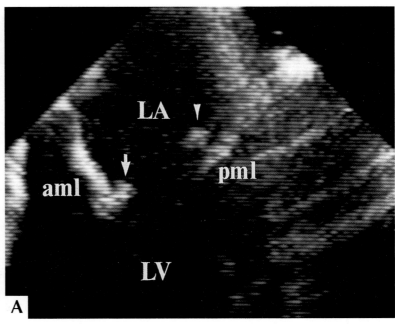

FIGURE 1-10. Libman-Sacks vegetation and mitral valve thickening in a patient with systemic lupus erythematosus (SLE). Transesophageal four-chamber echocardiographic view showing an irregular mass (*arrow*) of heterogeneous echodensity on the atrial side of the posterior mitral leaflet (pml). Diffuse thickening predominantly of the mid and tip portions of the anterior (aml) and posterior mitral leaflets can also be seen. Moderate mitral regurgitation was present. LA—left atrium; LV—left ventricle; RV—right ventricle. (*Adapted from* Roldan and coworkers [1]; with permission from the American College of Cardiology.)

FIGURE 1-11. Libman-Sacks vegetations and mitral valve thickening in a patient with systemic lupus erythematosus (SLE). **A,** Transesophageal four-chamber echocardiographic view showing a mass on the atrial side of the tip of the anterior mitral leaflet (aml; *arrow*). A second mass can be seen in the midportion of the posterior mitral leaflet (pml; *arrowhead*). Associated diffuse thickening of both mitral leaflets is also evident. (*continued*)

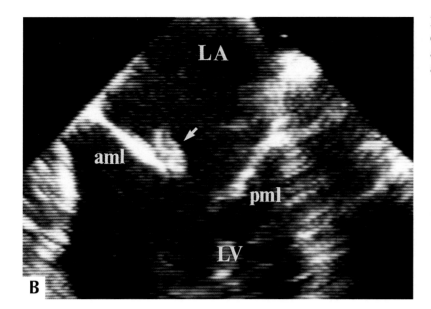

B

FIGURE 1-11. (*continued*) **B,** Transesophageal four-chamber echocardiographic view for defining better the large mass on the aml tip (*arrow*). Mild mitral regurgitation was detected. LA—left atrium; LV—left ventricle.

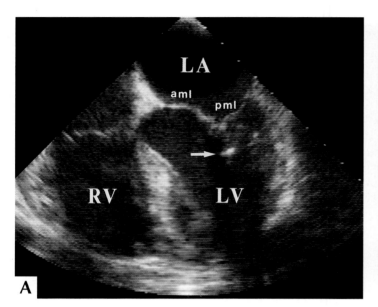

A

B

FIGURE 1-12. Mitral valve chordal Libman-Sacks vegetation in a patient with systemic lupus erythematosus (SLE). **A,** Transesophageal four-chamber echocardiographic view showing a large chordal mass (*arrow*) extending to the posterior tip and midportions of the posterior mitral leaflet (pml). **B,** Close-up transesopha-geal view of the mitral valve indicating a large mass (*arrow*) having irregular borders and homogeneous echodensity on the ventricular side and posterior to the posterior mitral leaflet. Associated mild mitral regurgitation was also evident. aml—anterior mitral leaflet; LA—left atrium; LV—left ventricle; RV—right ventricle.

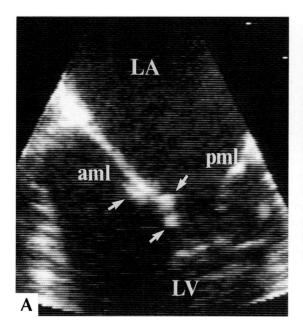

A

B

FIGURE 1-13. Mitral valve thickening and regurgitation in a patient with SLE. **A,** Transesophageal four-chamber echocardiographic view showing multinodular thickening (*arrows*) of the tip and midportions of the anterior mitral leaflet (aml). **B,** Transesophageal four-chamber view demonstrating on color Doppler flow mapping mild-to-moderate mitral regurgitation, with an eccentric jet directed to the atrial lateral wall (*small arrows*). LA—left atrium; LV—left ventricle; pml—posterior mitral leaflet.

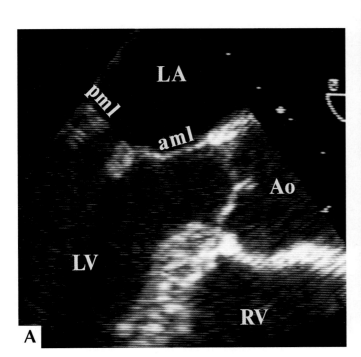

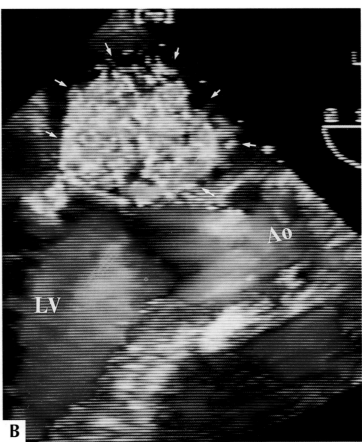

FIGURE 1-14. Mitral valve thickening and regurgitation in a patient with systemic lupus erythematosus (SLE). **A,** Transesophageal echocardiographic view, longitudinal to the left outflow tract, showing severe thickening of the tips of the anterior (aml) and posterior (pml) mitral leaflets. The aortic valve cusps appear normal. **B,** Transesophageal view, similar to that in *A*, demonstrating moderately severe mitral regurgitation on color Doppler flow mapping. Ao—aorta; LA—left atrium; LV—left ventricle; RV—right ventricle.

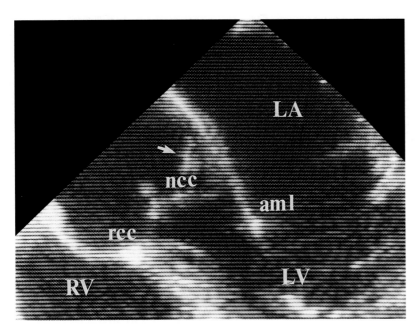

FIGURE 1-15. Aortic valve Libman-Sacks vegetation in a patient with systemic lupus erythematosus (SLE). Transesophageal echocardiographic view, longitudinal to the left outflow tract, showing a mass with irregular borders (*arrow*) and heterogeneous echodensity at the base of the noncoronary cusp (ncc) and posteromedial aortic root wall. No aortic regurgitation was seen. aml—anterior mitral leaflet; LA—left atrium; LV—left ventricle; RA—right atrium; rcc—right coronary cusp. (*Adapted from* Roldan and coworkers [1]; with permission from the American College of Cardiology.)

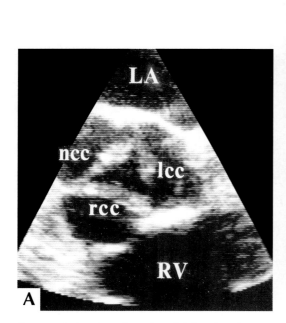

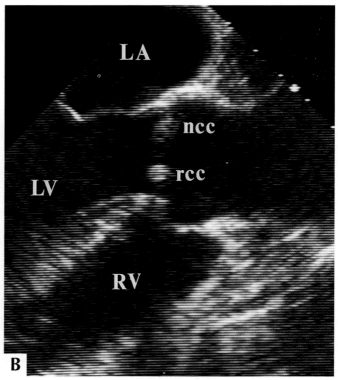

FIGURE 1-16. Aortic valve thickening in a patient with systemic lupus erythematosus (SLE). **A,** Transesophageal basilar short-axis echocardiographic view showing diffuse and marked thickening of the left (lcc), right (rcc), and noncoronary (ncc) aortic cusps. **B,** Transesophageal view, longitudinal to the left outflow tract, demonstrating severe thickening and retraction predominantly of the tip portions of the noncoronary and right coronary cusps. Note also in this view the normal appearance of the mitral valve leaflets. LA—left atrium; LV—left ventricle; RV—right ventricle. (Part A *adapted from* Roldan and coworkers [1]; with permission from the American College of Cardiology.)

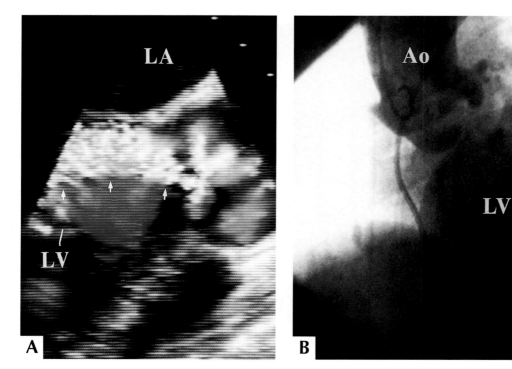

FIGURE 1-17. Aortic valve regurgitation in a patient with systemic lupus erythematosus (SLE). **A,** Transesophageal echocardiographic view, longitudinal to the outflow tract, revealing moderately severe aortic valve regurgitation (*arrows*) on color Doppler flow mapping. **B,** This degree of regurgitation was confirmed during aortography in the left anterior oblique view of the ascending aorta (Ao) and left ventricle (LV). These echocardiographic and angiographic findings correspond to those of the patient featured in Fig. 1-16. LA—left atrium.

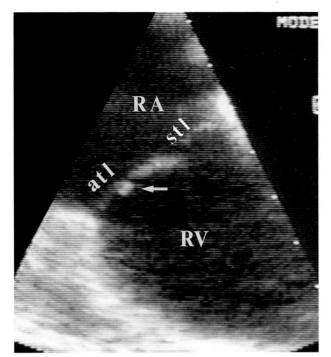

FIGURE 1-18. Tricuspid valve Libman-Sacks vegetation and thickening in a patient with systemic lupus erythematosus (SLE). Transesophageal echocardiographic horizontal view of the right heart chambers and tricuspid valve showing a small mass (*arrow*) on the ventricular side of the basal midportion of the anterior tricuspid valve leaflet (atl). Moderate thickening of the tip and midportions of the anterior leaflet can be seen. Mild tricuspid regurgitation was demonstrated on color Doppler flow mapping. RA—right atrium; RV—right ventricle; stl—septal tricuspid leaflet.

Pericarditis

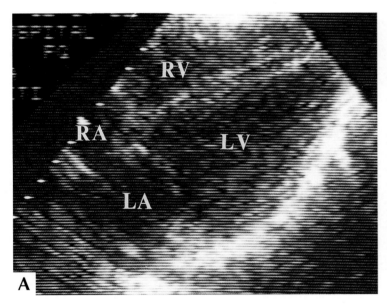

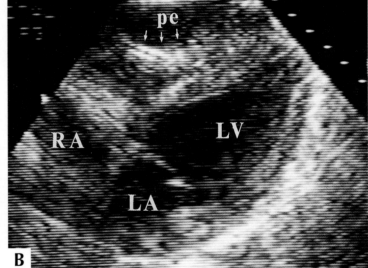

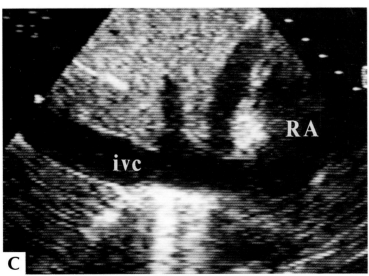

FIGURE 1-19. Pericarditis complicated by cardiac tamponade in a patient with systemic lupus erythematosus (SLE). **A,** This initial transthoracic subcostal four-chamber echocardiographic view in a 31-year-old woman with active and flaring SLE as well as symptoms and physical findings of pericarditis shows no evidence of pericardial effusion or thickening. **B** and **C,** These transthoracic subcostal four-chamber and inferior vena caval views obtained 5 days later show a large pericardial effusion (pe) with partial compression of the right ventricle (RV) during diastole (*small arrows* in *B*) and a severely plethoric inferior vena cava (ivc) indicative of increased right atrial (RA) pressure. These echocardiographic findings correlated with clinical evidence of cardiac tamponade. Urgent pericardiocentesis was performed and the pericardial fluid was found to be an exudate positive for antinuclear antibodies. (*continued*)

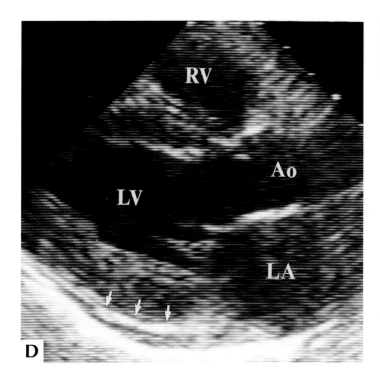

FIGURE 1-19. (*continued*) **D,** A follow-up echocardiogram in the long parasternal view reveals only minimal posterior pericardial effusion and moderate visceral pericardial thickening (*small arrows*). Ao—aorta; LA—left atrium; LV—left ventricle.

Myocarditis or Cardiomyopathy

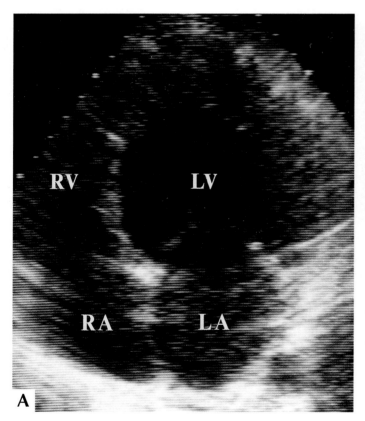

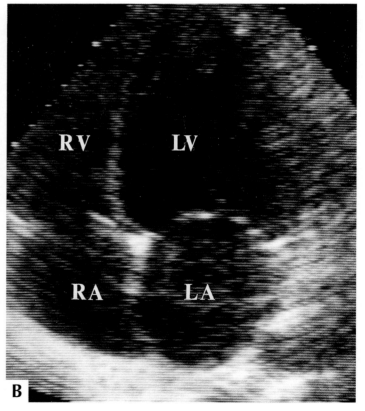

FIGURE 1-20. Severe systemic lupus erythematosus (SLE)–associated dilated cardiomyopathy in a 21-year-old man with severe and active SLE. These transthoracic four-chamber echocardiographic views at end diastole (**A**) and end systole (**B**) show severe four-chamber dilatation and poor biventricular contractile function. Diffuse left ventricular (LV) hypokinesis was noted. Radionuclide ventriculography demonstrated an ejection fraction of 24%. LA—left atrium; RA—right atrium; RV—right ventricle.

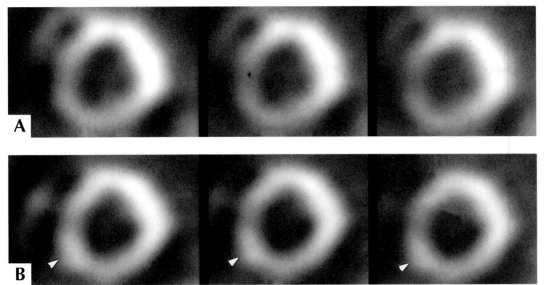

FIGURE 1-21. Severe nonischemic dilated cardiomyopathy in systemic lupus erythematosus (SLE). These thallium-201 single-photon emission computed tomographic (SPECT) cross-sectional images of the mid left ventricle show marked chamber dilatation similar to that seen in Fig. 1-20, as well as diffuse myocardial thinning and decreased uptake of radioisotope, predominantly by the septal, inferior, and inferolateral walls during exercise (**A**) and rest (**B**; *arrowheads*). Coronary arteriography revealed normal epicardial coronary arteries.

Coronary Artery Disease

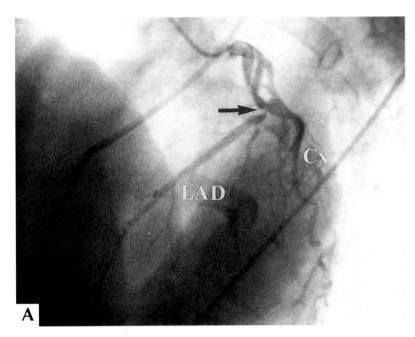

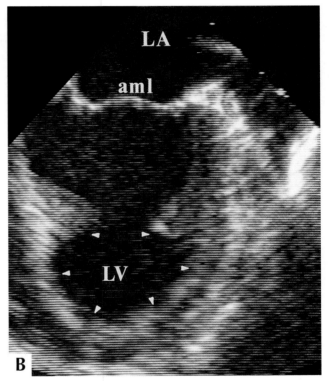

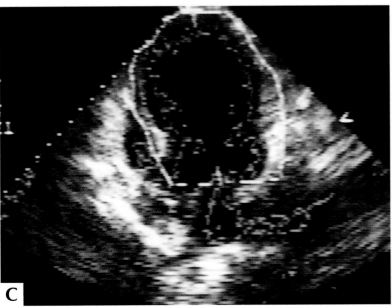

FIGURE 1-22. Anteroapical myocardial infarction in a patient with SLE. **A,** Cranial left anterior oblique view on arteriography showing severe proximal stenosis (*arrow*) of the left anterior descending (LAD) coronary artery that led into an anteroapical infarction in a 41-year-old woman with flaring SLE. **B,** Transesophageal two-chamber echocardiographic view showing thinning and dyskinesis of the apex and a well-defined, moderate-sized apical aneurysm (*arrowheads*). **C,** Transthoracic four-chamber echocardiographic view with endocardial acoustic quantification showing the anteroapical aneurysm. Left ventricular (LV) systolic function was severely depressed, with an ejection fraction of 27%. Because it was not possible to differentiate among atherosclerosis, coronary arteritis, and primary thrombosis in this young woman with active SLE and positive antiphospholipid antibodies, medical therapy with high-dose intravenous steroids, heparin, and nitrates was begun. aml—anterior mitral leaflet; Cx—circumflex artery.

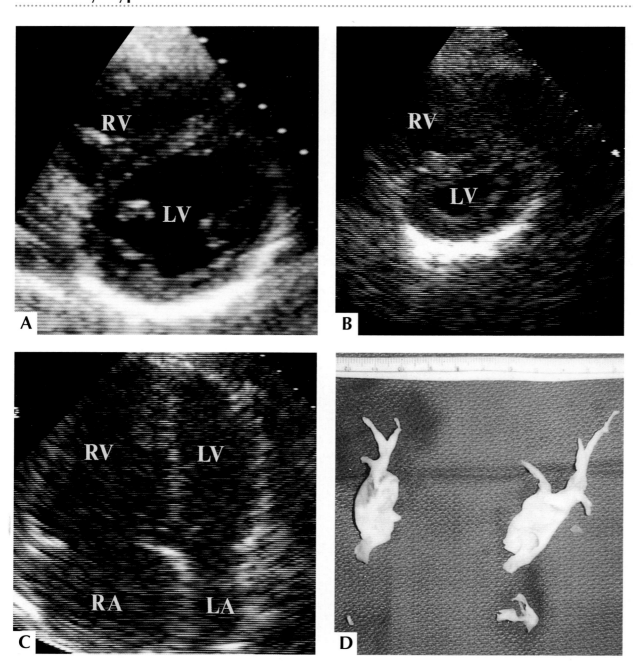

FIGURE 1-23. Severe pulmonary hypertension and cor pulmonale in a patient with systemic lupus erythematosus (SLE). **A,** Transthoracic parasternal short-axis echocardiographic view in a 22-year-old woman with inactive SLE, positive anticardiolipin antibodies, and documented previous pulmonary embolism and who was on warfarin therapy. The right ventricle (RV) is normal in size. Because of progressive dyspnea on exertion, she underwent repeat echocardiography 26 months after the initial study. **B** and **C,** Severe dilatation and hypertrophy of the RV as well as paradoxical septal motion were noted. By applying the simplified Bernoulli equation ($4V^2$) to the tricuspid valve regurgitation peak velocity of 4 m/s and adding an estimated right atrial (RA) pressure of 15 mm Hg, pulmonary artery systolic pressure was estimated to be 75 to 80 mm Hg. **D,** Bilateral pulmonary artery thromboendarterectomy was performed, resulting in remarkable resolution of clinical and echocardiographic abnormalities over a period of 3 months. LA—left atrium; LV—left ventricle.

CHARACTERISTICS OF CARDIOVASCULAR DISEASES ASSOCIATED WITH RHEUMATOID ARTHRITIS

PERICARDITIS	MYOCARDITIS	VALVE DISEASE	CORONARY ARTERY DISEASE

Rarely detected clinically (1%–10%) and generally uncomplicated	Clinical prevalence is low (<1%)	Etiologies
		  Inflammatory (nonspecific) is most common
		  Vasculitis
		  Granulomatous (3%–5%)
			Type
			  Atherosclerotic and inflammatory disease (arteritis)

Asymptomatic in 30% of cases	Types
	  Nonspecific and necrotizing (>50%)
	  Granulomatous (1%–11%)
	  Amyloid (rare)
		Granulomatous valve disease is unique to rheumatoid arthritis	Coronary arteritis is rare

Cardiac tamponade and constriction are rare (<2%)	Generally asymptomatic, mild, and uncomplicated	Valve granulomas affect mainly aortic and mitral valves and are generally focal	True clinical prevalence unknown but rare
Characteristically low glucose content in pericardial fluid	Myocardial perfusion scans frequently abnormal	Valve granulomas usually cause no valve dysfunction	Clinically and angiographically indistinguishable
NSAIDs and steroids are beneficial	Steroid therapy is beneficial	Effect of anti-inflammatory therapy is unknown	Steroids and cytotoxic agents beneficial for coronary arteritis

FIGURE 1-24. The cardiovascular diseases associated with rheumatoid arthritis are generally mild and uncomplicated. They are more common in patients with high titers of IgG and IgM rheumatoid factor and in those with active and nodular disease. Although they have no distinctive clinical or echocardiographic features, the presence of rheumatoid granules on histologic examination establishes the diagnosis of rheumatoid arthritis associated with heart disease. Pericarditis is the most common cardiovascular finding detected clinically and on echocardiography (in 1% to 50% of cases), while coronary arteritis is the least common. Steroid therapy is indicated for patients with pericarditis, myocarditis, and coronary arteritis.

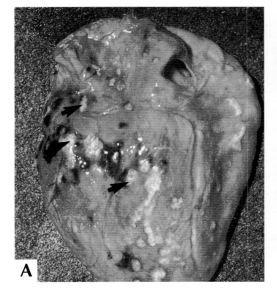
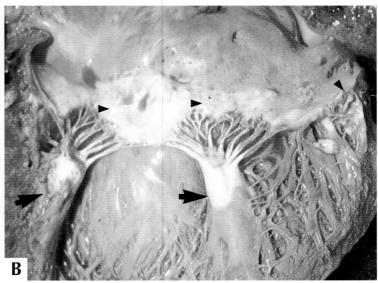

FIGURE 1-25. Rheumatoid nodular disease of the myocardium, mitral valve, and papillary muscles. **A,** Multiple, pale rheumatoid nodules (*arrows*) variable in size can be seen on the left ventricular and atrial posterior walls. **B,** Multiple nodules (*arrowheads*) are evident on the atrial side of the free margins of both mitral leaflets, the tips of the papillary muscles, and the basal portions of the left ventricular walls (*large arrows*). (*Adapted from* Farrer-Brown [26]; with permission.)

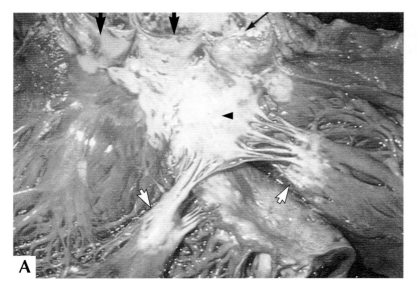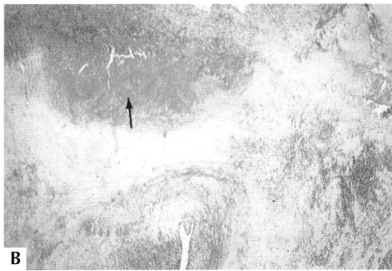

FIGURE 1-26. Mitral and aortic valve disease in a patient with rheumatoid arthritis. **A,** Coalescing rheumatoid nodules are noted on the tips of the papillary muscles (*white arrows*) and anterior mitral leaflet (*arrowhead*) extending up to the aortic valve. Because of rheumatoid valvulitis, the aortic valve cusps (*black arrows*) show contraction and thickening but no commissural adhesion. **B,** Microscopic appearance of the mitral valve. An area of fibrinoid necrosis, stained deep red (*arrow*), is surrounded by a blue-staining cellular infiltrate of mononuclear cells. The tissue stained pale pink is fibrotic. (Hematoxylin and eosin, × 55.) (*Adapted from* Farrer-Brown [26]; with permission.)

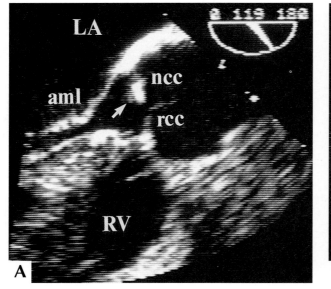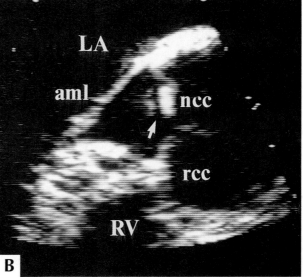

FIGURE 1-27. Aortic valve disease in a patient with rheumatoid arthritis. A transesophageal echocardiographic view longitudinal to the outflow tract (**A**) and the longitudinal close-up view of the aortic valve (**B**) show a well-localized nodularity with homogeneous but increased echodensity on the midportion of the aortic noncoronary cusp (ncc). Aortic valve regurgitation was not demonstrated. With the exception of this nodular abnormality, the other portions of the noncoronary cusp and the other two aortic valve cusps was normal. These findings are suggestive of an aortic valve granuloma. aml—anterior mitral leaflet; LA—left atrium; rcc—right coronary cusp; RV—right ventricle.

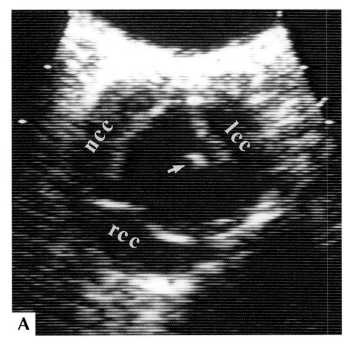

A

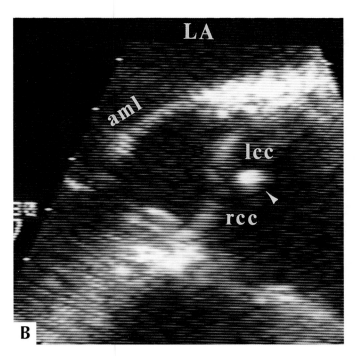

B

FIGURE 1-28. Aortic valve disease in a 63-year-old man with severe rheumatoid nodular disease. **A,** Transesophageal basilar short-axis close-up echocardiographic view of the aortic valve showing a small mass with irregular borders and homogeneous echodensity on the left coronary cusp (lcc) (*arrow*). **B,** Transesophageal view longitudinal to the left outflow tract of the aortic valve revealing the mass on the tip of the left coronary cusp (*arrowhead*). No valve regurgitation was detected. Note the otherwise normal appearance of the three aortic valve cusps. This aortic valve abnormality may correspond to a valve granuloma; however, even with no history of endocarditis, such a differentiation cannot be made from an old or healed vegetation. aml—anterior mitral leaflet; LA— left atrium; ncc—noncoronary cusp; rcc—right coronary cusp.

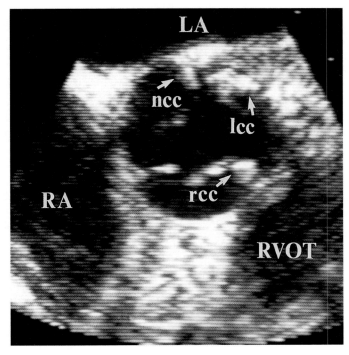

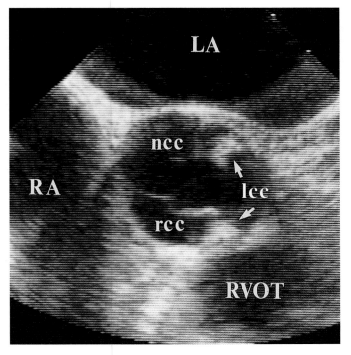

FIGURE 1-29. Aortic valve disease in a 42-year-old woman with rheumatoid arthritis and a high level of rheumatoid factor. This transesophageal basilar short-axis close-up echocardiographic view shows multiple, irregular, localized nodularities at the bases of the left (lcc), right (rcc), and noncoronary (ncc) cusps (*arrows*). These findings may reflect an immune-mediated valvulitis, with a subsequent fibrotic reparative process, or granulomatous valve disease. Mild aortic regurgitation was detected. LA—left atrium; RA—right atrium; RVOT—right ventricular outflow tract. (*Adapted from* Roldan and Crawford [28]; with permission.)

FIGURE 1-30. Aortic valve disease in a 52-year-old man with rheumatoid arthritis. This transesophageal basilar short-axis close-up echocardiographic view of the aortic valve demonstrates localized nodular thickening (*arrows*) at the base of the right coronary cusp (rcc) and especially of the left coronary cusp (lcc). Similar to the patient described in Fig. 1-29, the echocardiographic characteristics of aortic valve disease in this patient may reflect valvulitis, granulomatous deposition, or even age-related changes. LA—left atrium; ncc—noncoronary cusp; RA—right atrium; RVOT—right ventricular outflow tract.

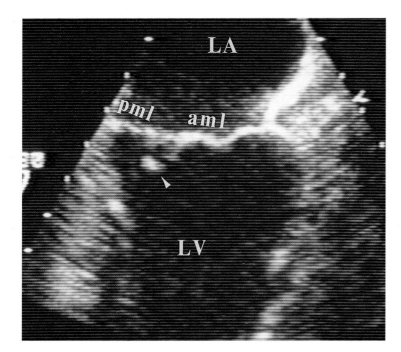

Figure 1-31. Mitral valve disease in a 63-year-old man with rheumatoid nodular disease. This transesophageal two-chamber echocardiographic view at a depth of 8 cm demonstrates a small nodular mass (*arrowhead*) with homogeneous echodensity at the tip and chordal junction of the posterior mitral leaflet (pml). Associated mild thickening of the posterior and anterior mitral leaflet (aml) tips can be seen. Mild mitral regurgitation was noted. This mitral valve mass is suggestive of a valve granuloma. LA—left atrium; LV—left ventricle.

SCLERODERMA

CHARACTERISTICS OF CARDIOVASCULAR DISEASES ASSOCIATED WITH SCLERODERMA

CORONARY ARTERY DISEASE	MYOCARDITIS	PERICARDITIS	VALVE DISEASE
Intramural fixed and dynamic (cardiac Raynaud's phenomena) are the most common	Most commonly due to recurrent intramyocardial ischemia; immune-mediated is rare	Unknown pathogenesis	Prevalence and pathogenesis unknown
Pathogenesis Immune-mediated endothelial injury and dysfunction	High association between peripheral myopathy and immune myocarditis	Clinical pericarditis is uncommon (5%–15%)	Rarely recognized clinically and generally uncomplicated
High association between peripheral and cardiac Raynaud's phenomena	Left ventricular systolic or asystolic dysfunction is common (10%–50%)	More common in limited cutaneous-type scleroderma	Characteristics are nonspecific
Epicardial coronary vasospasm can occur	Endomyocardial biopsy is nonspecific	Cardiac tamponade and constriction are rare	Mitral and aortic valve disease are most common
Myocardial perfusion abnormalities are common	Calcium-channel blockers are beneficial for ischemic type	Pericardial fluid characteristics are nonspecific	Mitral valve prolapse is common (up to 30%)
Calcium-channel blockers are beneficial	Effect of steroids for immune type is unknown	Steroids are generally not effective	Effect of steroids is unknown

Figure 1-32. The associated cardiovascular diseases are less frequent and less severe in patients with the cutaneous type of scleroderma than in those with the diffuse type. Cardiovascular diseases are the third most common cause of death after pulmonary and renal diseases in patients with scleroderma. The major causes of death are ischemic heart disease followed by refractory heart failure, sudden cardiac death, and pericarditis. Overall survival in these patients at 7 years is 20%. Valve disease is generally of no clinical or prognostic significance. Calcium-channel blockers and angiotensin-converting enzyme inhibitors for ischemic heart disease have proved beneficial in these patients.

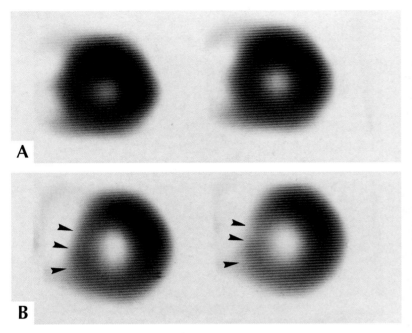

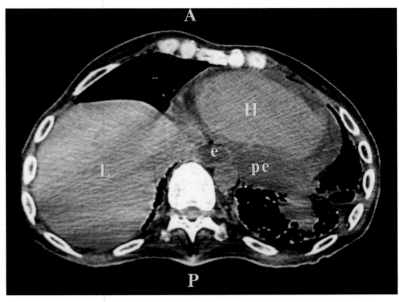

FIGURE 1-33. Intramural coronary artery disease in a 48-year-old man with diffuse cutaneous-type scleroderma and resting and exertional chest pain. These left ventricular short-axis resting (**A**) and postexercise (**B**) perfusion scans with SPECT Cardiolyte show completely reversible perfusion defects suggestive of ischemia of the septal and inferior walls (*arrowheads*). On coronary angiography, the epicardial coronary arteries were normal. The diagnosis of intramyocardial coronary artery disease or intramyocardial Raynaud's phenomenon was considered. The patient was treated successfully with calcium-channel blockers.

FIGURE 1-34. Pericarditis with pericardial effusion (pe) in a 35-year-old man with diffuse cutaneous-type scleroderma. This computed tomogram of the chest shows a large effusion located predominantly posteriorly. No pericardial thickening or calcification was detected. Esophageal dilatation (e) can be seen. A—anterior; H—heart; L—liver; P—posterior. (*Adapted from* Roldan and Crawford [28]; with permission.)

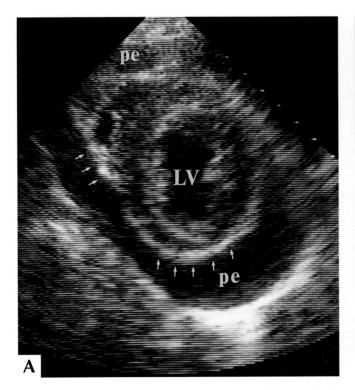

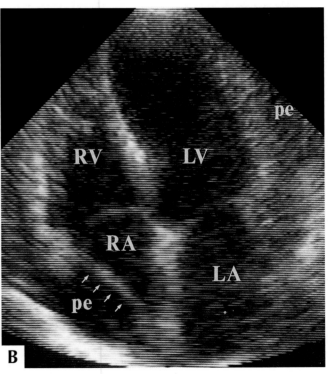

FIGURE 1-35. Pericarditis and pericardial effusion (pe) in a 72-year-old woman with scleroderma. **A,** Transthoracic short-axis echocardiographic view of a large anterior and predominantly posterior pericardial effusion. Posteroinferior visceral pericardial thickening (*arrows*) can also be seen. **B,** Transthoracic four-chamber view showing a pericardial effusion and right atrial (RA) compression (*arrows*) suggestive of cardiac tamponade. Mild right ventricular (RV) compression during diastole was also evident on the long parasternal view. Despite these echocardiographic findings, there was no clinical evidence of cardiac tamponade, and the patient was treated successfully with high doses of intravenous steroids. LA—left atrium; LV—left ventricle.

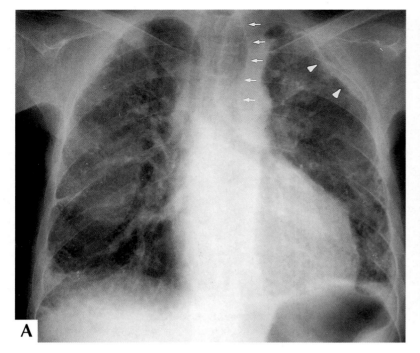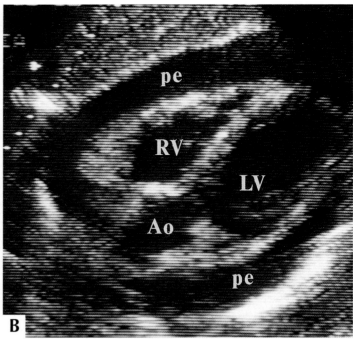

FIGURE 1-36. Pulmonary fibrosis, esophageal dilatation, cardiomegaly, and pericardial effusion in a 35-year-old man with diffuse cutaneous-type scleroderma. **A,** Anteroposterior chest radiograph showing diffuse bilateral interstitial changes predominantly in the lung bases. Associated pleural thickening (*arrowheads*) can be seen, as well as marked esophageal dilatation (*small arrows*) and cardiomegaly. **B,** A moderate pericardial effusion (pe) was demonstrated on echocardiography. At the time of these studies this patient was being treated with high oral doses of steroids. Ao—aorta; LV—left ventricle; RV—right ventricle.

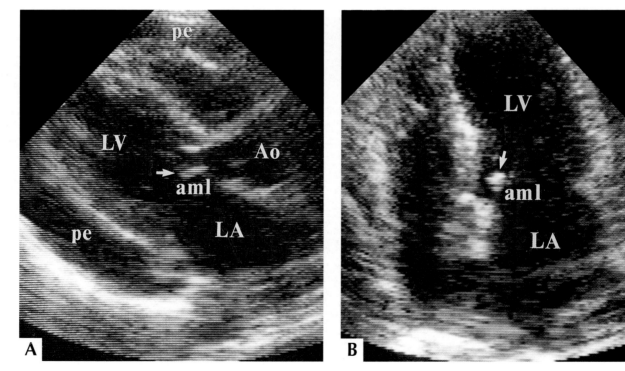

FIGURE 1-37. Mitral valve disease in a 72-year-old woman with scleroderma. Transthoracic long parasternal (**A**) and four-chamber (**B**) echocardiographic views showing an irregular, echodense nodularity or mass in the midportion of the anterior mitral leaflet (aml; *arrows*). Mild regurgitation was demonstrated. In spite of the patient's age, no degenerative changes were detected in the mitral or aortic valve. Therefore, this valve abnormality is most likely related to scleroderma, probably immune-mediated valve disease. Anterior and posterior pericardial effusion (pe) can be seen in the long parasternal view. Ao—aorta; LA—left atrium; LV—left ventricle.

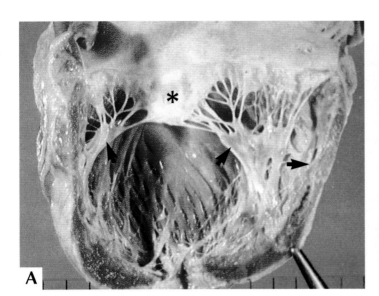
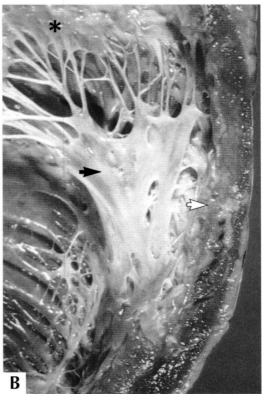

FIGURE 1-38. **A** and **B**, Myocardial disease in a 53-year-old woman with scleroderma. Myocardial degeneration is widespread, with fibrous tissue replacement leading to thinning of the papillary muscles (*black arrows*) and left ventricular wall (*white arrows*). The normally red myocardium has been replaced extensively by pale, pinkish-white fibrous tissue. *Asterisks* indicate the mitral valve. (*Adapted from* Farrer-Brown [26]; with permission.)

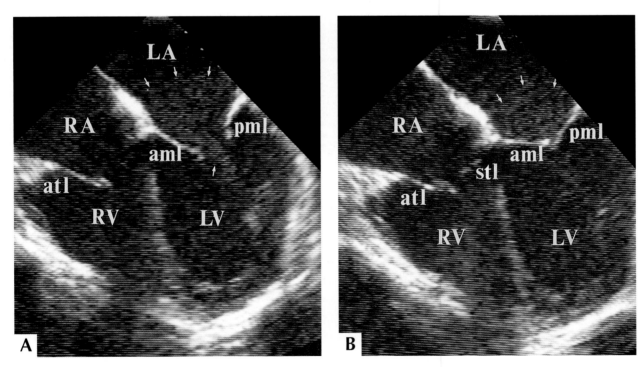

FIGURE 1-39. Dilated nonischemic cardiomyopathy in a 45-year-old man with diffuse cutaneous-type scleroderma. Transesophageal four-chamber echocardiographic views during end diastole (**A**) and end systole (**B**) show dilatation of all four chambers and depressed biventricular function. Left ventricular (LV) ejection fraction was estimated to be 35%. Moderate diffuse LV and right ventricular (RV) hypokinesis was seen, as was a moderate degree of pseudocontrast or "smoke" in the left atrium (LA; *arrows*). A recent myocardial perfusion scan showed no fixed or reversible defects. These findings suggest myocarditis associated with scleroderma, probably immune-mediated. This patient also has chronic atrial fibrillation. aml—anterior mitral leaflet; atl—anterior tricuspid leaflet; pml—posterior mitral leaflet; RA—right atrium; stl—septal tricuspid leaflet.

CHARACTERISTICS OF CARDIOVASCULAR DISEASES ASSOCIATED WITH ANKYLOSING SPONDYLITIS

AORTIC ROOT/VALVE DISEASE	CONDUCTION DISTURBANCES	MYOCARDITIS	PERICARDITIS
Proximal aortitis and regurgitation are characteristic of this disease	Most common after aortic root disease	Unknown pathogenesis; clinically rare	Unknown pathogenesis and prevalence
Aortic valve cusps are mildy affected	Due to subaortic fibrosis extending to basilar septum, His bundle, and AV node	Most commonly manifests as diastolic dysfunction (up to 53%)	Generally asymptomatic
Aortic regurgitation results mostly from aortic root and annulus dilatation	AV blocks are most common (50%–66%); complete heart block is rare	Systolic dysfunction is rare	Usually detected incidentally
Basilar thickening of the anterior mitral leaflet or "subaortic bump" results from extension of aortitis	Often associated with aortic root disease	No distinctive clinical or echocardiographic features	Pericardial thickening and/or small effusions on echocardiography (up to 45%)
Severe aortic regurgitation is rare	Anti-inflammatory therapy is of no benefit	No specific therapy is available	No specific therapy is available

FIGURE 1-40. The cardiovascular diseases associated with ankylosing spondylitis are more prevalent in patients who have had the disease for over 20 years, in those older than age 50 years, and in those with peripheral articular involvement. Aortitis and conduction disturbances are the most common and clinically important. Aortitis of the proximal aorta extends to the aortic cusps, to the aortomitral intervalvular fibrosa, producing the "subaortic bump," and into the basilar septum. This leads to aortic root thickening and dilatation, aortic and mitral regurgitation, and conduction disturbances. Myocardial and pericardial diseases are rare, generally asymptomatic, and of no clinical significance. AV—atrioventricular.

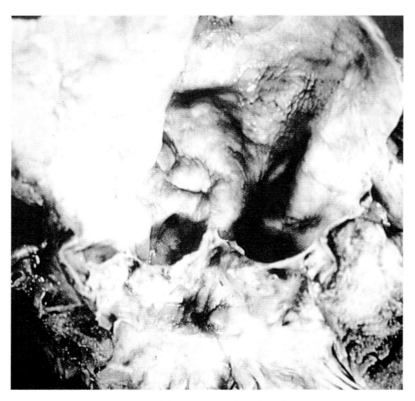

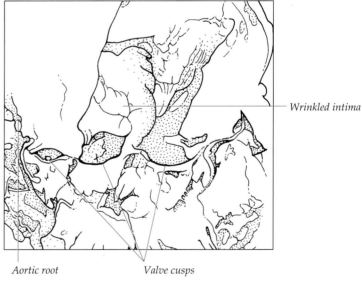

Wrinkled intima

Aortic root   *Valve cusps*

FIGURE 1-41. Aortic root dilatation and valve disease in ankylosing spondylitis. The aortic root wall is thickened and the intima wrinkled. The valve cusps are also thickened, retracted, and distorted. Aortic regurgitation was present. (*Adapted from* Sutton and Fox [29]; with permission.)

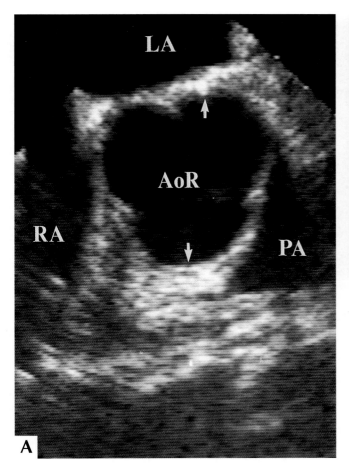

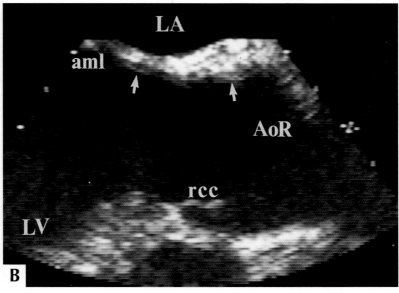

FIGURE 1-42. Disease of the aortic root (AoR) and aortic and mitral valves in a 31-year-old man with ankylosing spondylitis. **A,** Transesophageal basilar short-axis echocardiographic view showing marked thickening of the aortic root, predominantly of the posterolateral and anteromedial walls (*arrows*), with mild root dilatation. **B,** Transesophageal longitudinal close-up view of the aortic root showing marked thickening of the posterior wall (*arrows*) extending to the basal portion of the anterior mitral leaflet (aml). This basal anterior mitral valve abnormality, referred to as a "subaortic bump," is characteristic of ankylosing spondylitis. LA—left atrium; LV—left ventricle; PA—pulmonary artery; rcc—right coronary cusp. (*Adapted from* Roldan and Crawford [28]; with permission.)

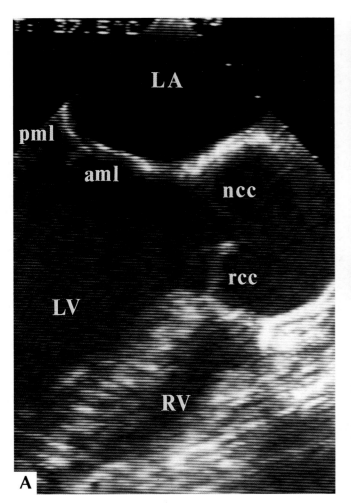

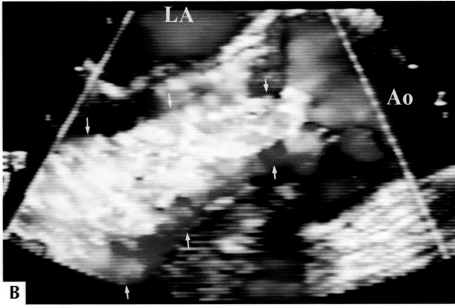

FIGURE 1-43. Aortic root disease and aortic valve regurgitation in the patient shown in Fig. 1-42. **A,** Transesophageal echocardiographic view longitudinal to the outflow tract showing thickening and dilatation of the aortic root and mild thickening of the tip of the right coronary cusp (rcc). **B,** Transesophageal longitudinal view showing moderately severe aortic regurgitation on color Doppler flow mapping (*arrows*). aml—anterior mitral leaflet; Ao—aorta; LA—left atrium; LV—left ventricle; ncc—noncoronary cusp; pml—posterior mitral leaflet; RV—right ventricle.

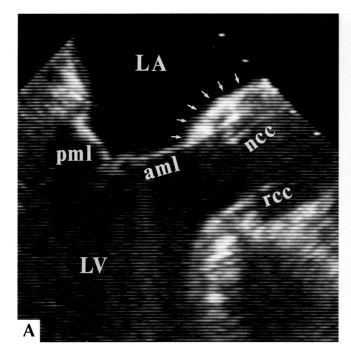

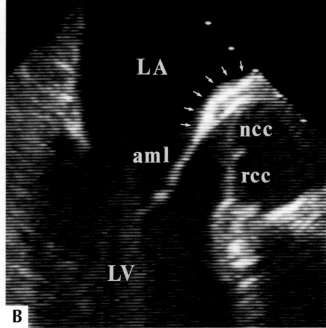

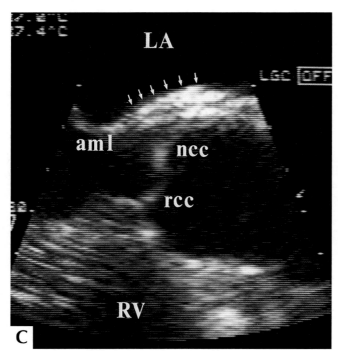

FIGURE 1-44. Aortic root disease and mitral "subaortic bump" (*small arrows*) in a 55-year-old man with ankylosing spondylitis. Transesophageal views longitudinal to the outflow tract during systole (**A**) and diastole (**B**), along with a close-up view (**C**), showing marked thickening of the proximal aortic root (predominantly of the posterior wall) that extends about 1 cm into the basal portion of the anterior mitral leaflet (aml) to produce the characteristic subaortic bump. Decreased mobility of the anterior mitral leaflet and mild mitral regurgitation were noted. The aortic cusps appeared normal. LA—left atrium; LV—left ventricle; ncc—noncoronary cusp; pml—posterior mitral leaflet; rcc—right coronary cusp; RV—right ventricle.

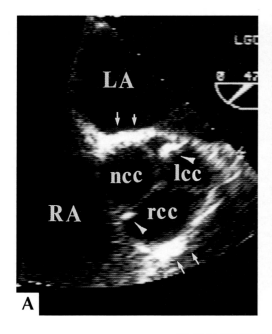

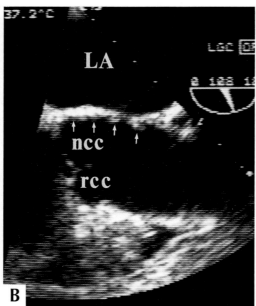

FIGURE 1-45. Aortic root and valve disease in a 46-year-old woman with ankylosing spondylitis. **A,** Transesophageal basilar short-axis echocardiographic view showing moderate thickening of the anterior and posterior aortic root walls (*arrows*) and localized nodular thickening (*arrowheads*) at the base of the left (lcc) and right (rcc) coronary cusps. **B,** Transesophageal longitudinal view of the ascending aorta further demonstrating moderate and irregular thickening of the first 3.5 cm of the posterior aortic root wall (*arrows*). No valve regurgitation was seen. LA—left atrium; ncc—noncoronary cusp; RA—right atrium.

POLYMYOSITIS-DERMATOMYOSITIS

CHARACTERISTICS OF CARDIOVASCULAR DISEASES ASSOCIATED WITH POLYMYOSITIS/DERMATOMYOSITIS

CONDUCTION DISTURBANCES/ARRHYTHMIAS	MYOCARDITIS	PERICARDITIS
High-grade AV blocks are rare (2%–6%)	More common in polymyositis	Unknown clinical prevalence but rare
Bundle branch and fascicular blocks are most common	Can mimic myocardial infarction	Generally asymptomatic and uncomplicated
AV blocks can progress despite remission of disease	Often associated with peripheral myositis	Cardiac tamponade and constriction are extremely rare
Arrhythmias, predominantly atrial tachyarrhythmias, are common	Systolic or diastolic failure occurs in 3%–44% of patients; dilated cardiomyopathy occurs in 3%–19%	More common in overlap syndrome than in isolated polymyositis or dermatomyositis
More common in polymyositis than dermatomyositis	Steroid therapy not proven beneficial	Steroid therapy not proven beneficial

FIGURE 1-46. Cardiovascular diseases are the third most common cause of death after malignant and infectious diseases in patients with polymyositis-dermatomyositis. They are more common in patients with polymyositis than in those with dermatomyositis, and their presence does not correlate with age or gender or with the duration, activity, or severity of disease. Myocarditis with left ventricular or biventricular diastolic or systolic dysfunction and associated arrhythmias or conduction disturbances is the most prevalent and clinically important. Anti-inflammatory therapy has not proved beneficial in these patients. AV—atrioventricular.

HERITABLE CONNECTIVE TISSUE DISEASES

MARFAN SYNDROME

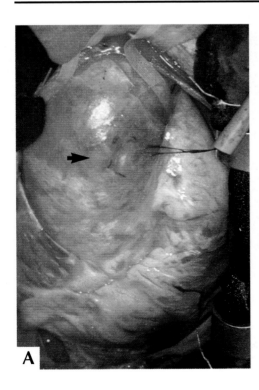

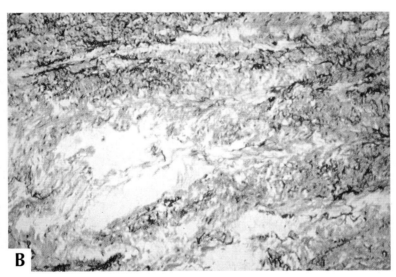

FIGURE 1-47. Aortic aneurysm and cystic medial degeneration in Marfan syndrome.
A, A fusiform aneurysm of the ascending aorta in a patient with Marfan syndrome (*arrow*).
B, Cystic medial degeneration with disruption of the normal structure, fragmentation, and disruption of the elastic fibers in the aortic media, particularly in areas of mucoid degeneration. Elastic tissue appears black, smooth muscle brown, and fibrous tissue red. (*continued*)

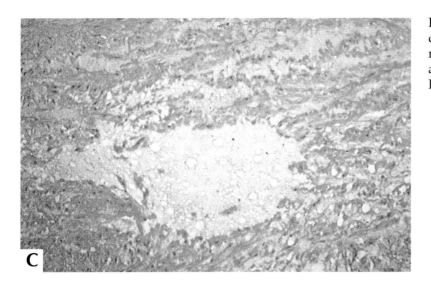

FIGURE 1-47. (*continued*) **C,** The medial layer of the aorta is also disrupted by a large basophilic pool of mucoid material. Cystic medial degeneration of the aorta leads to wall weakening and aneurysmal dilatation in Marfan syndrome. (*Adapted from* Farrer-Brown [26]; with permission.)

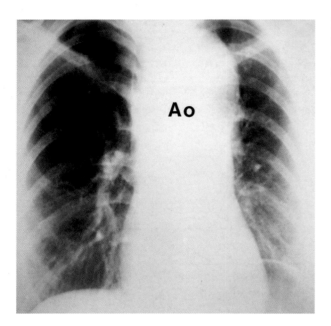

FIGURE 1-48. Posteroanterior chest radiograph showing dilatation of the ascending and descending thoracic aorta (Ao) in a 27-year-old man with Marfan syndrome. The cardiac silhouette appears normal. An aneurysmal ascending and descending aorta 6 cm in diameter was found on echocardiography.

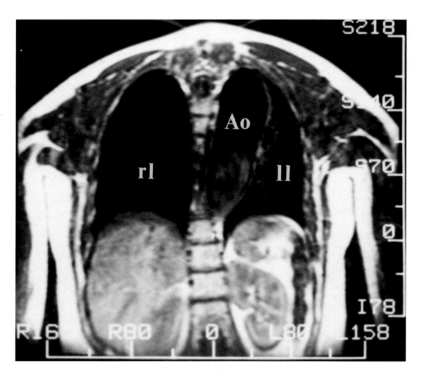

FIGURE 1-49. Aortic aneurysm in an asymptomatic 31-year-old man with Marfan syndrome. This sagittal nuclear magnetic resonance image of the thorax shows marked aneurysmal dilatation of the aorta (Ao) that begins distal to the arch and extends down through the thoracic aorta. Careful clinical and echocardiographic follow-up during β-blocker therapy has shown no progression of the aortic aneurysmal dilatation. rl—right lung, ll—left lung.

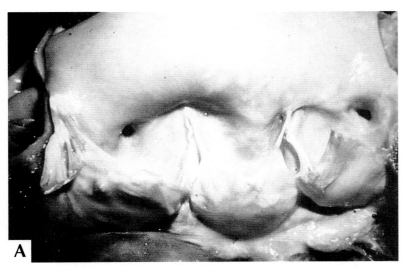

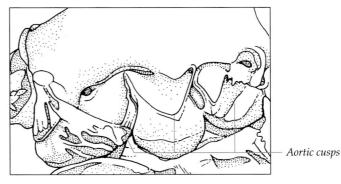
Aortic cusps

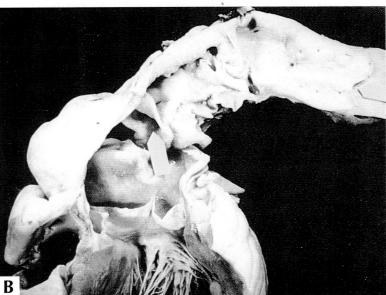

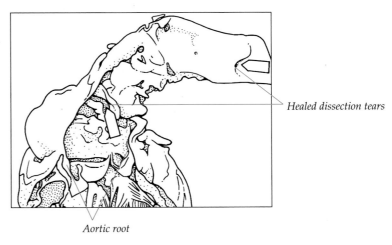
Healed dissection tears

Aortic root

FIGURE 1-50. Aortic root and valve disease in Marfan syndrome. **A,** Markedly dilated aortic root with ballooned, thin, and prolapsing aortic cusps leading to aortic regurgitation. **B,** Aortic root dila-

tation in a different patient showing two healed dissection tears. (*Adapted from* Sutton and Fox [29]; with permission.)

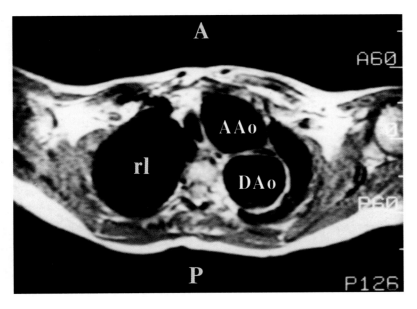

FIGURE 1-51. Aortic disease in a 22-year-old man with Marfan syndrome. Transverse nuclear magnetic resonance image at midthorax showing marked dilatation of the ascending (AAo) and descending (DAo) aorta of approximately 5 to 6 cm at the widest diameter. The aortic dilatation extended to the aortic annulus, and mild aortic regurgitation could be detected on cardiac auscultation. A—anterior; P—posterior; rl—right lung.

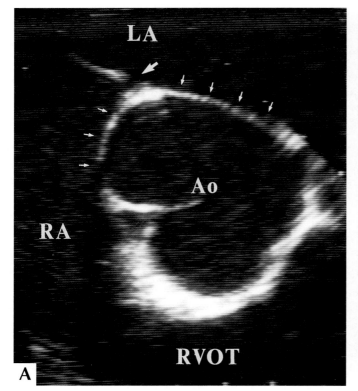

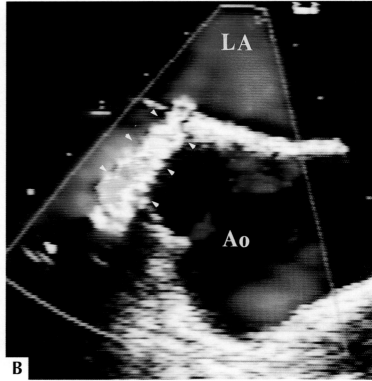

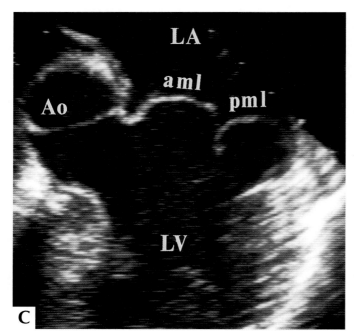

FIGURE 1-52. Aortic root dilatation and mitral valve prolapse in a 21-year-old man with Marfan syndrome. **A** and **B,** Transesophageal basilar short-axis echocardiographic view showing mild aortic root dilatation and characteristically thin aortic root walls (*small arrows* in *A*). Mild aortic regurgitation was present. A small secundum-type interatrial septal defect was noted incidentally (*large arrow* in *A*) with a left-to-right shunt (*arrowheads* in *B*). **C,** Transesophageal view longitudinal to the left ventricular (LV) outflow tract showing thin, elongated, and prolapsing anterior and posterior mitral leaflets. Mild eccentric mitral regurgitation was demonstrated. aml—anterior mitral leaflet; Ao—aorta; LA—left atrium; pml—posterior mitral leaflet; RA—right atrium; RVOT—right ventricular outflow tract.

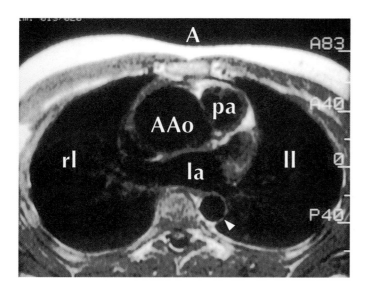

FIGURE 1-53. Disease of the aortic root and pulmonary artery (pa) in a 14-year-old boy with Marfan syndrome. Transverse nuclear magnetic resonance image at the superior thorax shows marked dilatation of approximately 10 cm of the ascending aorta (AAo). This is in contrast to the normal diameter of the descending aorta (*arrowhead*). Moderate dilatation of the pulmonary artery can also be seen. A—anterior; la—left atrium; ll—left lung; rl—right lung.

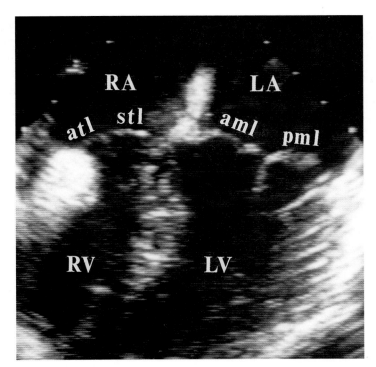

FIGURE 1-54. Mitral and tricuspid valve prolapse in a 27-year-old man with Marfan syndrome. Transesophageal four-chamber echocardiographic view showing mild prolapse of the anterior (aml) and posterior (pml) mitral leaflets. Moderate myxomatous thickening of the posterior mitral leaflet can be seen, as well as mild prolapse of the anterior (atl) and septal (stl) tricuspid valve leaflets. Mild mitral and tricuspid regurgitation was noted. LA—left atrium; LV—left ventricle; RA—right atrium; RV—right ventricle.

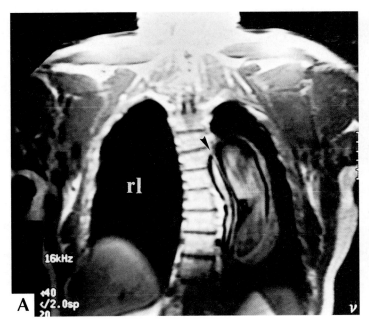

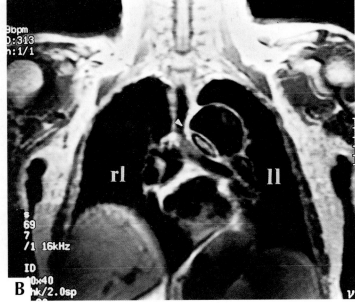

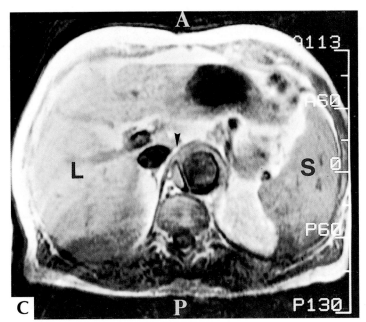

FIGURE 1-55. Aortic dissection in a 41-year-old man with Marfan syndrome. **A,** Sagittal nuclear magnetic resonance image of the posterior thorax shows moderate dilatation and type B dissection of the descending thoracic aorta. The entry site of the intimal tear, the intimal flap, and the small false lumen are well defined (*arrowhead*). **B** and **C,** Sagittal midthoracic and transverse abdominal nuclear magnetic resonance images in the same patient show aortic dilatation with dissection that begins just beyond the subclavian artery and extends to the abdominal aorta. The intimal flap and the false lumen are well demarcated (*arrowheads*). A—anterior; L—liver; ll—left lung; P—posterior; rl—right lung; S—spleen.

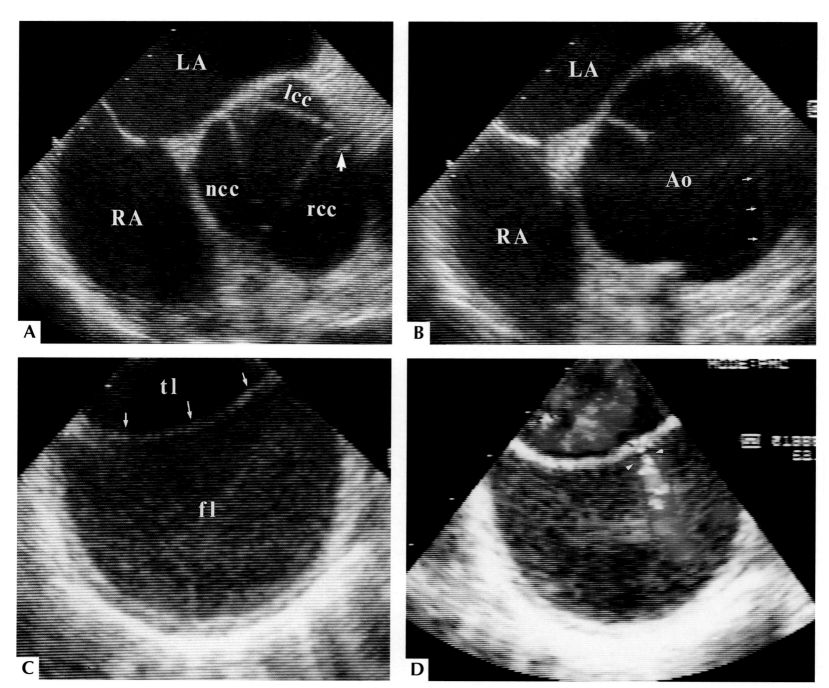

FIGURE 1-56. Aortic dissection in a 41-year-old man with Marfan syndrome. **A,** Transesophageal basilar short-axis echocardiographic view of the aortic valve showing aortic dilatation of 5.5-cm and normal aortic valve cusps. The possible entry site of an intimal tear close to the commissure of the right coronary cusp (rcc) (*arrow*) can be seen. **B,** View of ascending aorta further illustrating the marked dilatation along with an intimal flap in the lateral wall of the aorta (Ao; *small arrows*). **C,** Transesophageal basilar short-axis view of ascending aorta revealing an intimal flap (*arrows*), a small true lumen (tl), and a large false lumen (fl), with evidence of slow blood flow or pseudocontrast. **D,** Color Doppler flow mapping with jet originating from the true lumen and entering the false lumen through a tear in the intimal flap (*arrowheads*). LA—left atrium; lcc—left coronary cusp; ncc—noncoronary cusp; RA—right atrium.

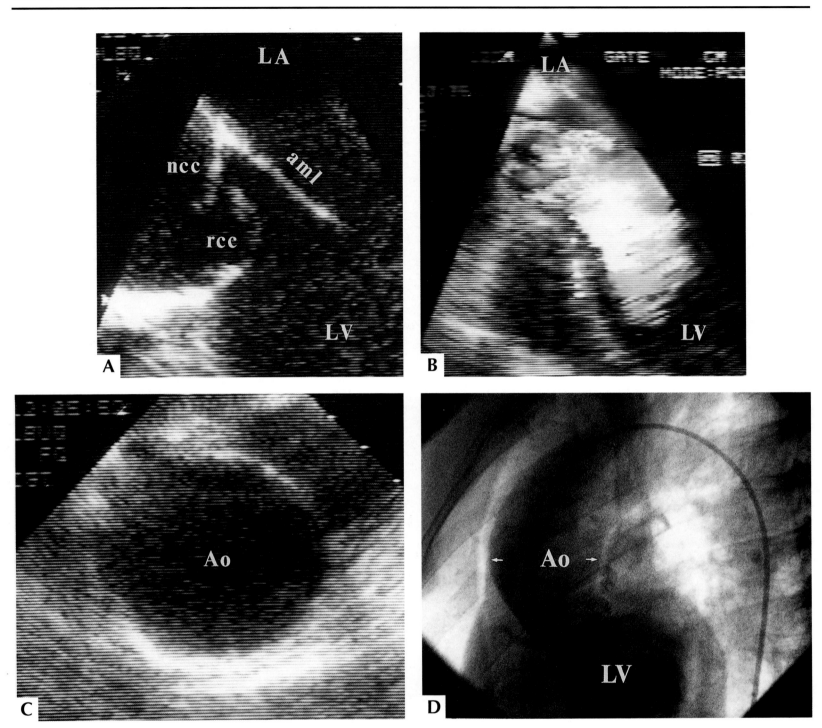

FIGURE 1-57. Aortic root and valve disease in a patient with osteogenesis imperfecta. **A** and **B,** Transesophageal longitudinal views to the outflow tract at a depth of 6 and 12 cm, respectively, demonstrating marked prolapse of the right coronary cusp (rcc) and severe aortic regurgitation. **C,** Transesophageal short-axis view showing moderate dilatation of the ascending aorta (Ao).

D, Left anterior oblique view during aortography revealing 4+ aortic regurgitation and moderate dilatation of the ascending aorta (*arrows*). This patient underwent valve replacement and the aortic valve was found to be bicuspid, with thickened and redundant cusps. aml—anterior mitral leaflet; LA—left atrium; LV—left ventricle; ncc—noncoronary cusp.

REFERENCES

1. Roldan CA, Shively BK, Gurule FT: Systemic lupus erythematosus valve disease by transesophageal echocardiography and the role of antiphospholipid antibodies. *J Am Coll Cardiol* 1992, 20:1127–1134.

2. Gleason CB, Stoddard MF, Wagner SG: A comparison of cardiac valvular involvement in the primary antiphospholipid syndrome versus anticardiolipin-negative systemic lupus erythematosus. *Am Heart J* 1993, 125:1123–1129.

3. Kahl LE: The spectrum of pericardial tamponade in systemic lupus erythematosus. Report of ten patients. *Arthritis Rheum* 1992, 35:1343–1349.

4. Sasson Z, Rasooly Y, Chow C-W: Impairment of left ventricular diastolic function in systemic lupus erythematosus. *Am J Cardiol* 1992, 69:1629–1634.

5. Petri M, Perez-Gutthann S, Spence D: Risk factors for coronary artery disease in patients with systemic lupus erythematosus. *Am J Med* 1992, 93:513–519.

6. Escalante A, Kaufman RL, Quismorio FP: Cardiac compression in rheumatoid pericarditis. *Semin Arthritis Rheum* 1990, 20:148–163.

7. Hara KS, Ballard DJ, Ilstrup DM: Rheumatoid pericarditis: clinical features and survival. *Medicine* 1990, 69:81–91.

8. Kelly CA, Bourke JP, Malcolm A: Chronic pericardial disease in patients with rheumatoid arthritis: a longitudinal study. *Q J Med* 1990, 75:461–470.

9. Mullins PA, Grace AA, Stewart SC: Rheumatoid heart disease presenting as acute mitral regurgitation [brief communication]. *Am Heart J* 1991, 122:242–245.

10. Anvari A, Graninger W, Schneider B: Cardiac involvement in systemic sclerosis. *Arthritis Rheum* 1992, 35:1356–1361.

11. Silver RM: Clinical aspects of systemic sclerosis (scleroderma). *Ann Rheum Dis* 1991, 50:854–861.

12. Kahan A, Devaux JY, Amor B: The effect of captopril on thallium-201 myocardial perfusion in systemic sclerosis. *Clin Pharmacol Ther* 1990, 47:483–489.

13. Follansbee WP, Zerbe TR, Medsger TA: Cardiac and skeletal muscle disease in systemic sclerosis (scleroderma): a high risk association. *Am Heart J* 1993, 125:194–203.

14. O'Neil TW: The heart in ankylosing-spondylitis. *Ann Rheum Dis* 1992, 51:705–706.

15. O'Neil TW, King G, Graham IH: Echocardiographic abnormalities in ankylosing spondylitis. *Ann Rheum Dis* 1992, 51:652–654.

16. Peeters AJ, Wolde S, Sedney MI: Heart conduction disturbance: an HLA-B27 associated disease. *Ann Rheum Dis* 1991, 50:348–350.

17. Tami LF, Bhasin S: Polymorphism of the cardiac manifestations in dermatomyositis. *Clin Cardiol* 1993, 16:260–264.

18. Buchpiguel CA, Roizenblatt S, Lucena-Fernandes MF: Radioisotopic assessment of peripheral and cardiac muscle involvement and dysfunction in polymyositis/dermatomyositis. *J Rheumatol* 1991, 18:1359–1363.

19. Byrnes TJ, Baethge BA, Wolf RE: Noninvasive cardiovascular studies in patients with inflammatory myopathy. *Angiology* 1991, 42:843–848.

20. Schwarz MI: Pulmonary and cardiac manifestations of polymyositis-dermatomyositis. *J Thorac Imaging* 1992, 7:46–54.

21. Simpson IA, de Belder MA, Treasure T: Cardiovascular manifestations of Marfan syndrome: improved evaluation by transesophageal echocardiography. *Br Heart J* 1993, 69:104–108.

22. Tahernia AC: Cardiovascular anomalies in Marfan syndrome: the role of echocardiography and beta blockers. *South Med J* 1993, 86:305–310.

23. Hwa J, Richards JG, Huang H: The natural history of aortic root dilatation in Marfan syndrome. *Med J Aust* 1993, 158:558–562.

24. Ohteki H, Ohtsubo S, Sakurai J, *et al.*: Aortic regurgitation and aneurysm of sinus of Valsalva associated with osteogenesis imperfecta. *Thorac Cardiovasc Surg* 1991, 39:294–295.

25. Takahashi T, Koide T, Yamaguchi H: Ehlers-Danlos syndrome with aortic regurgitation: dilatation of the sinuses of Valsalva and abnormal dermal collagen fibrils. *Am Heart J* 1992, 123:1709–1712.

26. Farrer-Brown G: *Color Atlas of Cardiac Pathology: Other Connective Disorders.* Chicago: Year Book Medical Publishers, 1977:107–109 and 137.

27. Robbins S: Diseases of immunity. In *Pathologic Basis of Disease*, ed 4. Edited by Robbins S. Philadelphia: WB Saunders Co, 1989:163–237.

28. Roldan CA, Crawford MH: Connective tissue diseases and the heart. In: *Current Diagnosis and Treatment in Cardiology.* Edited by Crawford MH. Norwalk, CT: Appleton & Lange, 1995:428–447.

29. Sutton GC, Fox KM: Valve disease. In *A Color Atlas of Heart Disease: Pathological, Clinical, and Investigatory Aspects.* Edited by Sutton GC, Fox KM. London: Current Medical Literature Ltd., 1990 (revised):107–173.

ENDOCRINE DISORDERS AND THE HEART

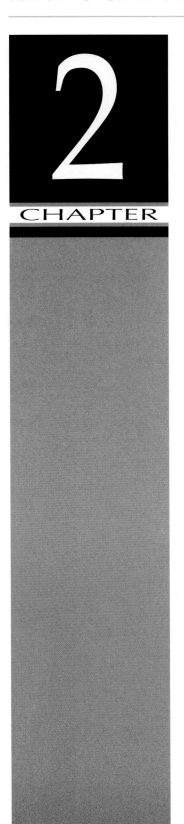

2

CHAPTER

B. Sylvia Vela

Endocrinology involves the study of hormones and the glands that secrete them. By definition, a hormone is a substance released into the circulation to exert its effects at distant target sites. These effects are often complex and may involve one or many tissues. The various hormones identified so far regulate reproduction, growth and development, homeostasis, and metabolism. Thus, the over- or underproduction of hormones can have numerous consequences and can affect every organ system, including the cardiovascular system.

Thyroid hormone is perhaps the best studied in terms of its profound effects on the cardiovascular system. By regulating the genetic expression of the myosin molecule in cardiac muscle, over- or underproduction of thyroid hormone leads to enhanced or diminished contractility, respectively. By contributing to the body's demand for efficient use and consumption of oxygen, thyroid hormone is linked inextricably to the cardiovascular system. All thyroid disorders can affect the heart, and certain cardiac conditions (such as thyrotoxic atrial fibrillation and myxedematous cardiomyopathy) can be reversed or cured through treatment of the underlying thyroid abnormality. Some conditions, such as unstable angina precipitated by thyrotoxicosis, are merely attenuated by thyroid hormone inhibition.

The adrenal gland can affect the cardiovascular system in several ways. Glucocorticoids regulate carbohydrate and lipid metabolism, while mineralocorticoids help govern electrolyte and water balance. Although cardiovascular effects are due mostly to mineralocorticoids, glucocorticoid receptors have been found on blood vessel walls, suggesting that they play a direct role in vascular physiology. Catecholamines, which are synthesized and stored in the adrenal medulla as well as in nerve endings throughout the nervous system, directly affect cardiac output, heart rate, and peripheral resistance. While the vasculature is regulated primarily by the sympathetic nerves supplying the heart, the adrenals can play a critical role in compensating for or augmenting impaired sympathetic responses. Indeed, excess adrenal catecholamines, as seen in pheochromocytoma, can have devastating cardiovascular effects.

Parathyroid conditions indirectly affect the heart through changes in serum calcium concentration. Both insulin resistance and insulin deficiency can accelerate atherosclerosis. Although acromegaly and carcinoid syndrome are relatively rare, both have specific cardiac sequelae that can result in severe and sometimes fatal heart disease.

Thus, many endocrinopathies can have important consequences on the cardiovascular system, usually detrimental ones. Recently, however, encouraging information has come to light concerning one class of hormones that may provide cardiovascular protection. Estrogens have been shown in epidemiologic studies to prolong life and decrease mortality and morbidity from cardiac disease in women. Although many questions remain regarding the mechanism by which estrogens confer such protection, these agents continue to represent an exciting link between hormones and the heart.

THYROID DISORDERS

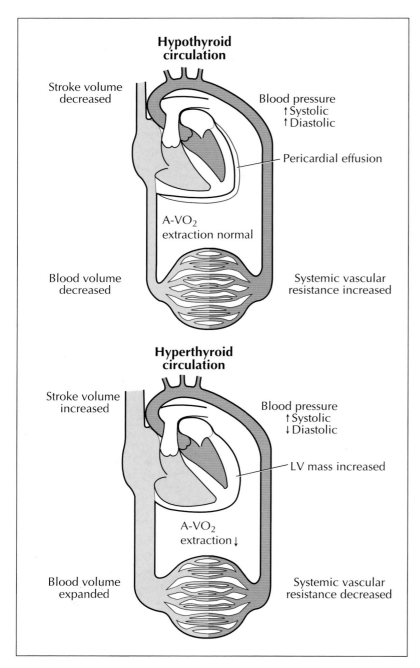

Hypothyroid circulation

Stroke volume decreased

Blood pressure
↑ Systolic
↑ Diastolic

Pericardial effusion

A-VO₂ extraction normal

Blood volume decreased

Systemic vascular resistance increased

Hyperthyroid circulation

Stroke volume increased

Blood pressure
↑ Systolic
↓ Diastolic

LV mass increased

A-VO₂ extraction ↓

Blood volume expanded

Systemic vascular resistance decreased

FIGURE 2-1. Comparison of cardiovascular hemodynamics in hypothyroid and hyperthyroid states [1]. More than any other hormone, thyroid hormone has profound effects on the cardiovascular system, regulating vascular tone, myocardial contractility, and the metabolic demands of the body. In general, thyroid hormone increases the basal metabolic rate by stimulating cellular oxygen consumption and substrate utilization. Diastolic and systolic performances are enhanced owing to the regulation of myosin, which augments cardiac contraction and increases calcium ATPase in the sarcoplasmic reticulum to regulate intracellular calcium concentration. Both these effects increase inotropy. Thus, the net effect of thyroid hormone on the heart is to increase cardiac output and decrease peripheral vascular resistance for optimal delivery of fuel and oxygen to the periphery [2]. A-VO₂—arteriovenous oxygen difference; LV—left ventricular. (*Adapted from* Klein [1]; with permission.)

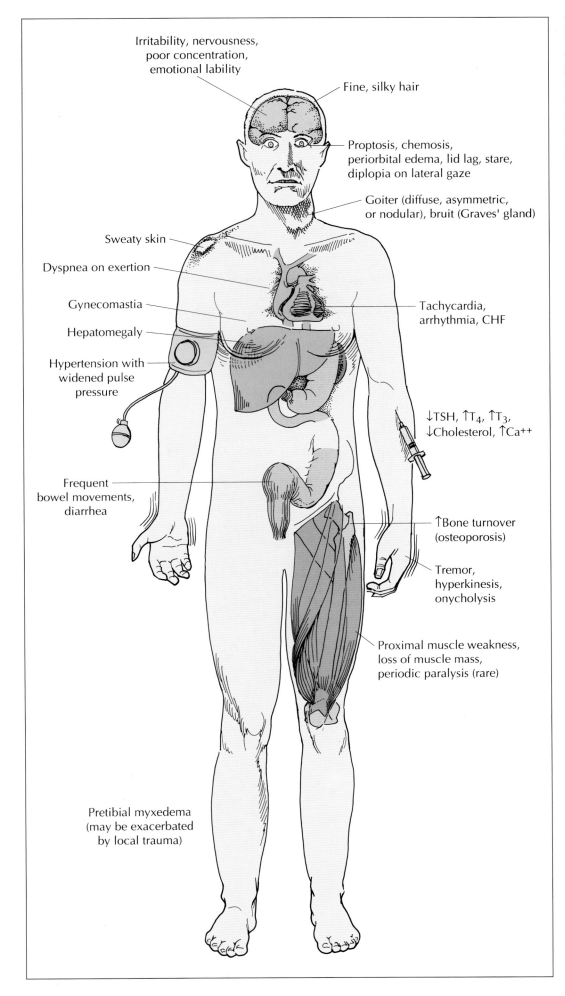

Irritability, nervousness, poor concentration, emotional lability

Fine, silky hair

Proptosis, chemosis, periorbital edema, lid lag, stare, diplopia on lateral gaze

Goiter (diffuse, asymmetric, or nodular), bruit (Graves' gland)

Sweaty skin

Dyspnea on exertion

Gynecomastia

Hepatomegaly

Hypertension with widened pulse pressure

Tachycardia, arrhythmia, CHF

$\downarrow$TSH, $\uparrow$T$_4$, $\uparrow$T$_3$, $\downarrow$Cholesterol, $\uparrow$Ca^{++}

Frequent bowel movements, diarrhea

$\uparrow$Bone turnover (osteoporosis)

Tremor, hyperkinesis, onycholysis

Proximal muscle weakness, loss of muscle mass, periodic paralysis (rare)

Pretibial myxedema (may be exacerbated by local trauma)

FIGURE 2-2. Signs and symptoms in hyperthyroidism. Patients with hyperthyroidism often complain of weight loss, nervousness, anxiety, irritability, insomnia, mood swings, heat intolerance, and more frequent bowel movements and/or diarrhea. In addition, a fine resting tremor of the hands, hyperreflexia, sweaty skin, proximal muscle weakness, and muscle wasting may be prominent. In most cases a goiter is present, although this may be minimal in the elderly. A hyperdynamic precordium and sinus tachycardia with a wide pulse pressure along with cardiac arrhythmias are typical findings. Atrial premature beats and atrial fibrillation are common. Ventricular arrhythmias usually indicate underlying cardiac disease. Uncommon findings include localized edema or "pretibial myxedema," usually on the shins; acropachy (subperiosteal resorption of the distal digits), which resembles clubbing; and onycholysis (lifting of the nail from the nail bed). Rarely, choreoathetosis and periodic paralysis occur. CHF—congestive heart failure; TSH—thyroid-stimulating hormone.

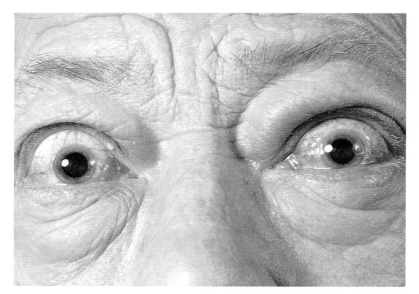

FIGURE 2-3. Eye findings in Graves' disease [2,3]. Stare, lid retraction, and lid lag may be present owing to the high-catecholamine-like state seen in thyrotoxicosis of all causes. Exophthalmos and diplopia on lateral gaze are due to extraocular muscle hypertrophy. Inflammatory changes include periorbital and lid edema, conjunctival chemosis, and injection. Diuretics, steroids, radiation therapy, or orbital decompression surgery may be employed once the patient becomes euthyroid [2]. (*Adapted from* Bahn and coworkers [3]; with permission.)

THYROID STORM

FACTORS PRECIPITATING THYROID STORM

Cerebrovascular accident	Pulmonary embolism
Congestive heart failure	Parturition
Diabetic ketoacidosis	Surgery
Infection	Trauma
Emotional stress	Hypoglycemia
Iodine-131 therapy	Iodinated contrast agents
Vigorous palpation of thyroid	Withdrawal of antithyroid medication

FIGURE 2-4. Factors that precipitate thyroid storm [4]. Although rare, thyroid storm is always fatal if not treated. It is characterized by systemic decompensation in a thyrotoxic patient, which often leads to vascular collapse, coma, and death. Patients present in a hypermetabolic state characterized by fever accompanied by sinus or supraventricular tachycardia disproportionate to the degree of fever. Encephalopathic changes may also be present. A symmetric goiter or exophthalmos is a clue to underlying Graves' disease. Routine thyroid function tests do not help discriminate patients with thyrotoxicosis from those with thyroid storm. Therefore, a high index of suspicion and prompt recognition of the underlying cause are central to successful therapy. Treatment is directed at counteracting systemic decompensation with supportive measures, reducing thyroid hormone action and production with antithyroid drugs, and controlling precipitating factors [5].

Onset is almost always abrupt in a patient with underlying thyrotoxicosis who is exposed to one of these factors. Infection, trauma, and surgery are the most common. The mechanism by which these factors lead to thyrotoxic decompensation is, however, unclear.

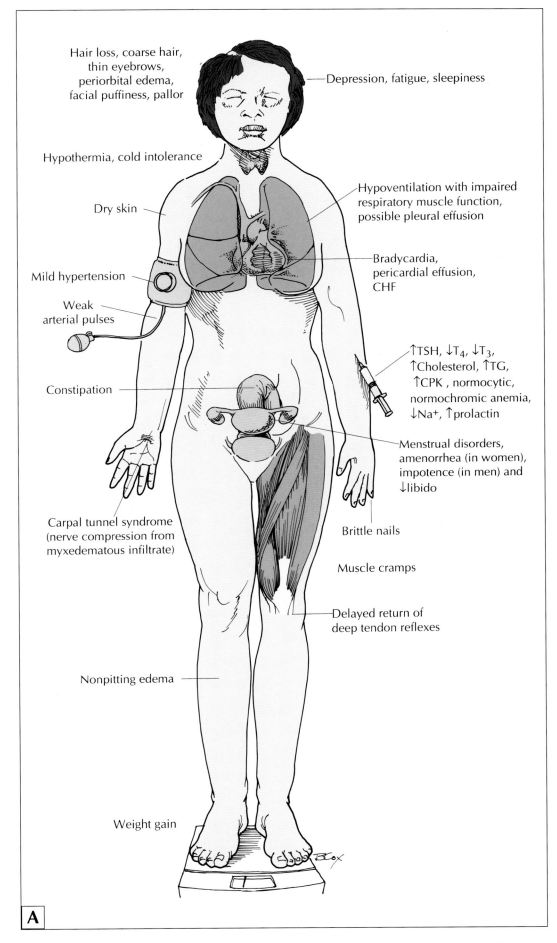

Hair loss, coarse hair, thin eyebrows, periorbital edema, facial puffiness, pallor

Depression, fatigue, sleepiness

Hypothermia, cold intolerance

Hypoventilation with impaired respiratory muscle function, possible pleural effusion

Dry skin

Bradycardia, pericardial effusion, CHF

Mild hypertension

Weak arterial pulses

$\uparrow$TSH, $\downarrow$T$_4$, $\downarrow$T$_3$, $\uparrow$Cholesterol, $\uparrow$TG, $\uparrow$CPK, normocytic, normochromic anemia, $\downarrow$Na$^+$, $\uparrow$prolactin

Constipation

Menstrual disorders, amenorrhea (in women), impotence (in men) and $\downarrow$libido

Carpal tunnel syndrome (nerve compression from myxedematous infiltrate)

Brittle nails

Muscle cramps

Delayed return of deep tendon reflexes

Nonpitting edema

Weight gain

A

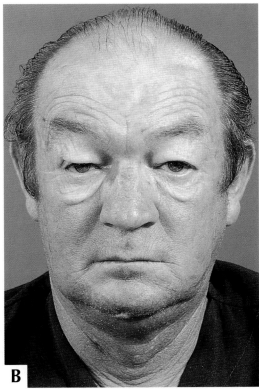

B

FIGURE 2-5. A, Clinical signs and symptoms in hypothyroidism. This insidious disease may be subtle in its presentation and progression. Typically patients complain of weight gain (although morbid obesity does not occur), weakness, lethargy, fatigue, depression, muscle cramps, constipation, cold intolerance, dry skin, and coarse hair. Women often have menstrual disorders (most commonly amenorrhea), and men may experience decreased libido and/or impotence. Hypothermia, bradycardia, weak arterial pulses, and mild hypertension are characteristic vital signs. Thyroid hormone replacement normalizes blood pressure in approximately one third of cases.

B, Periorbital edema, facial puffiness, and dry/coarse hair and skin are characteristic of hypothyroidism. Goiter is usually present. Reflexes are typically delayed during the return phase. Nonpitting edema may be seen. As the hypothyroidism worsens, congestive heart failure and high-protein pleural and pericardial effusions become prominent [6]. The effusions typically resolve within a year after thyroid hormone replacement. CHF—congestive heart failure; CPK—creatine phosphokinase; TG—triglycerides; TSH—thyroid-stimulating hormone.

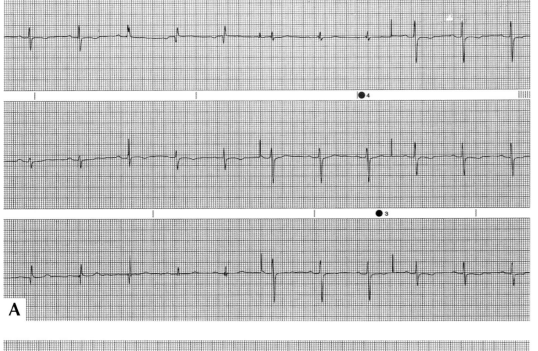

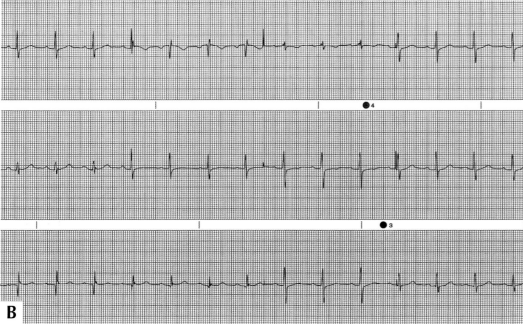

FIGURE 2-6. Electrocardiogram (ECG) in a hypothyroid patient with thyroid-stimulating hormone (TSH) above 60 mIU/mL (normal=0.5–4.5 mIU/mL). **A,** ECG changes include sinus bradycardia, prolonged P-R and Q-T intervals, low-voltage complexes, and flattened or inverted T waves. Many of these changes may be due to pericardial fluid. Atrial, ventricular, and intraventricular conduction delays are three times more likely in patients with hypothyroidism than in the general population. Systolic time intervals are altered, the pre-ejection period is prolonged, and the ratio of pre-ejection period to left ventricular ejection time is increased. **B,** The same patient's ECG 6 months later, when the TSH has normalized. The ECG changes often resolve by rendering the patient euthyroid.

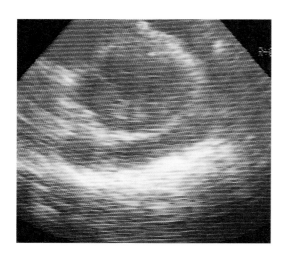 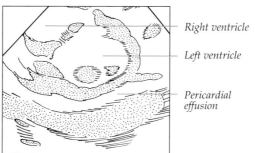

Right ventricle

Left ventricle

Pericardial effusion

FIGURE 2-7. Echocardiographic findings in hypothyroidism. Effusions are seen in as many as 30% of all hypothyroid patients. Note the increased echogenicity of the pericardial fluid, believed due to the increased protein and cholesterol content. Cardiac tamponade is unusual owing to the slow accumulation of fluid, which does not increase pericardial pressure excessively. Systolic anterior motion of the mitral valve and asymmetric septal hypertrophy with obstruction of the left ventricular outflow tract can occur, but these abnormalities disappear when the hypothyroidism is treated [7].

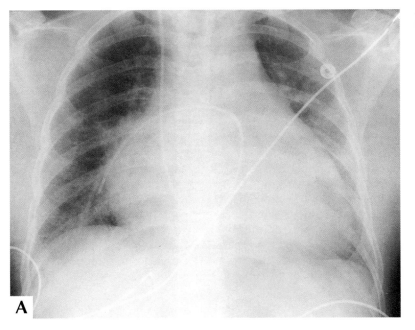

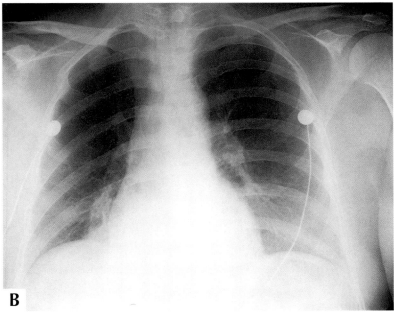

A

B

FIGURE 2-8. A, Chest radiograph in untreated hypothyroidism. An enlarged cardiac silhouette and pleural effusions may be seen owing to pericardial effusion and/or congestive heart failure (CHF) [8]. Myxedematous heart failure can be distinguished from CHF of other causes in that the myxedematous heart (1) responds to exercise with an increased heart rate, (2) improves with thyroid hormone replacement but not with digitalis and diuretics, (3) is rarely accompanied by pulmonary congestion, and (4) exhibits effusions with a high protein content. **B,** The same patient 4 months after thyroid hormone replacement. The cardiac silhouette is markedly smaller, and the lung fields are clear.

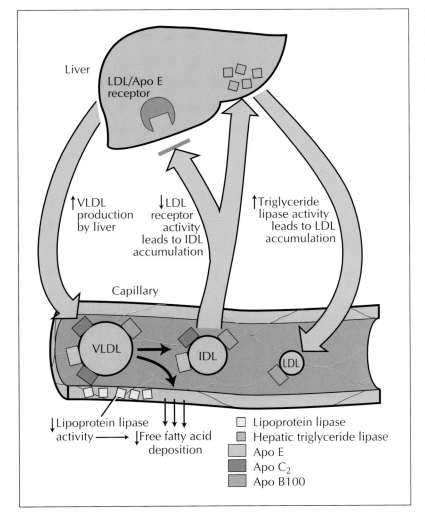

FIGURE 2-9. Hyperlipidemia of hypothyroidism. Hypothyroidism is associated with accelerated atherosclerosis, probably as a result of the accompanying hyperlipidemia. The pattern of hyperlipoproteinemia secondary to hypothyroidism is variable owing to a multitude of defects in lipoprotein metabolism [9,10]. Overproduction of very-low-density lipoprotein (VLDL) cholesterol by the liver can result in hypertriglyceridemia. Reduced lipoprotein lipase activity in the capillary wall or abnormal apolipoprotein (Apo) C_2, which is ineffective in activating lipoprotein lipase, will interrupt triglyceride hydrolysis and subsequent deposition of free fatty acids into the parenchyma. Hypertriglyceridemia results from the accumulation of VLDL. Reduced low-density lipoprotein (LDL) B100/Apo E receptor activity can cause intermediate-density lipoprotein (IDL) cholesterol to accumulate, resulting in hypercholesterolemia and hypertriglyceridemia. Alternatively, with increased triglyceride lipase activity in the liver, LDL can accumulate, resulting in hypercholesterolemia. Thyroid hormone replacement reverses these hyperlipoproteinemias.

CLINICAL FEATURES OF MYXEDEMA COMA

Hypothermia
Stupor or coma
Hypoventilation and respiratory failure
Congestive heart failure
Hyponatremia
Hypotension
Seizures
Hypoglycemia

FIGURE 2-10. Clinical features of myxedema coma [11]. Myxedema coma usually develops in hypothyroid patients subjected to a stress such as infection, surgery, congestive heart failure, stroke, seizure, trauma, or the administration of sedatives. Typically patients present with altered thermoregulation (hypothermia) and mental status (stupor or coma). Like thyroid storm, this condition is fatal if untreated. Even when it is recognized and treated promptly, mortality approaches 60%. Virtually all organ systems may be involved, but the respiratory and cardiovascular systems are predominantly affected. Respiratory failure occurs as a result of neuromuscular dysfunction and a blunted response to hypercapnia and hypoxemia. Cardiac failure may occur, especially in the setting of myocardial infarction. Frank anasarca is often seen. If congestive heart failure is present, pitting edema may be superimposed on the nonpitting edema of myxedema. Treatment must be provided in an intensive-care setting to treat the respiratory depression, shock, and hypothermia. Various amounts of thyroid hormone are advocated by different authors [12], for example, high-dose (400 µg) versus low-dose (100 µg). In all cases thyroid hormone should be given intravenously, with each patient considered individually.

HYPERPARATHYROIDISM

CLINICAL MANIFESTATIONS OF HYPERPARATHYROIDISM

Muscle weakness	Arthralgias
Easy fatigability	Gout or pseudogout
Headache	Peptic ulcer
Weight loss	Pancreatitis
Depression	Polyuria
Renal colic	Polydipsia
Bone pain and/or fracture	Constipation
Pruritus	Ectopic calcification
Hypertension	

FIGURE 2-11. Common clinical manifestations in hyperparathyroidism [13]. Many patients with chronic hyperparathyroidism (most commonly due to a parathyroid adenoma) are asymptomatic; others complain of nonspecific symptoms such as fatigue and vague aches and pains, polyuria, polydipsia, constipation, ulcer, mental status changes, and pruritus (from calcium deposition in the skin). Patients may present with nephrolithiasis, osteoporosis, and occasionally pancreatitis and peptic ulcer. Calcium may also be deposited in the cornea (band keratopathy), soft tissues, joints, and heart, including the valves and coronary arteries [14]; this finding is especially common in patients with renal failure. Hypertension occurs in 20% to 60% of patients; although the mechanism is unknown, it may be due to nephrocalcinosis, hyperreninemia, or the hypercalcemia itself.

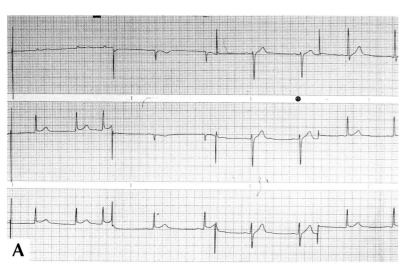

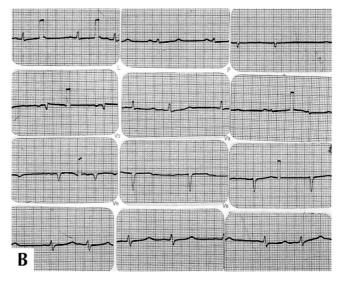

FIGURE 2-12. A, Electrocardiogram (ECG) in hyperparathyroidism. Arrhythmias are uncommon, but acute hypercalcemia can cause bradycardia, first-degree heart block, and hypertension. Hypercalcemia decreases the plateau phase of the cardiac action potential, reflected in shortening of the ST segment and Q-T interval. The Q-Tc interval (ie, corrected for heart rate) is probably the most reliable ECG index of hypercalcemia. B, ECG findings in hypocalcemia, which are the opposite of those in A, with prolongation of the ST segment and Q-T interval.

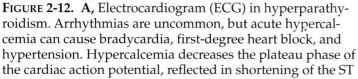

PHEOCHROMOCYTOMA

FINDINGS SUGGESTIVE OF PHEOCHROMOCYTOMA

Sustained hypertension resistant to treatment

Unusual lability of blood pressure

Paroxysms of any kind (especially hypertension and tachycardia, headache, palpitations, pallor, perspiration)

Apprehension or sense of impending doom

Signs of hypermetabolism (fever, weight loss)

Orthostatic hypotension

Nervousness

Chest pain or myocardial infarction in absence of coronary disease

Pressor response to anesthesia, surgery, or trauma

Diagnosis of neurofibromatosis

Diagnosis of multiple endocrine neoplasia (MEN) II syndrome

FIGURE 2-13. Findings suggestive of pheochromocytoma [15,16]. The hypersecretion of catecholamines from this tumor usually causes paroxysms of headache, palpitations, tachycardia, and sweating. Patients may complain of nervousness, irritability, an impending sense of doom, mild abdominal or chest pain, and constipation. Most pheochromocytomas secrete predominantly norepinephrine; about 15% secrete predominantly epinephrine. The effects of catecholamines on the heart are mediated by β_1-adrenergic receptors and include increased heart rate, enhanced contractility, augmented conduction velocity, and increased cardiac output. In 85% of patients, hypertension may be either paroxysmal or sustained and is usually resistant to treatment. Although many patients may have orthostatic hypotension, lightheadedness and syncope are rare.

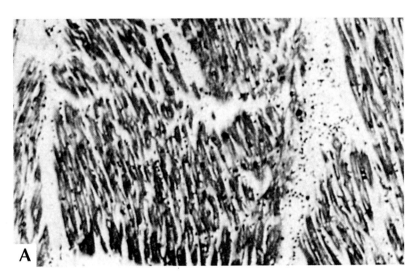

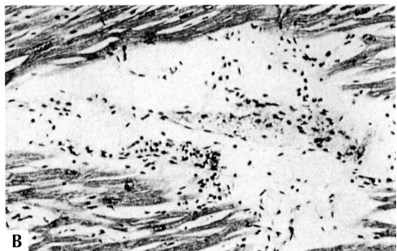

FIGURE 2-14. Myocarditis with contraction band necrosis in a patient with a pheochromocytoma. Both dilated and hypertrophic cardiomyopathies as well as myocarditis with contraction band necrosis and fibrosis have been associated with this tumor [17,18].

The myocarditis is characterized by diffuse infiltration by inflammatory cells (**A**), perivascular inflammation (**B** and **C**), and contraction band necrosis of myocytes (**D**) (hematoxylin and eosin, × 20 [*A*], × 45 [*B*], × 540 [*C*], and × 330 [*D*]). (*continued*)

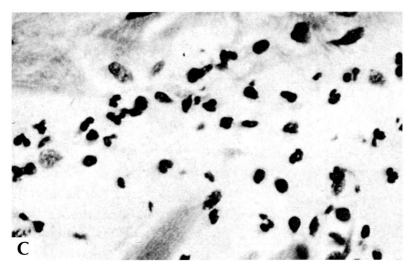

C

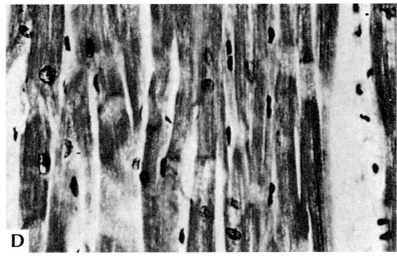

D

FIGURE 2-14. (*continued*) These changes are reversible if detected before extensive replacement fibrosis occurs. Chest pain, angina, and acute myocardial infarction may occur in the absence of coronary artery occlusive disease as a result of coronary spasm or myocarditis. Cardiac arrhythmias such as atrial and ventricular fibrillation occur, with sudden death. Pulmonary edema and shock may also be seen in association with myocarditis or infarction or following a hypertensive crisis. (*Adapted from* McManus and coworkers [18]; with permission.)

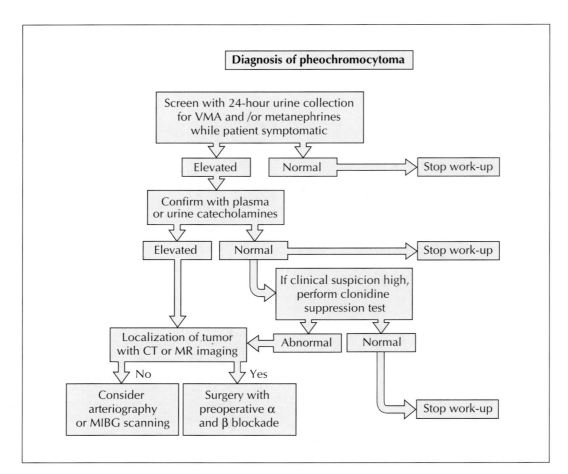

FIGURE 2-15. Diagnosis of pheochromocytoma. Screening consists of a 24-hour urine sample to measure vanillylmandelic acid (VMA) and/or metanephrines. If these values are elevated, the diagnosis can be confirmed by the finding of elevated plasma or urine catecholamines. In equivocal cases or if clinical suspicion is very high despite normal values, a clonidine suppression test may be useful [19]. Clonidine will suppress sympathetic outflow in normal persons but has a negligible effect in patients with a pheochromocytoma. After the biochemical diagnosis has been made, computed tomography (CT) or magnetic resonance (MR) imaging should be used to localize the tumor. If CT or MR imaging results are negative, arteriography or radionuclide scanning with ^{131}I-metaiodobenzylguanidine (MIBG) can be performed.

DRUGS USED PREOPERATIVELY

CLINICAL SETTING	DRUG	PROBLEMS AND SIDE EFFECTS
Hypertension	Phenoxybenzamine 10 mg PO bid to start 40 mg PO qid maximum	Nasal congestion Hypotension Drowsiness Miosis
	Prazosin 1 mg PO bid to start 5 mg PO tid maximum	Hypotension Dizziness Headache
	Metyrosine 250 mg PO qid to start 1 g PO qid maximum	Sedation Crystalluria Diarrhea Extrapyramidal reaction Psychic disturbance
Tachycardia and ventricular and atrial arrhythmias	Propranolol—to be started after α-blockade 10 mg PO tid to start 80 mg PO tid maximum	Paroxysmal hypertension Bradycardia Fatigue Exacerbation of bronchospasm

FIGURE 2-16. Treatment guidelines for preoperative adrenergic blockade pheochromocytoma [20]. α-Blockers should be given initially until the blood pressure is normalized for 2 weeks; this should be followed by β-blockers if the patient has tachycardia or arrhythmias prior to removal of the catecholamine-producing tumor. Instituting β-blockade without prior α-blockade can cause significant hypertension because of unopposed α-adrenergic–mediated vaso-constriction. Phentolamine and phenoxy-benzamine have been the mainstays of treatment. bid—twice daily; PO—by mouth; qid—four times daily; tid—three times daily. (*Adapted from* Malone and coworkers [20]; with permission.)

DRUGS COMMONLY USED INTRAOPERATIVELY

CLINICAL SETTING	DRUG	INDICATION (SIDE EFFECTS)
Hypertension	Sodium nitroprusside bolus, 250 µg; continuous drip (100 mg in 500 mL D₅W*)	Onset immediate, duration 3 min, potent vasodilator
	Phentolamine bolus, 1–5 mg (1 mg/mL); continuous drip (5, 40, or 80 mg in 500 mL D₅W*)	No tachycardia or tachyphylaxis, duration 5–10 min
Arrhythmia	Lidocaine bolus, 50–100 mg	Especially good for ventricular extrasystole and tachycardia, effect gone in 10–20 min, not useful in supraventricular arrhythmias (occasional convulsions and hypotension)
	Propranolol bolus, 0.10–0.25 mg	Use less than total of 5 mg during operation, may repeat if arrhythmia unresponsive
Hypotension	Volume expanders (red blood cells, 6% albumin, dextran)	May give 2 U of blood preoperatively
	Phenylephrine or norepinephrine (rarely needed), 8 mg/mL or 64 µg/mL	Purely adrenergic without causing catecholamine release or myocardial instability

*D₅W=5% dextrose in water for injection.

FIGURE 2-17. Treatment guidelines for intraoperative adrenergic blockade in pheochromocytoma [20]. The drugs used to control hypertension, arrhythmias, and hypotension are listed. Surgical removal of a pheochromocytoma is a high-risk procedure that requires an experienced surgeon and anesthesiologist. Induction of anesthesia and manipulation and removal of the tumor can cause pressor responses, hypotension, and fluid plasma volume shifts that can ultimately lead to arrhythmia or infarction. Careful cardiac monitoring is required. (*Adapted from* Malone and coworkers [20]; with permission.)

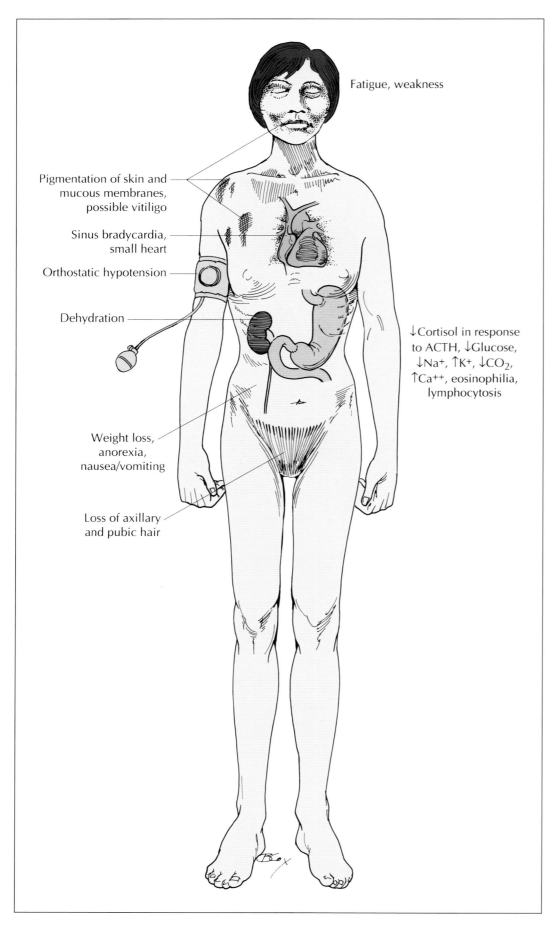

Fatigue, weakness

Pigmentation of skin and mucous membranes, possible vitiligo

Sinus bradycardia, small heart

Orthostatic hypotension

Dehydration

↓Cortisol in response to ACTH, ↓Glucose, ↓Na⁺, ↑K⁺, ↓CO₂, ↑Ca⁺⁺, eosinophilia, lymphocytosis

Weight loss, anorexia, nausea/vomiting

Loss of axillary and pubic hair

FIGURE 2-18. A, Signs and symptoms of adrenal insufficiency [21]. Glucocorticoid deficiency causes fatigue, anorexia, nausea, vomiting (and therefore weight loss), hypotension, and hypoglycemia. Mineralocorticoid or aldosterone deficiency leads to renal sodium and bicarbonate wasting, resulting in hyponatremia, hyperkalemia, acidosis, and profound dehydration. As a result, the heart is small, peripheral pulses are thready and diminished, and diastolic hypotension ensues. Overproduction of adrenocorticotropic hormone (ACTH) due to primary adrenal failure causes hyperpigmentation of the skin and mucous membranes, whereas this effect is not seen in secondary adrenal insufficiency due to pituitary failure. Vitiligo may accompany the adrenal insufficiency of autoimmune causes. Electrocardiographic changes include slow atrioventricular conduction and low voltage. The diagnosis of adrenal failure can be documented by the failure to produce endogenous cortisol in response to ACTH stimulation [22]. A normal cortisol response would be a doubling of the baseline value to above 18 mg/dL.

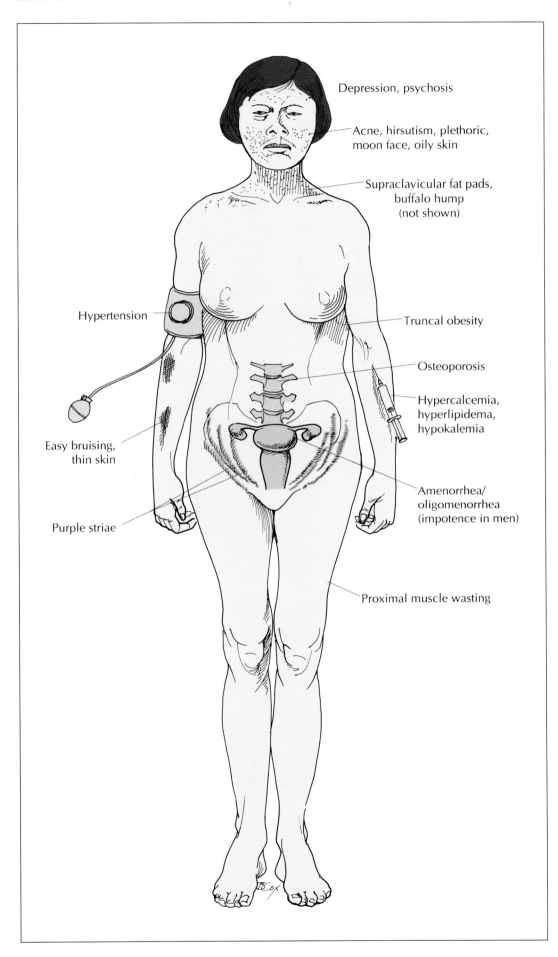

Depression, psychosis

Acne, hirsutism, plethoric, moon face, oily skin

Supraclavicular fat pads, buffalo hump (not shown)

Hypertension

Truncal obesity

Osteoporosis

Hypercalcemia, hyperlipidema, hypokalemia

Easy bruising, thin skin

Amenorrhea/ oligomenorrhea (impotence in men)

Purple striae

Proximal muscle wasting

FIGURE 2-19. Classic features of Cushing's syndrome. "Cushing's syndrome" refers to the chronic state of excess cortisol in the circulation, whereas "Cushing's disease" refers specifically to the state of hypercortisolemia due to an adrenocorticotropic hormone (ACTH)–producing pituitary adenoma. Other causes of Cushing's syndrome include ectopic ACTH production from tumors such as small cell carcinoma of the bronchus, adrenal tumors that secrete glucocorticoids, bilateral adrenal hyperplasia, and exogenous use of steroids. Excess cortisol causes truncal obesity, facial plethora, hypertension, purple striae, osteoporosis, proximal muscle weakness, interscapular adipose tissue ("buffalo hump"), depression, hyperglycemia, and hypokalemia. Androgen excess may cause oily skin, acne, and hirsutism in women. The facial features (rounding of the face, acne, hirsutism) generally revert to normal after treatment [25]. Since patients with Cushing's syndrome typically have central obesity, hypertension, hyperlipidemia, and hyperglycemia, they are at risk for progressive atherosclerosis.

Atherosclerotic cardiovascular disease is a major cause of morbidity and mortality when this syndrome goes untreated. A 5-year mortality rate as high as 50% has been reported in the past, before early detection and newer treatment modalities became available. The majority of these deaths were due to cardiac failure, cerebrovascular accidents, and renal insufficiency. These complications can be prevented by controlling the hypertension, hypokalemia, and hyperlipidemia.

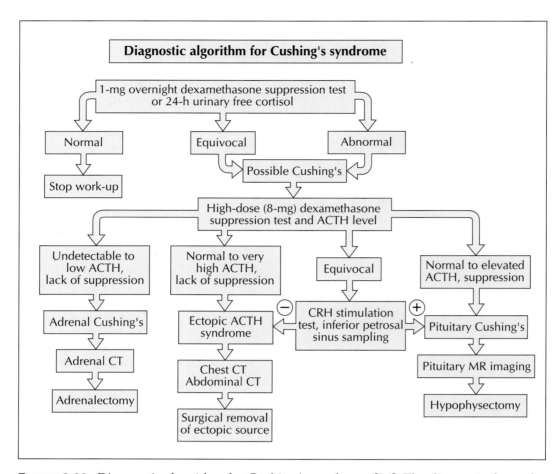

FIGURE 2-20. Diagnostic algorithm for Cushing's syndrome [26]. The diagnosis depends on the failure of dexamethasone to suppress cortisol secretion appropriately. After clinical suspicion, the best screening test is to measure 24-hour urinary free cortisol. In the vast majority of patients with Cushing's syndrome, this level will be elevated. The next step is to confirm the hypercortisolemia by demonstrating a lack of cortisol suppression with high-dose (8 mg) dexamethasone and to determine whether or not the process is dependent on adrenocorticotropic hormone (ACTH). Treatment depends on the specific cause, although surgery is generally performed. ACTH-producing pituitary tumors may also require radiation therapy. CRH—cortisol-releasing hormone; CT—computed tomography; MR—magnetic resonance. (*Adapted from* Kaye and Crapo [26]; with permission.)

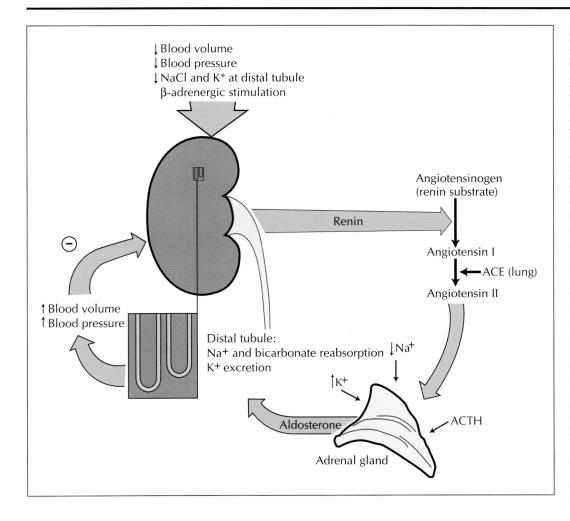

FIGURE 2-21. Aldosterone regulation [27]. Increased and autonomous production of aldosterone by the adrenal gland is known as primary hyperaldosteronism. Secondary hyperaldosteronism occurs when stimulators of renin secretion, such as decreased plasma volume or sodium depletion, cause excessive secretion of aldosterone. The four predominant stimuli to aldosterone secretion are angiotensin II, hyponatremia, hyperkalemia, and adrenocorticotropic hormone (ACTH). Consequences of excessive aldosterone production include sodium retention, with plasma volume expansion and hypertension; renal loss of potassium and hydrogen ion, causing hypokalemia and alkalosis; and suppression of renin and angiotensin. Hyperaldosteronism is believed to account for 0.5% to 2.0% of all cases of hypertension. The diagnosis should be suspected in hypertensive patients with spontaneous hypokalemia or that which is easily provoked by diuretic therapy or sodium ingestion. The heart is usually only modestly enlarged; congestive heart failure is rarely seen. Electrocardiographic changes include those seen in left ventricular hypertrophy and hypokalemia. ACE—angiotensin-converting enzyme. (*Adapted from* Young and Klee [27]; with permission.)

LABORATORY DIAGNOSIS OF PRIMARY HYPERALDOSTERONISM

PRIOR TO ADMISSION FOR TESTING:

1. Discontinue spironolactone (6 wk), diuretics (4 wk), and sympathetic inhibitors (1 wk).
2. Allow unrestricted sodium intake (1 wk).

ADMISSION AND TESTING PROCEDURES:

Day 1

Admit patient to hospital on liberal sodium diet (100 mEq). Replace potassium and keep patient recumbent overnight.

Day 2

Draw blood samples to measure supine (8:00 AM) and 4-h upright (noon) plasma aldosterone, plasma renin activity, and 18-hydroxycortisone. Start 24-h urine collection to measure aldosterone or tetrahydroaldosterone.

Day 3

Complete 24-h urine analysis.

FIGURE 2-22. The diagnosis of primary hyperaldosteronism is suspected when aldosterone excess and suppression of plasma renin activity are seen in the setting of hypertension and hypokalemia. Confirmation involves salt and/or volume loading to demonstrate the lack of aldosterone suppression. This is most commonly done on an inpatient basis, as described here [28]. (*Adapted from* Melby [28]; with permission from The Endocrine Society, © 1989.)

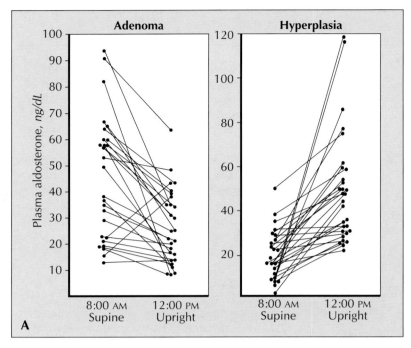

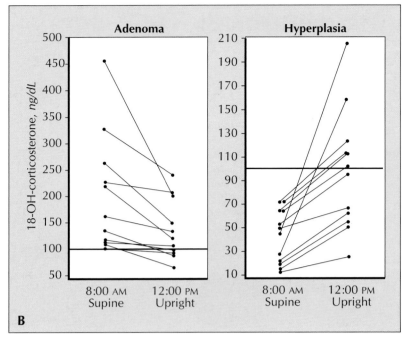

FIGURE 2-23. Characteristic response of aldosterone (**A**) and 18-hydroxycorticosterone (**B**) levels to postural changes in patients with aldosterone-producing adenoma versus adrenal hyperplasia [29]. Assessing these responses to the supine and upright positions can help determine the etiology of primary hyperaldosteronism. Aldosterone-producing adenomas paradoxically cause a fall in aldosterone and 18-hydroxycorticosteroids, whereas hyperplasia causes a characteristic rise. Adenomas typically produce over 100 ng/dL of 18-hydroxycorticosterone, whereas hyperplasia does not.

The surgical treatment of primary hyperaldosteronism depends on the cause. Surgical resection of an aldosterone-producing adenoma is successful in the majority of patients. In as many as 70%, the hypertension and hypokalemia are cured. On the other hand, bilateral adrenalectomy improves hypertension in only one third of patients with hyperplasia and is no longer recommended. Medical therapy for unresectable tumors or for patients with hyperplasia includes the aldosterone antagonist spironolactone (100 to 200 mg/d), amiloride (10 to 40 mg/d), and calcium-channel blockers. (*Adapted from* Melby [29]; with permission.)

ACROMEGALY

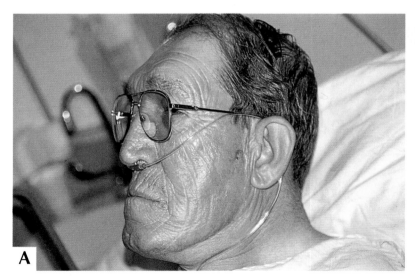

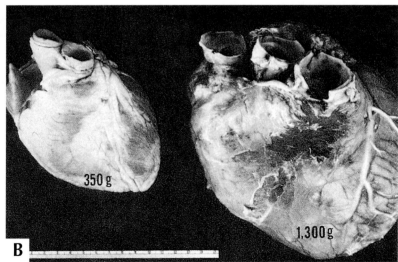

FIGURE 2-24. Acromegaly is caused by the excessive secretion of growth hormone (GH). Excessive GH mediated through insulin-like growth factor-1 (IGF-1) or somatomedin C causes soft tissue, bony, and visceral overgrowth. **A,** The typical prominent jaw and frontal sinuses and the coarsened facial features in acromegaly. **B,** Extreme cardiomegaly (1300 vs 350 g for the normal heart) is out of proportion to the generalized organomegaly otherwise seen,

and, even in the absence of hypertension, suggests a direct effect of growth hormone on the myocyte. Cardiac dysfunction and heart failure are a major cause of death, and the coexistence of hypertension and/or diabetes in this condition likely contributes to cardiovascular mortality. (Part B *adapted from* Lie and Grossman [30]; with permission.)

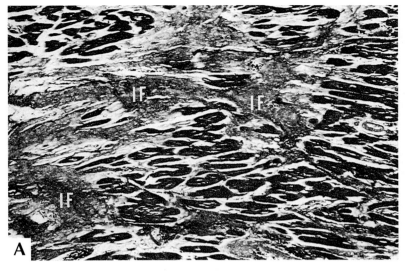

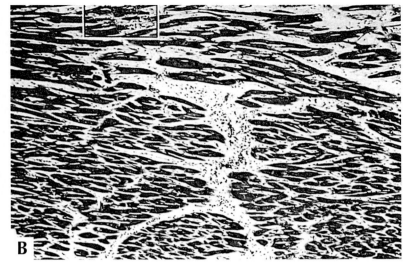

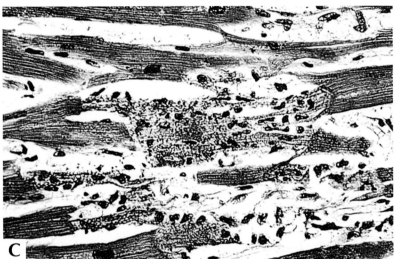

FIGURE 2-25. Histologic findings in acromegalic myocarditis. **A,** Myocardial fiber hypertrophy and interstitial fibrosis (IF) are commonly seen, although these changes are relatively nonspecific (Mallory-Heidenhain, × 120) [30]. **B,** Myocarditis, focal or diffuse, may also be seen. The inset in *B* (× 48) is shown at higher magnification in **C** (× 300), revealing necrosis of individual myocytes and a lymphomononuclear cell infiltrate (hematoxylin and eosin). Both symmetric and asymmetric cardiac hypertrophy have been noted on echocardiography. Electrocardiographic abnormalities include ST-segment depression and nonspecific T-wave changes, intraventricular conduction disturbances, and the changes seen in left ventricular hypertrophy. Cardiac arrhythmias are relatively common and include ventricular premature beats and atrial fibrillation/flutter. (*Adapted from* Lie and Grossman [30]; with permission.)

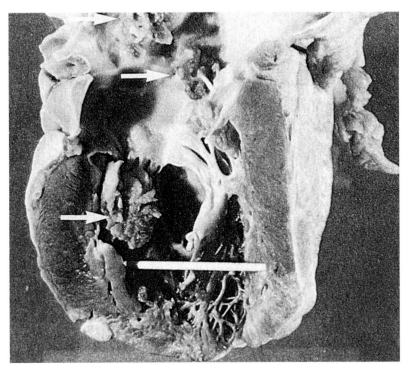

FIGURE 2-26. Carney's myxoma in association with acromegaly. A rare condition known as Carney's syndrome (or Carney's complex) involves growth hormone–secreting pituitary tumors in the setting of atrial myxoma, Sertoli cell tumors, cutaneous hyperpigmentation, hypothyroidism, and pigmented nodular adrenocortical disease [31]. Cardiac myxomas are found in 76% of patients with Carney's complex. The myxomas differ from other cardiac myxomas in that they occur in young individuals, are usually multiple, and may involve more than one chamber. Three masses are evident on the interatrial septum, papillary muscle, and chordae of the anterior leaflet of the mitral valve (*arrows*). (*Adapted from* Wallace and coworkers [31]; with permission.)

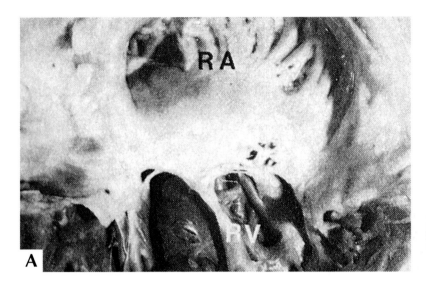

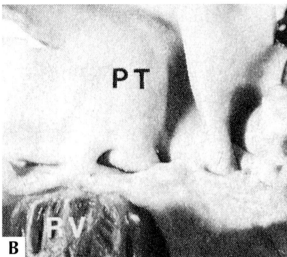

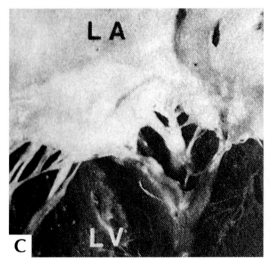

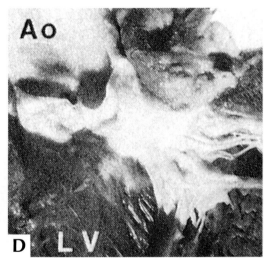

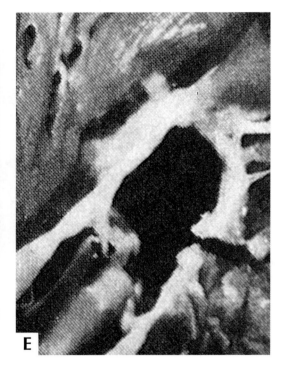

FIGURE 2-27. Gross pathologic findings in carcinoid [32]. Carcinoid tumors are neuroendocrine tumors that contain vasoactive secretagogues found in the gastrointestinal tract or pulmonary bronchioles. They can secrete numerous hormones including adrenocorticotropic hormone (ACTH) and growth hormone–releasing hormone (GHRH), but most commonly they secrete serotonin and its metabolites. Symptoms associated with carcinoid include flushing of the head and neck, diarrhea (if liver metastases are present), and bronchospasm (in pulmonary carcinoid only). A unique endocrine effect of carcinoid tumors is the deposition of fibrotic, plaque-like thickenings on the endocardium of the atria and ventricles (**A** and **C**), pulmonic valves (**B**), sometimes the mitral and aortic valves (**C** and **D**), and the tricuspid valve (**E**). The tricuspid valve is fixed and incompetent. Deposition may also be seen on the superior and inferior vena cava and pulmonary artery and in the coronary sinus. Although the right side of the heart is affected predominantly, left-sided heart disease may be seen in as many as 30% of cases, although it is less significant. Ao—opened aorta; LA—left atrium; LV—left ventricle; PT—pulmonary trunk; RA—right atrium; RV—right ventricle. (*Adapted from* Ross and Roberts [32]; with permission.)

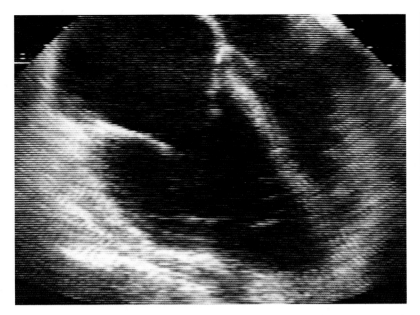

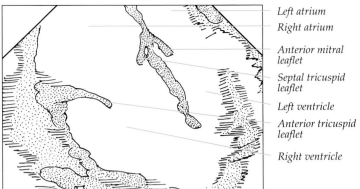

Left atrium
Right atrium
Anterior mitral leaflet
Septal tricuspid leaflet
Left ventricle
Anterior tricuspid leaflet
Right ventricle

FIGURE 2-28. Transesophageal four-chamber echocardiogram at end diastole in a patient with metastatic carcinoid tumor and refractory right-sided heart failure [33]. Diffuse thickening of the valves caused severe tricuspid regurgitation and pulmonic stenosis with decreased mobility of the anterior and septal tricuspid leaflets. The right atrium and right ventricle are markedly enlarged. Elaboration of serotonin by tumor metastases to the liver is believed to mediate the valvular fibrosis; however, lowering serotonin levels does not lead to regression of the plaques. All patients diagnosed with carcinoid should undergo echocardiography regularly to look for cardiac involvement. Once right-sided heart failure occurs, especially if it cannot be controlled medically, valvular surgery should be considered. Postoperative complications such as flushing, bronchoconstriction, and hyperperistalsis can be prevented by treatment with somatostatin. (*Adapted from* Samaan and Roldan [33]; with permission.)

DIABETIC CARDIOMYOPATHY

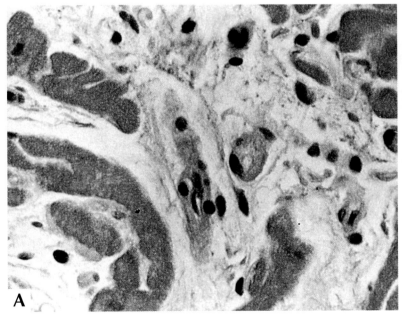

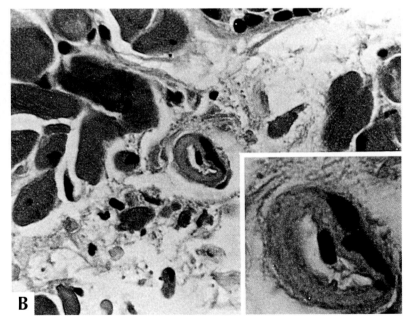

FIGURE 2-29. Histologic changes in diabetic myocardium. Autopsy studies [34] have shown hypertrophy, interstitial fibrosis (**A**), capillary microaneurysms, and hyalinization of arterioles (**B**) (hematoxylin and eosin, × 300; *inset*, × 750). Echocardiographic studies have shown abnormal systolic and diastolic function with diffuse hypokinesis and decreased stroke volume and ejection fraction [35]. The diabetic patient is twice as likely to be affected by coronary artery disease as the nondiabetic. This increased incidence is due in part to the accompanying hypertension, hyperlipidemia, hyperglycemia, and hyperinsulinemia (type II diabetes). However, the diabetic heart can also be affected by an autonomic neuropathy and a cardiomyopathy, resulting in nonischemic heart failure. The autonomic neuropathy manifests initially as sympathetic denervation and a fixed tachycardia, followed by lowering of the heart rate with complete denervation [36]. Diabetic cardiomyopathy does not have a clear pathogenesis [37] and may be related to small-vessel disease, metabolic abnormalities, or a combination of factors. In addition to the nonischemic form of diabetic cardiomyopathy, ischemic heart failure occurs more frequently in diabetics than in nondiabetics with coronary disease of similar extent. Potential explanations include multiple myocardial infarcts and poor contractile performance of the diabetic nonischemic myocardium. (*Adapted from* Sutherland and coworkers [34]; with permission.)

TREATMENT OF HEART DISEASE IN THE DIABETIC PATIENT

1. Be vigorous with antihypertensive therapy. Choose a lipid-neutral drug. Avoid diuretics. ACE inhibitors are probably the drug of choice for hypertension.
2. Be vigorous with lipid-lowering drugs. Good choices are gemfibrozil plus a resin or an HMG CoA reductase inhibitor.
3. Try to maintain good glucose control. Aim to keep glycosylated hemoglobins below 8%.
4. Encourage weight loss, exercise, and smoking cessation.
5. During the peri-infarction period, use insulin to control blood glucose level. Keep blood glucose between 150 and 250 mg/dL to avoid counter-regulatory catecholamine release.
6. Avoid hypoglycemia, especially if the patient is on a β-blocker, which would hinder detection of hypoglycemia.

FIGURE 2-30. The treatment of coronary heart disease in diabetics is similar to that for nondiabetics. However, particular attention to treating hypertension and diabetic dyslipidemia is warranted. Early, vigorous antihypertensive therapy with angiotensin-converting enzyme (ACE) inhibitors is recommended. Diuretics and β-blockers will aggravate dyslipidemia and should not be prescribed as first-line therapy for hypertension. In addition, β-blockers will potentiate hypoglycemia, since catecholamines are a counter-regulatory hormone for hypoglycemia and may mask hypoglycemic episodes. While hospitalized, diabetics may require insulin therapy in order to keep blood glucose levels between 150 and 250 mg/dL. This rather liberal range is preferred because hypoglycemia will lead to catecholamine release, which should be avoided in the peri-infarction period. HMG CoA—hepatic hydroxymethyl glutaryl coenzyme A.

POSTMENOPAUSAL ESTROGEN REPLACEMENT THERAPY

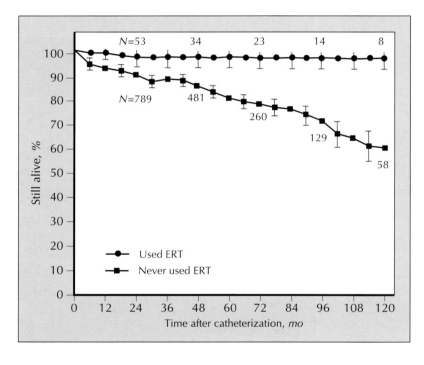

FIGURE 2-31. Ten-year survival of women with left main or three-vessel disease based on whether or not they received estrogen replacement therapy (ERT) [38]. At 10 years, 97% of the users were still alive, while only 60% of the nonusers had survived (P=0.007). Ischemic heart disease is the leading cause of death in post-menopausal women. Postmenopausal status or premature menopause without ERT is now considered a risk factor for coronary artery disease [39]. Observational studies like the Nurses' Health Study [40] have shown that women receiving ERT live longer than their counterparts without ERT and show less atherosclerosis on cardiac catheterization [41]. Postmenopausal hormone replacement therapy appears to reduce a woman's risk for myocardial infarction by as much as 50% in some studies, especially in women known to have extensive coronary disease. Estrogen therapy lowers mortality from all causes combined, including deaths from endometrial and breast carcinoma. Despite the convincing epidemiologic evidence, no prospective, randomized, double-blind study has been carried out to date. (*Adapted from* Sullivan and Vander Zwaag [38]; with permission from the American Medical Association, Inc.)

ORAL CONTRACEPTIVES AND RISK FOR MYOCARDIAL INFARCTION

PAST ORAL CONTRACEPTIVE USE AND MYOCARDIAL INFARCTION RISK

STUDY	DESIGN	RR FOR MI, 95% CI	UNADJUSTED RR
Mann et al., 1975	Case-control	1.1 (0.4–3.0)*	
Mann 1975, 1976	Case-control	1.1 (0.6–2.0)*†	
Jick et al., 1978	Case-control	3.6 (0.6–20.6)*	
Petitti et al., 1979	Prospective	0.8 (0.3–2.1)*	
Shapiro et al., 1979	Case-control	1.2 (0.8–1.7)	
Rosenberg et al., 1980	Case-control	0.9 (0.6–1.4)	1.0
Adam and Thorogood, 1981	Case-control	1.1 (0.6–1.8)*	
Slone et al., 1981	Case-control	1.1 (0.9–1.4)	1.2
La Vecchia et al., 1987	Case-control	1.9 (0.8–4.7)	1.8
Rosenberg et al., 1988	Case-control‡		
	1-4 y duration	1.2 (0.8–1.7)*	
	5-9 y duration	1.2 (0.8–1.9)*	
	10+ y duration	1.3 (0.7–2.4)*	
Stampfer et al., 1988	Prospective	0.8 (0.6–1.0)	0.9
Croft and Hannaford, 1989	Case-cohort§	1.0 (0.7–1.6)	1.3

Meta-analyses:

1. Without adjustment for confounding, 1.05 (0.94–1.17)
2. Limited only to cohort studies, 0.85 (0.69–1.05)
3. With adjustment for confounding, 1.01 (0.91–1.13)

*Adjusted for age alone or crude data within a limited age range but unadjusted for confounders.

†Includes results from both studies without duplication.

‡There were 675 cases, but the number of exposed cases is not given.

§Case-control study nested in a prospective cohort.

FIGURE 2-32. Summary of reports on past use of oral contraceptives (OCs) in relation to risk for myocardial infarction [42]. OCs have long been considered risk factors for thrombotic events, including myocardial infarction, deep venous thrombosis, and stroke. In general, the high risk reported in the past was increased among current users of OCs, especially in women who were cigarette smokers. In addition, the OC preparations used in most of these studies contained high doses of estrogens; those used currently contain low doses of estrogen (50 μg), and some contain progestin only. Meta-analyses that analyzed studies through 1990 yielded a relative risk (RR) for myocardial infarction of 1.05, 0.85 in the three cohort studies, and 1.01 in those which adjusted for confounding factors. Therefore, otherwise healthy women who are not diabetic, hypertensive, or smokers are not at increased risk from OC use. CI—confidence interval. (*Adapted from* Stampfer and coworkers [42]; with permission from The CV Mosby Co.)

REFERENCES

1. Klein I: Thyroid hormone and the cardiovascular system. *Am J Med* 1990, 88:633–637.

2. Woeber KA: Thyrotoxicosis and the heart. *N Engl J Med* 1992, 327:94–97.

3. Bahn RS, Garrity JA, Gorman CA: Diagnosis and management of Graves' ophthalmopathy. *J Clin Endocrinol Metab* 1990, 71:559–563.

4. Wartofsky L: Thyrotoxic storm. In *Werner and Ingbar's The Thyroid*, ed 6. Edited by Braverman LE, Utiger RD. Philadelphia: JB Lippincott; 1991:871–879.

5. Mackin JF, Canary JJ, Pittman CS: Thyroid storm and its management. *N Engl J Med* 1974, 291:1396–1397.

6. Ladenson PW: Recognition and management of cardiovascular disease related to thyroid dysfunction. *Am J Med* 1990, 88:638–639.

7. Santos AD, Miller PR, Puthenpurakal KM, *et al.*: Echocardiographic characterization of the reversible cardiomyopathy of hypothyroidism. *Am J Med* 1980, 68:675–682.

8. Gottehrer A, Roa J, Stanford GG, *et al.*: Hypothyroidism and pleural effusions. *Chest* 1990, 98:1130–1132.

9. Nikkila EA, Kekki M: Plasma triglyceride metabolism in thyroid disease. *J Clin Invest* 1972, 51:2103–2114.

10. Kutty KM, Bryant DG, Farid NR: Serum lipids in hypothyroidism: a re-evaluation. *J Clin Endocrinol Metab* 1978, 46:55–56.

11. Nicoloff JT: Thyroid storm and myxedema coma. *Med Clin North Am* 1985, 69:1005–1017.

12. Hylander B, Rosenqvist U: Treatment of myxoedema coma: factors associated with fatal outcome. *Acta Endocrinol (Copenh)* 1985, 108:65–71.

13. Heath H III: Primary hyperparathyroidism: recent advances in pathogenesis, diagnosis and management. *Adv Intern Med* 1991, 37:275–293.

14. Roberts WC, Waller BF: Effect of chronic hypercalcemia on the heart: an analysis of 18 necropsy patients. *Am J Med* 1981, 71:371–384.

15. Benowitz NL: Pheochromocytoma. *Adv Intern Med* 1990, 35:195–220.

16. Greene JP, Guay AT: New perspectives in pheochromocytoma. *Urol Clin North Am* 1989, 16:487–503.

17. Stenstrom G, Holmberg S: Cardiomyopathy in phaeochromocytoma: report of a case with a 16 year follow-up after surgery and review of the literature. *Eur Heart J* 1985, 316:539–544.

18. McManus BM, *et al.*: Fatal catecholamine crisis in pheochromocytoma: curable cause of cardiac arrest. *Am Heart J* 1981, 102:930–935.

19. Sjoberg RJ, Simcic KJ, Kedd GS: The clonidine suppression test for pheochromocytoma. *Arch Intern Med* 1992, 152:1193–1197.

20. Malone MJ, Libertino JA, Tsapatsaris NP, *et al.*: Preoperative and surgical management of pheochromocytoma. *Urol Clin North Am* 1989, 16:567–582.

21. Nerup J: Addison's disease—clinical studies: a report of 108 cases. *Acta Endocrinol (Copenh)* 1974, 76:127–141.

22. Oelkers H, Diederich S, Bahr V: Diagnosis and therapy surveillance in Addison's disease: rapid ACTH test and measurement of plasma ACTH, renin activity and aldosterone. *J Clin Endocrinol Metab* 1992, 75:259–264.

23. Stoffer SS: Addison's disease: how to improve patients' quality of life. *Postgrad Med* 1993, 93:265–266.

24. Chin R: Adrenal crisis. *Crit Care Clin* 1991, 7:23–42.

25. Sheeler LR: Cushing's syndrome—1988. *Cleve Clin J Med* 1988, 55:329–337.

26. Kaye TB, Crapo L: The Cushing syndrome: an update on diagnostic tests. *Ann Intern Med* 1990, 112:434–444.

27. Young WF Jr, Klee GG: Primary aldosteronism: diagnostic evaluation. *Endocrinol Metab Clin North Am* 1988, 17:367–395.

28. Melby JC: Endocrine hypertension. *J Clin Endocrinol Metab* 1989, 69:697–703.

29. Melby JC: Diagnosis and treatment of primary hyperaldosteronism and isolated hypoaldosteronism. In *Endocrinology*. Edited by DeGroot LJ. Philadelphia: WB Saunders Co; 1989: 1709–1711.

30. Lie JT, Grossman SJ: Pathology of the heart in acromegaly: anatomic findings in 27 autopsied patients. *Am Heart J* 1980, 100:41–48.

31. Wallace TM, Levin HS, Ratliff NB, *et al.*: Evaluation and management of Carney's complex: an illustrative case. *Cleve Clin J Med* 1991, 58:248–256.

32. Ross EM, Roberts WC: The carcinoid syndrome: comparison of 21 necropsy subjects with carcinoid heart disease to 15 necropsy subjects without carcinoid disease. *Am J Med* 1985, 79:339–354.

33. Samaan SA, Roldan CA: Echocardiography in carcinoid heart disease. *Video J Echocard* 1992, 2:137–144.

34. Sutherland CGC, *et al.*: Endomyocardial biopsy pathology in insulin-dependent diabetic patients with abnormal ventricular function. *Histopathology* 1989, 14:593–602.

35. Ruddy TD, Shumak SL, Liu PP, *et al.*: The relationship of cardiac diastolic dysfunction to concurrent hormonal and metabolic status in type I diabetes mellitus. *J Clin Endocrinol Metab* 1988, 66:113–118.

36. Dillman WH: Diabetes and thyroid hormone induced changes in cardiac function and their molecular basis. *Annu Rev Med* 1989, 40:373–393.

37. Regan TJ, Lyons MM, Ahmed SS, *et al.*: Evidence for cardiomyopathy in familial diabetes mellitus. *J Clin Invest* 1977, 60:884–899.

38. Sullivan JM, Vander Zwaag R, Hughes MA, *et al.*: Estrogen replacement and coronary artery disease: effect on survival in postmenopausal women. *Arch Intern Med* 1990, 150:2557–2562.

39. Summary of the Second Report of the National Cholesterol Education Program (NCEP) Expert Panel on the Detection, Evaluation, and Treatment of High Blood Cholesterol in Adults (Adult Treatment Panel II). *JAMA* 1993, 269:3015–3023.

40. Stampfer MJ, Colditz GA, Willett WC, *et al.*: Postmenopausal estrogen therapy and cardiovascular disease: 10 year follow-up from the Nurses' Health Study. *N Engl J Med* 1991, 325:756–762.

41. Sullivan JM, Vander Zwaag R, Lemp GF, *et al.*: Postmenopausal estrogen use and coronary atherosclerosis. *Ann Intern Med* 1988, 108:358–362.

42. Stampfer MJ, Willett WC, Colditz GA, *et al.*: Past use of oral contraceptives and cardiovascular disease: a meta-analysis in the context of the Nurses' Health Study. *Am J Obstet Gynecol* 1990, 163:285–291.

HEMATOLOGIC DISORDERS AND THE HEART

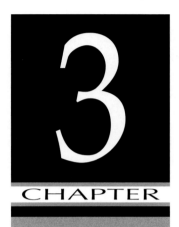

CHAPTER 3

Stuart J. Hutchison, J. Lawrence Hutchison, and P. Anthony N. Chandraratna

Numerous elements of the hematologic system are associated with protean cardiovascular complications. These elements include the marrow, lymph, cells, and serum and their abnormal states: excesses and deficiencies, benign or malignant growth, and the effects of diverse modes of therapy such as chemotherapy and/or radiation therapy.

Although functional disturbances of the cardiovascular system secondary to hematologic diseases and their treatment are less common than anatomic disturbances, the former are more important clinically. For example, in an autopsy series of 196 patients with lymphoma, cardiac metastases occurred in 48 cases, 41 of which were to the pericardium [1]. Pericardial compression, the major clinical cardiovascular manifestation of lymphoma, is less common. Only three patients in this series had evidence of this syndrome.

Often a patient may have more than one cardiovascular disturbance attributable to hematologic disease and/or its therapy [1]. Some cardiovascular complications are common, such as hemochromatosis/cardiomyopathy complicating severe thalassemia; while others are rare, such as coronary artery stenosis following mediastinal irradiation [2].

In some cases, complications of therapy are manifest acutely, such as myopericarditis following high-dose cyclophosphamide administration [3], whereas others may be delayed for years, such as fibrosis that develops after mediastinal irradiation [4]. Many are idiosyncratic, but a few can be predicted, such as dose-related anthracycline myotoxicity [5].

Some of these cardiovascular complications are potentially curable or may resolve spontaneously, and some may be satisfactorily managed, while others invariably will be fatal. For example, myocardial dysfunction due to hemochromatosis may vary in severity [6], may improve with phlebotomy (primary hemochromatosis) or chelation therapy (thalassemia-associated hemochromatosis) [7], or eventually may prove fatal despite therapy. In most cases, cardiovascular complications of hematologic disease are best managed by specific therapy. Therefore, prompt recognition of these complications with appropriate intervention may prove beneficial. For example, pericardial tamponade has been managed successfully at the time of presentation in acute leukemia [8], after bone marrow transplantation [9], and when it has occurred as a complication of other hematologic diseases and treatments.

The presence of hematologic disease can tax the cardiovascular system. For example, cardiac output must increase to compensate for severe anemia (hemoglobin < 7 g/dL). More frequent, if not common, is the burden imposed on the cardiovascular system by complications of treatment, such as myelosuppression after chemotherapy or radiotherapy with febrile neutropenic states and anemia, in which a high cardiac output regularly occurs. Thus, complications may occur against a background of increased cardiovascular demands and may be poorly tolerated.

By carefully evaluating a patient's cardiovascular system, the clinician may identify characteristics that will influence the selection of therapy for the hematologic disease. Subnormal left ventricular function mitigates against the use of anthracyclines [5]. Patients with significant preexisting cardiovascular disease may not tolerate more potent forms of chemotherapy that are likely to lead to remission of malignancy but are also more cardiotoxic. In such cases treatment may be selected that is less likely to achieve long-term success but is also less likely to decompensate the cardiovascular system in the short term.

Older patients may have concurrent significant heart disease, such as coronary artery disease, hypertension, or valvular disease, that is unrelated to but possibly exacerbated by hematologic disease and/or the complications of its treatment. In fact, anemia may precipitate unstable angina. Patients with anemia, particularly in the presence of underlying heart disease [10] or even alone if the hemo-globin is less than 4 or 5 g/dL, may develop congestive heart failure.

With better supportive therapy and knowledge about drug dose responsiveness [11], the treatment of hematologic disorders, particularly marrow and lymphoid tissue malignancies, has become more intensive over the last 20 years [12]. Induction therapy [13] and postinduction therapy [11,14] for the acute leukemias, such as acute myelogenous leukemia, has intensified, with beneficial clinical results. Similarly, chronic myelogenous leukemia is currently treated with more aggressive therapy, including bone marrow transplantation [12]. Although bone marrow transplants have been used increasingly over the last 10 years [15], they are associated with acute cardiotoxicity—an important limiting factor that may be fatal [16]—as well as with cardiac abnormalities both at rest and on exercise, even in children and young adults [17].

Depending on the general condition and prognosis of patients with hematologic disorders, aggressive management of cardiovascular complications is warranted when the underlying hematologic disease can potentially be controlled or cured. It is crucial for the cardiovascular consultant to know these possible complications and to interact closely with the hematologist in order to make the diagnosis and arrive at a course of therapy tailored to the needs and anticipated course of the individual patient.

In this chapter we review these cardiovascular complications through case examples that include the anemias, sickle cell disease, hemochromatosis, hypercoagulable states, acute leukemias, lymphomas, malignant myeloma, myeloproliferative syndromes, chemotherapy, and radiation therapy.

COMPLICATIONS OF ANEMIA

CARDIOVASCULAR COMPLICATIONS OF AND ASSOCIATIONS WITH ANEMIA

HEMODYNAMIC COMPLICATIONS

Increased preload (increased venous return)

Increased diastolic dimensions

Decreased afterload (reduced wall stress and SVR)

Reduced viscosity

Increased stroke volume

Increased contractility

"Eccentric hypertrophy"

Increased cardiac output at rest
  with hemoglobin < 7 g/dL

Normal plasma volume

Hemodynamic intolerance to transfusions (common)

PHYSICAL EXAMINATION

Hyperactive precordium

Systolic flow murmurs

Mid-diastolic rumble

OTHER COMPLICATIONS

Decreased cardiovascular reserve/exercise tolerance

May precipitate unstable angina

Electrocardiography: repolarization abnormalities

Congestive heart failure
  Usually with underlying structural heart disease
  May be present without underlying heart disease when
    hemoglobin < 4 g/dL

Without decreased blood viscosity, increase in cardiac output is smaller

FIGURE 3-1. Cardiovascular complications of and associations with anemia: general clinical findings [10,18,19]. SVR—systemic vascular resistance.

CARDIOVASCULAR COMPLICATIONS OF INTRAVASCULAR HEMOLYSIS

May occur in the presence of normal or hemolysis-prone erythrocytes (eg, hemoglobin SS, thalassemia, other)

May occur in patients with

Prosthetic valve dysfunction (ball-in-cage > tilting disk > bioprosthesis)

Native valve disease

Hypertrophic cardiomyopathy with or without mitral valve prolapse, endocarditis

Mitral valve repair

Repaired congenital defect

Cardiac surgery (on bypass)

Left ventricular assist devices

When erythrocytes are normal, the common denominator is usually turbulence causing excessive shear force that ruptures red cells

May be worse with increased activity of patient, increased circulation, causing increased shearing

May occur after cardiac surgery; consider above causes and transfusion incompatibility

FIGURE 3-2. Intravascular hemolysis, whether due to a primary hematologic abnormality (*eg*, hemoglobinopathy), a cardiovascular abnormality (as listed here), or both, may lead to anemia, with its attendant demands on the cardiovascular system (*see* Fig. 3-1) [18,20].

HEMOLYTIC ANEMIA

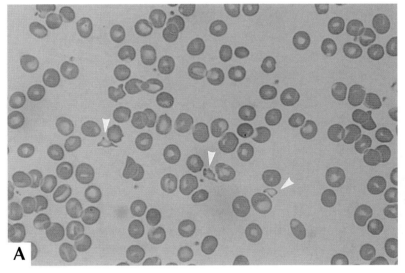
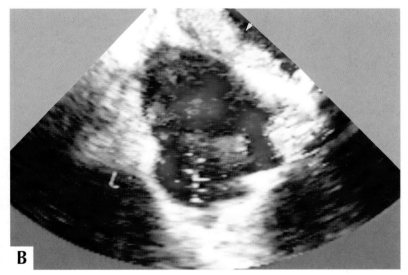

FIGURE 3-3. Intravascular hemolysis due to dysfunction of a mechanical mitral valve prosthesis. A 53-year-old woman with mitral stenosis initially presented with atrial fibrillation and peripheral arterial emboli to the legs. The mitral valve was surgically replaced by a St. Jude prosthesis. Postoperatively, she showed persistent anemia, with hyperbilirubinemia (total bilirubin=2.3 mg/dL, direct=1.6 mg/dL), elevated lactic dehydrogenase and serum hemoglobin, and low serum haptoglobin (<48 mg/dL),

consistent with intravascular hemolysis. **A,** Peripheral blood smears revealed fragmented red blood cells (*arrowheads*). **B,** Severe paravalvular mitral insufficiency, originating from several sites, was noted on transesophageal echocardiography (*arrow*). The patient underwent repeat mitral valve surgery, with insertion of another St. Jude prosthesis. Postoperatively, the hemolytic anemia resolved, but encephalopathy developed as a result of the prolonged surgery.

CARDIOVASCULAR COMPLICATIONS OF SICKLE CELL ANEMIA

HEMODYNAMIC COMPLICATIONS

Increased cardiac output
  (greater than in other anemias)
Increased preload
Decreased afterload
Increased stroke volume
Systemic hypertension, with renal disease
Flow murmurs in most patients,
  especially children

PULMONARY COMPLICATIONS

Pulmonary hypertension/cor
  pulmonale
RV hypertrophy
Pulmonary artery thrombosis
Pulmonary infarction
Pulmonary embolism
Fat and bone necrosis and
  embolism

MYOCARDIAL COMPLICATIONS

Increased mass—"eccentric hypertrophy"
Abnormalities during relaxation
Intrinsic cardiomyopathy (controversial)
Hemochromatosis in transfused patients
Abnormal response of EF to exercise

SICKLE CRISIS

Chest pain
Focal changes
  Wall motion abnormalities
  Thallium defects
Diffuse ventricular dilatation
Reduced EF
Elevated filling pressures
Elevated pulmonary artery pressures
ECG abnormalities
  Nonspecific
  Typical of ischemia
  Arrhythmias
Ischemia possible
MI uncommon

CORONARY ARTERY COMPLICATIONS

Angina
MI with angiographically normal
  coronaries (rare)
Papillary muscle infarction
Fibromuscular dysplasia of coronaries

OTHER COMPLICATIONS

ECG
  Normal or abnormalities at rest
    (nonspecific)
  Septal Q waves
  LV hypertrophy
  First-degree AV block
MVP (? associated)
Conduction system degeneration
Sudden death

FIGURE 3-4. Sickle cell anemia is associated with a variety of cardio-vascular abnormalities in addition to the general hemodynamic effects on the cardiovascular system that are common to any chronic anemia [10,21–29]. Unique among anemias, sickle disease is associated with tissue infarction because of vascular occlusion by abnormal erythrocytes. Notable are the occurrence of pulmonary vascular disease, with its burden on the right heart, and sickle (tissue infarction) crisis, which may directly affect the heart. AV—atrioventricular; EF—ejection fraction; LV—left ventricular; MI—myocardial infarction; MVP—mitral valve prolapse; RV—right ventricular.

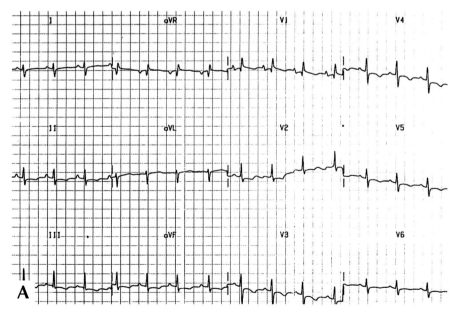

FIGURE 3-5. Clinical findings in sickle cell trait and pulmonary hypertension secondary to recurrent pulmonary emboli in a 57-year-old woman who presented with a 1-year history of dyspnea on exertion and orthopnea. She was found to have severe pulmonary hypertension, with evidence of an organizing central pulmonary artery embolus, and was admitted to the hospital for elective pulmonary endarterectomy. On admission, examination showed elevated jugular venous pressure, peripheral edema, hepatomegaly, and a murmur of tricuspid insufficiency. **A,** Electrocardiography revealed right axis deviation, high voltages in the right precordial leads compatible with right ventricular hypertrophy, and diffuse repolarization abnormalities. (*continued*)

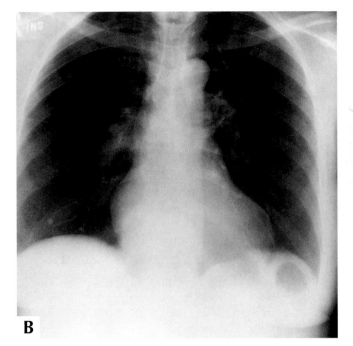

B

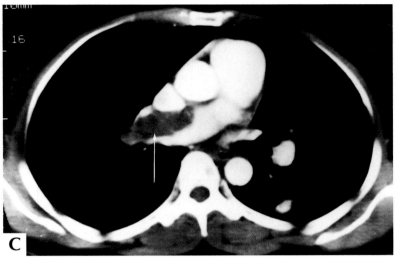

C

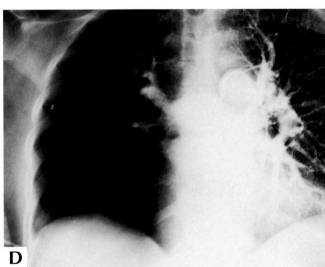

D

FIGURE 3-5. (*continued*) **B,** Chest radiography revealed cardiomegaly, prominence of the right atrial contour, and large central pulmonary arteries. Hemoglobin electrophoresis indicated 48% sickle hemoglobin. **C,** Computed tomography with contrast showed a large filling defect within the right pulmonary artery (*arrow*), consistent with an embolus. **D,** Contrast pulmonary angiography confirmed severely reduced flow to the right lower lung. Exchange transfusions were performed in preparation for surgery, reducing the amount of sickle hemoglobin to 30%. A few hours before the scheduled operation, the patient suffered a cardiac arrest (electromechanical dissociation). With a presumed diagnosis of a critical pulmonary embolus, urgent thoracotomy was performed, and fresh thrombus was found in the right main pulmonary artery, which was removed. The patient did not survive. (Courtesy of Benoit de Varrennes, MD, Royal Victoria Hospital, McGill University, Montreal, Canada.)

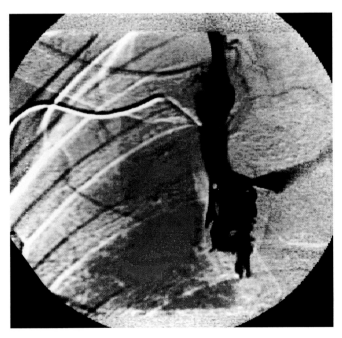

FIGURE 3-6. Thrombotic superior vena caval (SVC) obstruction in a 21-year-old man with known sickle cell disease. The patient presented with gross swelling of the head, neck, and arms several months after a permanent indwelling catheter was inserted into the SVC via subclavian puncture. Upper extremity digital subtraction venography revealed complete obstruction of the SVC, with no dye entering the right atrium. At thoracotomy, the inferior portion of the SVC was completely obstructed and was ligated to prevent thrombus from entering the heart. Synthetic grafts were placed from the innominate and subclavian veins into the right atrium. One shunt became blocked within several days; the other became blocked later during warfarin therapy, but since extensive collaterals had formed and the patient was relatively well, further surgery has not been performed. (Courtesy of Milton J. Herba, MD, Montreal General Hospital, McGill University, Montreal, Canada.)

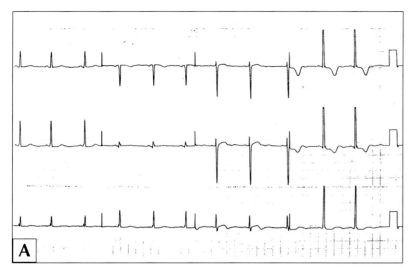

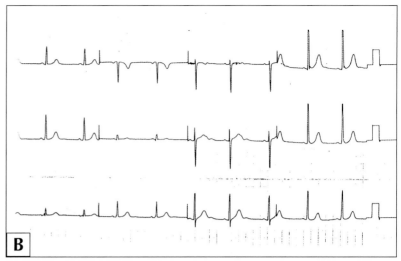

FIGURE 3-7. Sickle cell disease with possible myocardial ischemia in a 19-year-old man with hemoglobin SS who developed a severe sickling crisis, with worsening anemia and chest pain. He had a history of strokes and leg ulcers. **A,** On admission, the electrocardiogram (ECG) revealed repolarization abnormalities consistent with ischemia or left ventricular hypertrophy with strain. Enzyme levels (peak/trough) were as follows: creatine phosphokinase, 110/32 IU; lactic dehydrogenase, 2710/370 IU; alanine transaminase, 1670/10 IU; and aspartate transaminase, 2050/21 IU. **B,** On a follow-up ECG obtained 3 weeks later, repolarization had normalized. (Courtesy of L. Julian Haywood, MD, Los Angeles County/University of Southern California Medical Center, Los Angeles, CA.)

COMPLICATIONS OF HEMOCHROMATOSIS AND THALASSEMIA

CARDIOVASCULAR COMPLICATIONS OF HEMOCHROMATOSIS AND THALASSEMIA

MYOCARDIAL COMPLICATIONS

Early
  Normal internal chamber dimensions
  Thickened ventricular walls
  "Bright" ventricular walls on echocardiography
  May be asymptomatic
  May have preclinical LV dysfunction
Late
  Overt LV dysfunction
  CHF
  Dilated/restrictive cardiomyopathy
CHF is the leading cause of death in inherited hemochromatosis
LV function and survival may improve with iron removal therapy
  (phlebotomy or iron chelation)

ELECTRICAL ABNORMALITIES

Bradycardia
Atrioventricular nodal disease
Supraventricular tachycardia
Late: decreased voltages
Nonspecific repolarization abnormalities

OTHER COMPLICATIONS

Thalassemia
  Concurrent burden of anemia
  Pericarditis occurs in 50% of cases and is often recurrent
  Ascorbic acid, used with desferrioxamine therapy,
    may be acutely cardiotoxic

FIGURE 3-8. Cardiovascular complications associated with hemochromatosis and thalassemia [7,30–32]. CHF—congestive heart failure; LV—left ventricular.

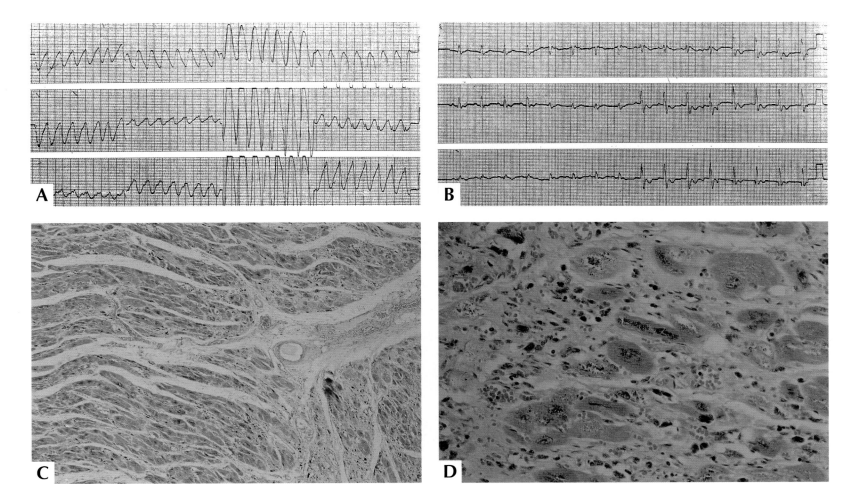

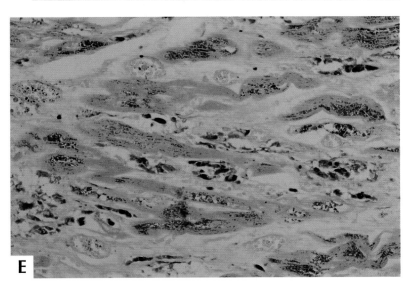

FIGURE 3-9. Hemochromatosis secondary to transfusions in an 18-year-old man with thalassemia who had received transfusions and desferrioxamine since birth. **A,** The patient presented with biventricular congestive heart failure and ventricular tachycardia. **B,** The resting 12-lead electrocardiogram revealed sinus tachycardia, right bundle branch block, and nonspecific repolarization abnormalities. The patient died of complications of sepsis. **C** to **E,** Necropsy revealed gross cardiomegaly, thrombi in the left atrium and ventricle, and myocardial fibrosis with intracellular and intercellular iron pigment seen on staining with both hematoxylin and eosin (*panels C and D*) and Prussian blue (*panel E*). (Parts C, D, and E courtesy of William P. Duguid, MD, Montreal General Hospital, McGill University, Montreal, Canada.)

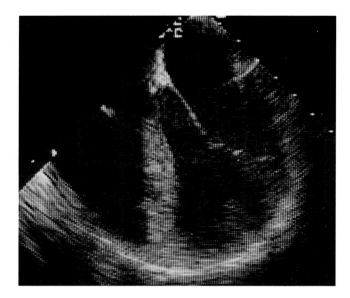

FIGURE 3-10. Transesophageal echocardiogram of a 31-year-old man with primary hemochromatosis. At low gain settings, the myocardial tissue is bright and reflective.

COMPLICATIONS OF HYPERCOAGULABLE STATES

CARDIOVASCULAR COMPLICATIONS OF HYPERCOAGULABLE STATES

MOLECULAR DEFICIENCIES			ANTI-PHOSPHOLIPID ANTIBODY
ANTITHROMBIN III DEFICIENCY	PROTEIN S DEFICIENCY	PROTEIN C DEFICIENCY	
MI	MI	MI	MI
Valve prosthesis thrombosis	Pulmonary hypertension	Intracardiac thrombus	Intracardiac thrombus
Pulmonary embolism	Pulmonary embolism	Valvular vegetations	Valvular vegetations
Intracardiac thrombus	Intracardiac thrombus	Arterial thrombosis	Pulmonary hypertension
			Thromboembolism
			In situ thrombosis

FIGURE 3-11. Cardiovascular complications associated with hypercoagulable states, including deficiencies of antithrombin III or proteins S and C and the presence of antiphospholipid antibody [33–38]. MI—myocardial infarction.

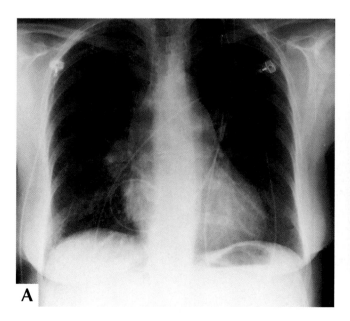

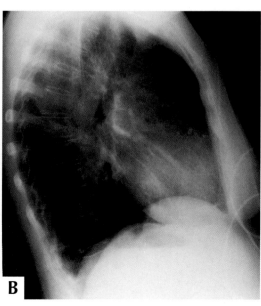

FIGURE 3-12. Pulmonary thromboemboli of the microvasculature related to anticardiolipin antibody in a 60-year-old woman who presented with worsening dyspnea. Physical findings were consistent with pulmonary hypertension. **A** and **B,** The chest radiographs revealed cardiomegaly with large central pulmonary arteries. (*continued*)

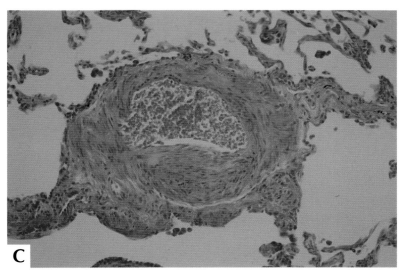

FIGURE 3-12. (*continued*) **C,** A lung biopsy showed medial hypertrophy and intimal sclerosis of the small pulmonary arteries. Pulmonary emboli were not detectable on pulmonary arteriography. Cardiac catheterization indicated pulmonary artery pressures of 95/25 mm Hg, a mean pulmonary capillary wedge pressure of 15 mm Hg, and a cardiac output of 4.2 L/min. With prostacyclin challenge, there was little change in the pulmonary pressures, but cardiac output doubled. The anticardiolipin antibody test was strongly positive. The patient has been managed with warfarin, nifedipine, and oxygen therapy. (Courtesy of David Langleben, MD, Sir Mortimer B. Davis/Jewish General Hospital, McGill University, Montreal, Canada.)

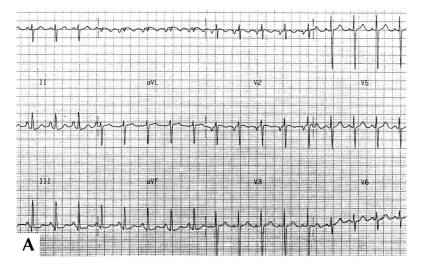

FIGURE 3-13. Pulmonary thromboemboli of the macrovasculature related to anticardiolipin antibody in an 18-year-old woman with recurrent deep venous thromboses of the lower extremities who was positive for this antibody. The patient presented with dyspnea and cardiovascular collapse due to submassive and chronic pulmonary embolism. **A,** The electrocardiogram revealed sinus tachycardia, right axis deviation, and P-pulmonale. **B** and **C,** Chest radiography showed cardiomegaly with enlargement of the right ventricle and central pulmonary arteries. (*continued*)

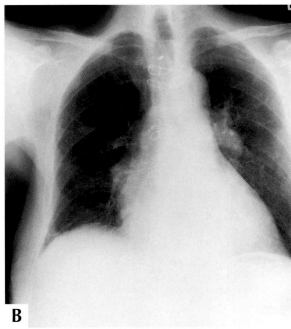

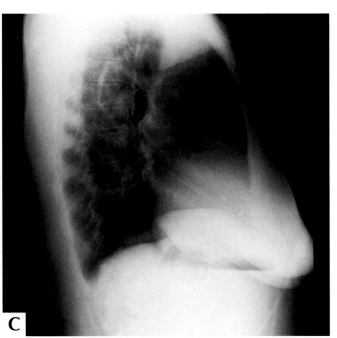

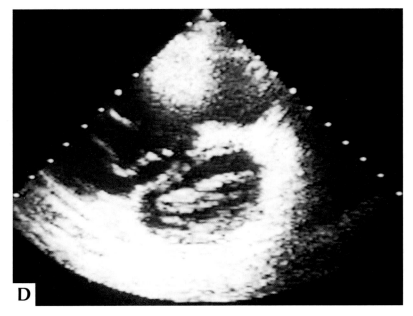

Right ventricle

Left ventricle

FIGURE 3-13. (*continued*) **D,** This parasternal short-axis echocardiographic view confirmed the markedly enlarged right ventricle, revealing a "D-shaped" interventricular septum consistent with elevated right ventricular pressure.

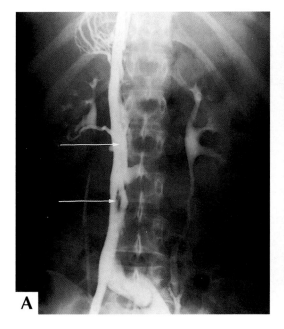

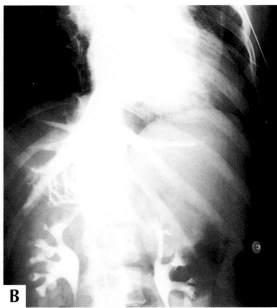

FIGURE 3-14. Cardiac catheterization in the patient with chronic pulmonary thromboemboli secondary to anticardiolipin antibody described in Fig. 3-13 revealed pulmonary artery pressures of about 100/40 mm Hg, a mean pulmonary capillary wedge pressure of 10 mm Hg, and a cardiac output of 3.3 L/min. Lower extremity venograms were positive bilaterally, and contrast injection of the inferior vena cava detected a long, linear thrombus (*arrows*; **A**), a dilated caval system, and tricuspid regurgitation with opacification of the hepatic venous system with contrast (**B**).

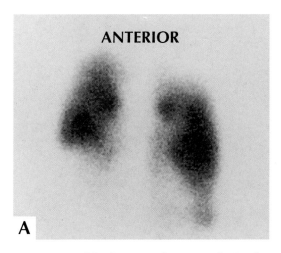

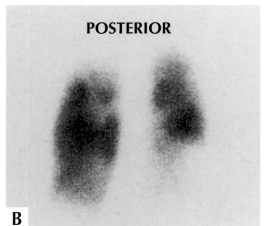

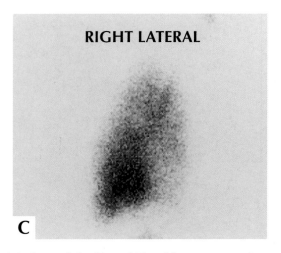

FIGURE 3-15. Nuclear ventilation-perfusion lung scans in the same patient (*see* Figs. 3-13 and 3-14) with chronic pulmonary thromboemboli secondary to anticardiolipin antibody revealed a segmental perfusion defect in the right lower lobe (**A** and **B**), with near-normal ventilation (**C**). (*continued*)

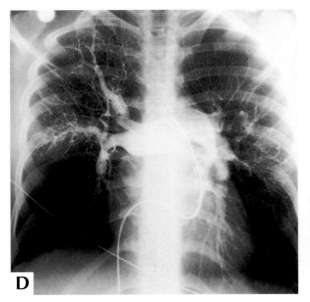

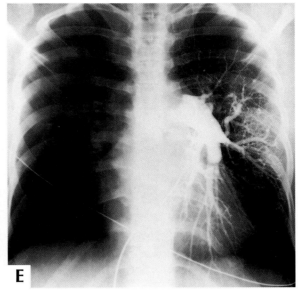

FIGURE 3-15. (*continued*) Pulmonary arteriography revealed complete blockage of the artery to the right lower lobe (**D**) as well as some reduction in flow to the left lower lobe (**E**). Successful pulmonary thromboendarterectomy revealed extensive fresh and organizing thrombus, mainly in the right pulmonary artery. Lung biopsy showed interstitial pneumonitis and medial hypertrophy of the pulmonary artery. (Courtesy of Milton J. Herba, MD.)

D

E

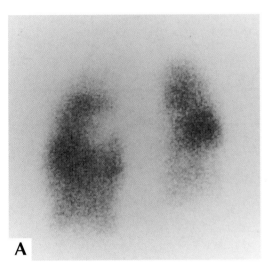

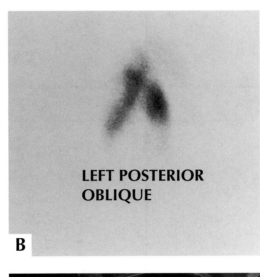

LEFT POSTERIOR OBLIQUE

A

B

FIGURE 3-16. Postoperative nuclear perfusion lung scanning in the same patient described in Figs. 3-13 to 3-15 with chronic pulmonary thromboemboli secondary to anticardiolipin antibody revealed increased perfusion of the right lower lobe (**A**) but also a new segmental defect in the left lower lobe or lingula (**B**). A repeat pulmonary angiogram confirmed that flow to the right lower lobe had improved (**C**), but now flow to the left lower lobe was reduced (**D**). Over time, clinical and arteriographic evidence indicated that pulmonary thromboembolism had recurred. The patient underwent a second pulmonary thromboendarterectomy and remains well several years later on long-term oral anticoagulant therapy. (Courtesy of Milton J. Herba, MD.)

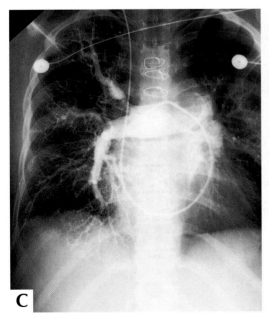

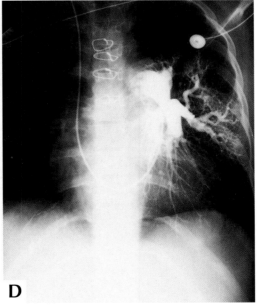

C

D

COMPLICATIONS OF HEMATOLOGIC MALIGNANCIES

LEUKEMIA

CARDIOVASCULAR COMPLICATIONS OF ACUTE LEUKEMIAS

MYOCARDIAL COMPLICATIONS	PERICARDIAL COMPLICATIONS	ENDOCARDIAL COMPLICATIONS	ELECTRICAL COMPLICATIONS	OTHER COMPLICATIONS
Infiltration	Infiltration	Valvular infiltration with insufficiency	Nonspecific or intraventricular conduction delays	Myocardial infarction
Intramyocardial hemorrhage	Hemorrhage	Valvular vegetations	Repolarization abnormalities	Hyperviscosity from increased cells
Focal myocardial necrosis	Effusions			
Congestive heart failure	Tamponade			
Rupture				

FIGURE 3-17. Cardiovascular complications of the acute leukemias [39–41].

MALIGNANT LYMPHOMA

CARDIOVASCULAR COMPLICATIONS OF MALIGNANT LYMPHOMAS

MYOCARDIAL COMPLICATIONS	PERICARDIAL COMPLICATIONS	ENDOCARDIAL COMPLICATIONS	VASCULAR COMPLICATIONS	OTHER COMPLICATIONS
Nodules	Nodules	Valvular infiltration	Superior vena cava syndrome	Myocardial infarction from coronary ostial narrowing
Masses	Masses	Valvular vegetations		Hyperviscosity from dysproteinemia
Diffuse infiltration	Effusions			
	Tamponade			

FIGURE 3-18. Cardiovascular complications of malignant lymphomas [1,42].

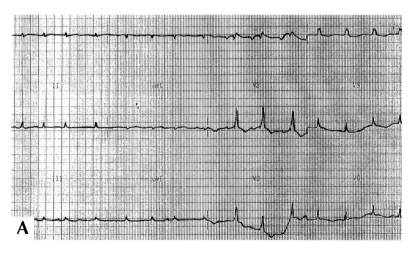

FIGURE 3-19. Cardiac tamponade associated with lymphoma in a 77-year-old man who presented with a mass in the tongue, initially diagnosed as anaplastic carcinoma. Sixteen months after he was treated with local irradiation, the patient suffered weight loss and dyspnea and, later, peripheral edema. Examination showed tachycardia, elevated jugular venous pressure, hepatomegaly, peripheral edema, dullness at the lung bases, distant heart sounds, and a pericardial friction rub. Cardiomegaly was evident on the chest radiograph. **A,** The electrocardiogram revealed low voltages, first-degree atrioventricular block, and right bundle branch block. A gated scan revealed mildly depressed left ventricular function, with evidence of a mass adjacent to the right ventricle. (*continued*)

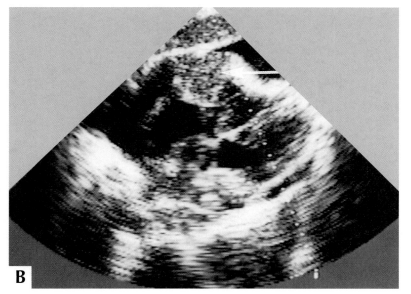

FIGURE 3-19. (*continued*) **B,** Transthoracic echocardiography showed a moderate-sized pericardial effusion and a large mass in the pericardial space, situated within the right atrioventricular groove and extending over the epicardium (*arrow*). Pericardiocentesis evacuated sanguineous fluid. Computed tomography revealed anterior mediastinal adenopathy. A bone marrow aspirate showed increased plasma cells. Re-evaluation of the tongue biopsy specimen led to a revised diagnosis: widespread large-cell lymphoma. Despite a course of combination chemotherapy (cyclophosphamide, doxorubicin, vincristine, and prednisone [CHOP]), this patient died of neutropenic sepsis and acute respiratory distress syndrome.

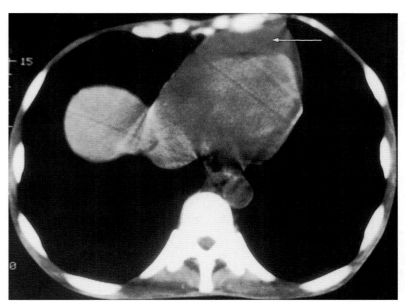

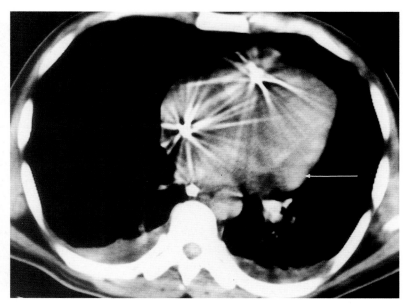

FIGURE 3-20. Lymphoma involving the pericardium in a patient with human immunodeficiency virus (HIV) disease. Computed tomography revealed soft tissue anterior to the heart (*arrow*), consistent with lymphomatous involvement in a patient with known widespread immunoblastic lymphoma, HIV disease, and multiple infections. (Courtesy of William D. Boswell, MD, Norris Cancer Hospital, University of Southern California, Los Angeles, CA.)

FIGURE 3-21. Pericardial involvement in a patient with widespread lymphoma. Computed tomography revealed nodular masses posterior and lateral to the left ventricle (*arrow*), consistent with lymphomatous involvement. The artifacts in the right atrium and right ventricular outflow tract are from a pulmonary artery catheter. (Courtesy of William D. Boswell, MD.)

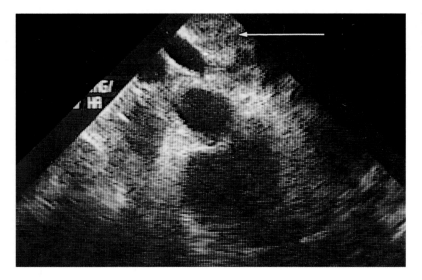

FIGURE 3-22. Lymphoma posterior to the left atrium. A horizontal plane transesophageal echocardiogram at the level of the aortic valve reveals a soft tissue mass extending to the left atrium (*arrow*).

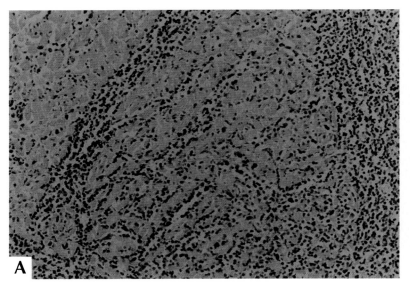

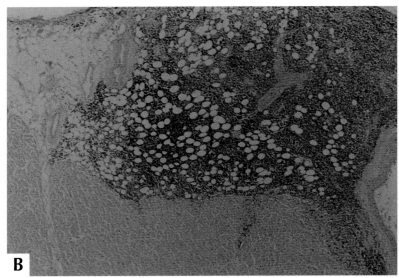

FIGURE 3-23. Lymphoma involving the myocardium in a 33-year-old man who presented with severe dyspnea, respiratory insufficiency, sepsis, and widespread non-Hodgkin's lymphoma. The patient died within 2 days of admission, and gross necropsy findings disclosed extensive lymphomatous involvement throughout the chest, including the pericardium and myocardium. Histologically, the myocardium was infiltrated with lymphoma cells (**A**), with infiltration extending through the epicardium into the pericardial space, around the coronary arteries (**B**).

MULTIPLE MYELOMA

CARDIOVASCULAR COMPLICATIONS OF MULTIPLE MYELOMA

MYOCARDIAL COMPLICATIONS	PERICARDIAL COMPLICATIONS	ELECTROPHYSIOLOGIC COMPLICATIONS	HEMODYNAMIC COMPLICATIONS
Nodules	Nodules	Sick sinus syndrome	Hyperviscosity due to dysproteinemia
Masses	Masses	Atrioventricular block	"High-output" state, especially with widespread bone disease
Restrictive cardiomyopathy due to amyloidosis	Effusions	Intraventricular conduction delays	Congestive heart failure
Amyloid cardiomyopathy with hypertrophic-obstructive picture	Tamponade		
Sensitivity to anthracyclines			

FIGURE 3-24. Cardiovascular complications of multiple myeloma [43–45].

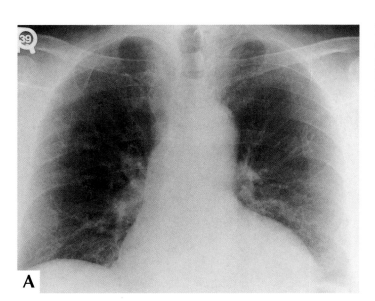

FIGURE 3-25. Myeloma, dysproteinemia, and congestive heart failure in a 60-year-old man who presented initially with dyspnea and an episode of amaurosis fugax. He had a history of hypertension and angina on effort, both well controlled. **A,** The chest radiograph revealed cardiomegaly and pulmonary vascular redistribution. (*continued*)

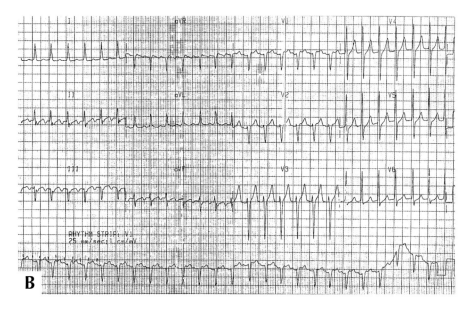

FIGURE 3-25. (*continued*) **B,** He developed atrial flutter with 2:1 block, which resolved spontaneously. Subsequently, he experienced prolonged chest pain and had a small myocardial infarction (creatine phosphokinase, 300 U). The left ventricular ejection fraction by gated scan was 64%. Renal insufficiency, anemia, and back pain suggested multiple myeloma, confirmed on bone marrow aspiration, with an associated monoclonal immunoglobulin G gammopathy. Serum hyperviscosity was marked (7.2 times water; normal, < 2.0). Plasmapheresis reversed the dysproteinemia and hyperviscosity and improved the congestive heart failure. The hyperviscosity had no cerebral or cardiac sequelae.

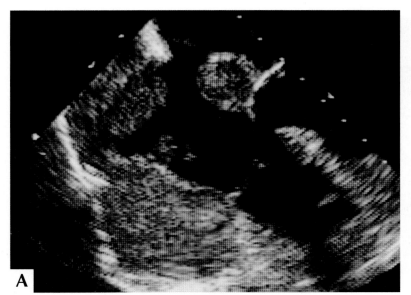

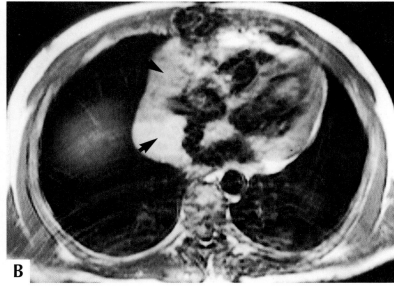

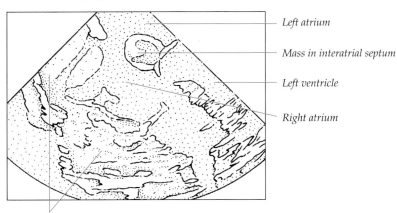

Left atrium

Mass in interatrial septum

Left ventricle

Right atrium

Large mass posterior and lateral to right atrium

FIGURE 3-26. Myeloma and cardiac masses in a man who presented with severe hypotension, pulmonary edema, and central cyanosis. The quality of the transthoracic echocardiographic study was poor. **A,** He was intubated, and a horizontal four-chamber view on transesophageal echocardiography revealed masses within the epicardial space, the left and right atria, and the interatrial septum other than the fossa ovalis. These masses were debulked surgically and were found on histologic examination to be consistent with multiple myeloma. **B,** Postoperative magnetic resonance imaging disclosed thickening of the atrial walls, with masses anterior to the right ventricle (*top arrow*) and lateral and posterior to the right atrium (*bottom arrow*). The patient was subsequently treated with chemotherapy. (Courtesy of Tahir Tak, MD, Los Angeles County Hospital/University of Southern California Medical Center, Los Angeles, CA.)

CARDIOVASCULAR COMPLICATIONS OF MYELOPROLIFERATIVE SYNDROMES

POLYCYTHEMIA VERA	ESSENTIAL THROMBOCYTOSIS	CHRONIC MYELOGENOUS LEUKEMIA	MYELOID METAPLASIA
Angina	MI	MI	Valvular thickening
MI	Valvular thickening	Tamponade	Valvular vegetations
Systemic hypertension	Valvular vegetations		
Pulmonary hypertension			
Valvular thickening			
Valvular vegetations			
Hyperviscosity			

FIGURE 3-27. Cardiovascular complications of the myeloproliferative syndromes [46,47]. MI—myocardial infarction.

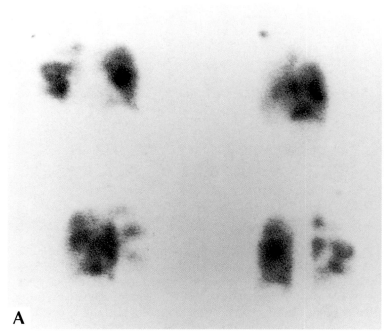

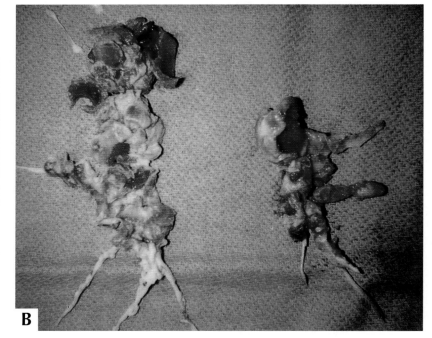

A   **B**

FIGURE 3-28. Primary thrombocytosis and anticardiolipin antibody in a 67-year-old man who presented with worsening dyspnea. He had a history of two episodes of deep venous thrombosis of the lower extremity. Physical findings were consistent with pulmonary hypertension. The platelet count was 600,000/mm^3. PO$_2$ on room air was 45 mm Hg. Perfusion lung scanning revealed defects consistent with severe pulmonary emboli (**A**). Cardiac catheterization showed a pulmonary artery pressure of 85/34 mm Hg, a mean pulmonary capillary wedge pressure of 12 mm Hg, and cardiac output of 5 L/min. Pulmonary angiography revealed extensive thromboemboli. Thromboendarterectomy was successful (**B**), with a postoperative systolic pulmonary pressure of 37 mm Hg. On warfarin and hydroxyurea the patient's condition worsened, and subsequent testing confirmed recurrent thromboembolism. (Courtesy of David Langleben, MD.)

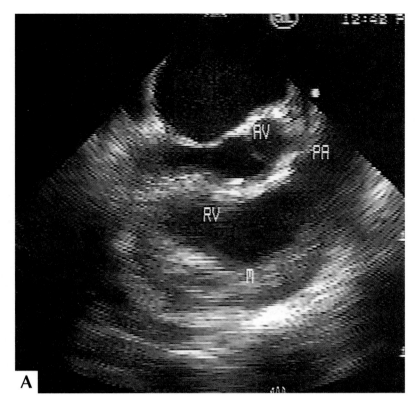

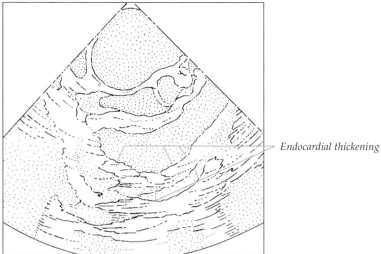

Endocardial thickening

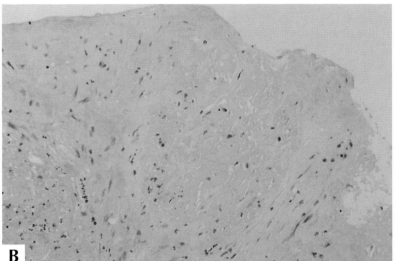

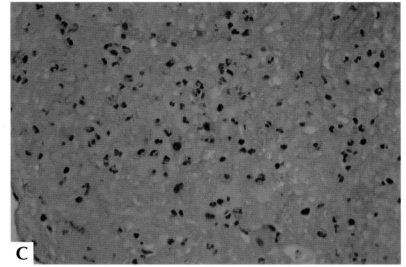

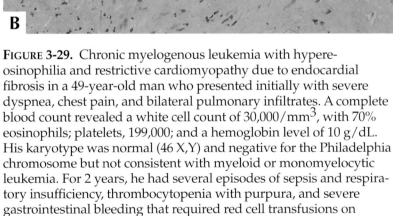

FIGURE 3-29. Chronic myelogenous leukemia with hypereosinophilia and restrictive cardiomyopathy due to endocardial fibrosis in a 49-year-old man who presented initially with severe dyspnea, chest pain, and bilateral pulmonary infiltrates. A complete blood count revealed a white cell count of 30,000/mm^3, with 70% eosinophils; platelets, 199,000; and a hemoglobin level of 10 g/dL. His karyotype was normal (46 X,Y) and negative for the Philadelphia chromosome but not consistent with myeloid or monomyelocytic leukemia. For 2 years, he had several episodes of sepsis and respiratory insufficiency, thrombocytopenia with purpura, and severe gastrointestinal bleeding that required red cell transfusions on several occasions. The hypereosinophilia was treated with hydrox-

yurea and prednisone. Over time, jugular venous distension, peripheral edema, and ascites developed. **A,** A vertical plane image along the right ventricular outflow tract on transesophageal echocardiography demonstrated prominent thickening of the endocardium that extended from the tricuspid to the pulmonic valve (valves not shown). Cardiac catheterization revealed elevated diastolic pressures in the pulmonary artery (PA), right ventricle (RV), and right atrium. A semiorganized thrombus was found on surgical resection. Histologically, the endocardial thickening consisted of thrombus and fibrous tissue (**B**), with eosinophils (**C**). AV—aortic valve; M—endocardial mass. (Courtesy of Benjamin L. Rosin, MD, Torrance Medical Center, Los Angeles, CA.)

CARDIOVASCULAR COMPLICATIONS OF CHEMOTHERAPY

ANTHRACYCLINES

Acute
  Pericarditis
  Myocarditis
  MI
  Electrocardiographic changes/arrhythmias
  Sudden death
Chronic
  Dose-related dysfunction
  Restrictive and dilated cardiomyopathy
  ↑CHF
Prior radiation therapy may contribute
Schemes for grading toxicity
  Ejection fraction
  Hemodynamics
  Endomyocardial biopsy

CYCLOPHOSPHAMIDE

At high doses
  Myopericarditis
  Pericardial effusions
  Pericardial tamponade
  CHF

OTHER AGENTS

5-Fluorouracil
  MI
  Angina
Vincristine
  MI
  Angina
Mitoxantrone
  LV dysfunction
  CHF

BMT

Involves different protocols
  of potent chemotherapy and
  whole-body irradiation
Patients often had prior chemotherapy
  or radiotherapy, increasing the
  cardiotoxicity of BMT
5%–10% of patients develop CHF,
  pericarditis, or arrhythmias
Subclinical LV dysfunction
  may persist

FIGURE 3-30. Cardiovascular complications of chemotherapy and bone marrow transplantation (BMT) [5,15,48–51]. CHF—congestive heart failure; LV—left ventricular; MI—myocardial infarction.

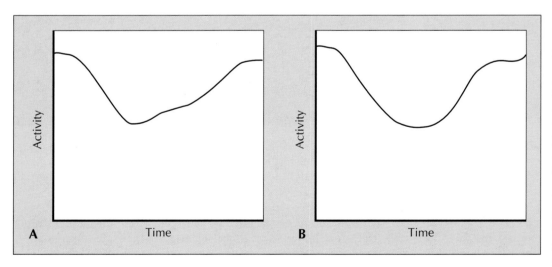

FIGURE 3-31. Anthracycline cardiotoxicity with severe diastolic and mild systolic dysfunction in a 44-year-old woman who presented initially with a stage IA Hodgkin's lymphoma (mixed cellularity) involving the left cervical area. She received mantle irradiation to a dose of 36 Gy (linear accelerator) over 5 weeks, with a boost of 4 Gy to the neck mass. Complete remission followed. Five years later, the patient relapsed with left supraclavicular adenopathy. A 6-month course of ABVD (doxorubicin, bleomycin, vinblastine, and dacarbazine) was given to a total dose of doxorubicin of 300 mg/m^2, and complete remission was again achieved. Two years later she presented with dyspnea and fatigue of gradual onset. A blood pool gated scan revealed mildly depressed left ventricular systolic function (ejection fraction, 44%) and a markedly abnormal (slow) diastolic filling pattern (**A**) but no wall motion abnormality. A thallium-201 scan revealed a reversible defect. The patient was treated with diltiazem and improved markedly. A follow-up blood pool gated scan obtained 2 years later was normal (**B**). The patient continues to be well and free of lymphoma. (Courtesy of Mark A. Rabinovitch, MD, Montreal General Hospital, McGill University, Montreal, Canada.)

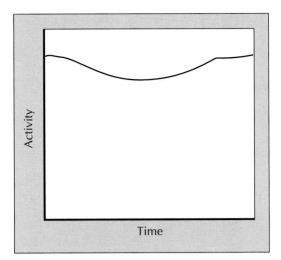

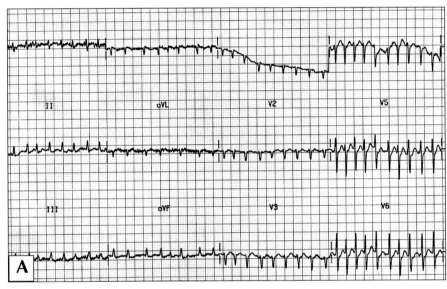

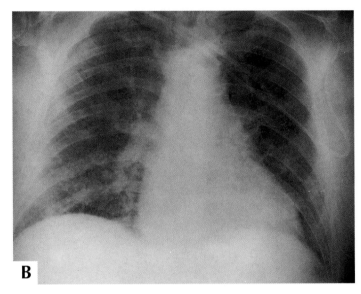

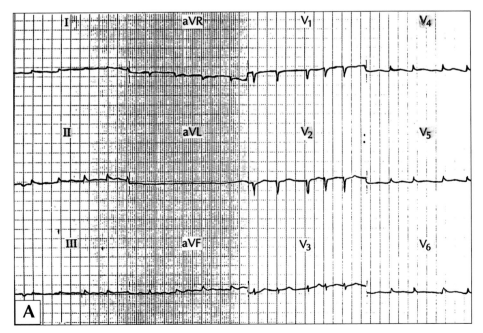

FIGURE 3-32. Anthracycline cardiotoxicity with severe, irreversible systolic dysfunction in a 61-year-old woman who was treated with doxorubicin. She developed severe dilated cardiomyopathy, with an ejection fraction of 15% on blood pool gated scan, and successfully underwent cardiac transplantation. (Courtesy of Mark A. Rabinovitch, MD.)

FIGURE 3-33. Acute anthracycline cardiotoxicity in a 66-year-old man with acute leukemia, a history of chronic but well controlled atrial fibrillation, and a baseline left ventricular ejection fraction (LVEF) of 62% on gated scan. **A,** After receiving two doses of doxorubicin (30 mg/m^2), he experienced severe dyspnea, and atrial fibrillation ensued, with a rapid ventricular response (increasing to 180 bpm), widespread repolarization abnormalities, and low voltages in the limb leads. **B,** The chest radiograph revealed cardiomegaly and interstitial pulmonary edema. LVEF fell to 50% on gated scan. Over the next week, the pulmonary edema cleared, and a follow-up gated scan revealed an LVEF of 64%.

FIGURE 3-34. Cyclophosphamide myopericarditis, tamponade, and congestive heart failure in a 55-year-old woman with acute myelogenous leukemia. The patient was treated initially with cytosine arabinoside for 7 days and daunorubicin (45 mg/m^2) for 3 days. Seven weeks later she received etoposide (50 mg/kg intravenously) for 4 days and cyclophosphamide (50 mg/kg intravenously) for 4 days. Within several days, she experienced dyspnea. **A,** The electrocardiogram showed atrial fibrillation, with low voltages in the limb and precordial leads. (*continued*)

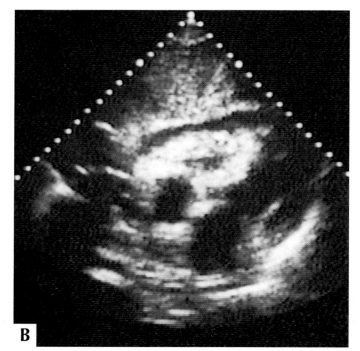

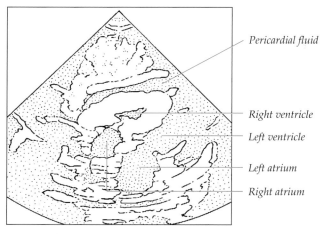

Pericardial fluid

Right ventricle

Left ventricle

Left atrium

Right atrium

FIGURE 3-34. (*continued*) **B,** The subcostal view on transthoracic echocardiography revealed a moderate-sized pericardial effusion with evidence of cardiac compression, increased left ventricular (LV) wall thickness, and moderately depressed LV systolic function. Pericardiocentesis resulted in transient improvement; the subsequent creation of a pericardial window led to a lasting remission. Pathologic examination disclosed reactive pericarditis. On follow-up study, LV wall thickness and systolic function had improved.

COMPLICATIONS OF RADIATION THERAPY

CARDIOVASCULAR COMPLICATIONS OF RADIATION THERAPY

MYOCARDIAL COMPLICATIONS	PERICARDIAL COMPLICATIONS	CORONARY ARTERY COMPLICATIONS	ELECTROPHYSIOLOGIC COMPLICATIONS	OTHER COMPLICATIONS
Early	Early	Fibrosis/atherosclerosis of the ostial/proximal coronary arteries	Acute	Sternal deformity/frailty
Inflammation	Inflammation		Nonspecific repolarization changes	Pulmonary hypertension from radiation-induced fibrosis
Left ventricular dysfunction	Pericarditis	Angina	Chronic	
Late	Effusion	Myocardial infarction	Complete atrioventricular block	
Fibrosis/hypertrophy	Tamponade	Sudden death		
Cardiomyopathy (restrictive, dilated)	Late			
Congestive heart failure	Constrictive pericarditis			
	Pericardial thickening			

FIGURE 3-35. Cardiovascular complications of radiation therapy [52].

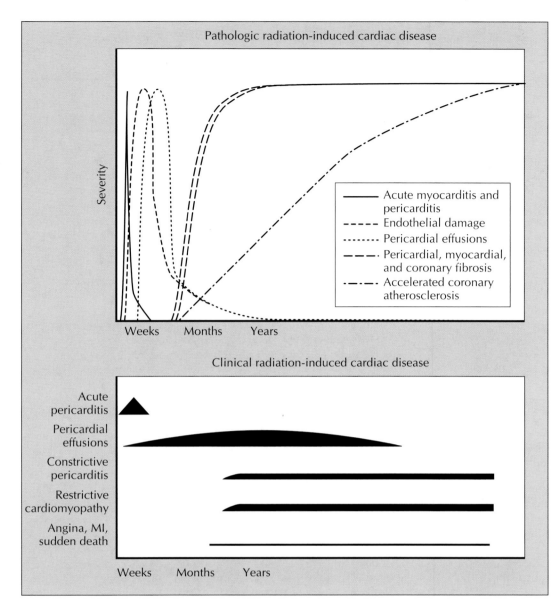

FIGURE 3-36. After radiation injury to the tissues of the heart, inflammatory and, later, fibrotic processes may ensue. The earliest pathologic changes are inflammatory and, correspondingly, the earlier clinical syndromes are of myopericarditis. In some patients inflammation may evolve into fibrosis, leading to the late clinical sequelae of pericardial constriction, restrictive cardiomyopathy, and coronary events. MI—myocardial infarction.

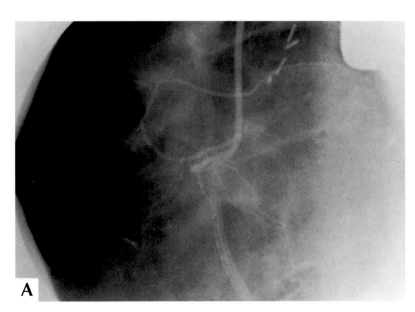
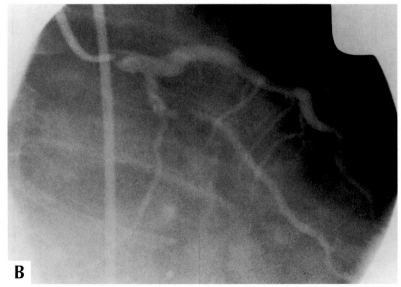

FIGURE 3-37. Proximal coronary stenosis after radiation therapy in a 43-year-old man with a history of Hodgkin's lymphoma and mediastinal radiation therapy at age 23 years. The patient presented with an anterior myocardial infarction, with postinfarction angina. **A,** Coronary arteriography revealed complete obstruction of the proximal right coronary artery; the faint ringlike density in the hilar area is a calcified lymph node. **B,** Angioplasty to relieve severe stenosis of the first obtuse marginal branch was successful, although it required higher pressures and longer periods of inflation than usual.

REFERENCES

1. Roberts WC, Glancy DL, DeVita VT Jr: Heart in malignant lymphoma (Hodgkin's disease, lymphosarcoma, reticulum cell sarcoma, and mycosis fungoides). A study of 196 cases. *Am J Cardiol* 1968, 22:85–107.

2. Grollier G, Commeau P, Mercier V, *et al.*: Post-radiotherapeutic left main coronary ostial stenosis: clinical and histological study. *Eur Heart J* 1988, 9:567–570.

3. Gottdiener JS, Appelbaum FR, Ferrans VJ, *et al.*: Cardiotoxicity associated with high dose cyclophosphamide therapy. *Arch Intern Med* 1981, 141:758–763.

4. Applefield MM, Wiernik PH: Cardiac disease after radiation therapy for Hodgkin's disease: analysis of 48 patients. *Am J Cardiol* 1983, 51:1679–1681.

5. Alexander J, Dainiak N, Berger HJ, *et al.*: Serial assessment of doxorubicin cardiotoxicity with quantitative radionuclide angio-cardiography. *N Engl J Med* 1979, 300:278–283.

6. Cecchetti G, Binda A, Piperno A, *et al.*: Cardiac alterations in 36 consecutive patients with idiopathic haemochromatosis: poly-graphic and echocardiographic evaluation. *Eur Heart J* 1991, 12:224–230.

7. Candell-Riera J, Lu L, Seres L, *et al.*: Cardiac hemochromatosis: beneficial effects of iron removal therapy. An echocardiographic study. *Am J Cardiol* 1983, 52:824–829.

8. Liepman MK, Goodlerner S: Surgical management of pericardial tamponade as a presenting manifestation of acute leukemia. *J Surg Oncol* 1981, 17:183–188.

9. Angelucci E, Mariotti E, Lucarelli G, *et al.*: Sudden cardiac tamponade after chemotherapy for marrow transplantation in thalassaemia. *Lancet* 1992, 339:287–289.

10. Varat MA, Adolph RJ, Fowler NO: Cardiovascular effects of anemia. *Am Heart J* 1972, 83:415–426.

11. Mayer RJ, Davis RB, Schiffer CA, *et al.*: Intensive postremission chemotherapy in adults with acute myeloid leukemia. *N Engl J Med* 1994, 331:896–903.

12. Silberman G, Crosse MG, Peterson EA, *et al.*: Availability and appropriateness of allogeneic bone marrow transplantation for chronic myeloid leukemia in 10 countries. *N Engl J Med* 1994, 331:1063–1067.

13. Bishop JF, Young GA, Szer J, *et al.*: Randomized trial of high dose cytosine arabinoside (ara-C) combination in induction in acute myeloid leukemia (AML) [Abstract]. *Progr Proc Am Soc Clin Oncol* 1992, 11:260.

14. Clift RA, Buckner CD, Thomas ED, *et al.*: The treatment of acute non-lymphoblastic leukemia by allogeneic marrow transplanta-tion. *Bone Marrow Transplant* 1987, 2:243–258.

15. Armitage JO: Bone marrow transplantation. *N Engl Med J* 1994, 330:827–838.

16. Cazin B, Gorin NC, Laporte JP, *et al.*: Cardiac complications after bone marrow transplantation. A report on a series of 63 consecu-tive transplantations. *Cancer* 1986, 53:2061–2069.

17. Larsen RL, Barber G, Heise CT, *et al.*: Exercise assessment of cardiac function in children and young adults before and after bone marrow transplantation (Part 2). *Pediatrics* 1992, 89:722–729.

18. Graettinger JS, Parsons RL, Campbell JA: A correlation of clinical and hemodynamic studies in patients with mild and severe anemia with and without congestive heart failure. *Ann Intern Med* 1963, 58:617–626.

19. Reisner SA, Rinkevich D, Markiewicz W, *et al.*: Cardiac involve-ment in patients with myeloproliferative disorders. *Am J Med* 1992, 93:498–504.

20. Skoularigis J, Essop MR, Skudicky D, *et al.*: Frequency and severity of intravascular hemolysis after left-sided cardiac valve replace-ment with Medtronic Hall and St. Jude medical prostheses, and influence of prosthetic type, position, size and number. *Am J Cardiol* 1993, 71:587–591.

21. Gerry JL, Bulkley BH, Hutchins GM: Clinicopathologic analysis of cardiac dysfunction in 52 patients with sickle cell anemia. *Am J Cardiol* 1978, 42:211–216.

22. Lewis JF, Maron BJ, Castro O, *et al.*: Left ventricular diastolic filling abnormalities identified by Doppler echocardiography in asympto-matic patients with sickle cell anemia. *J Am Coll Cardiol* 1991, 17:1473–1478.

23. Alpert BS, Dover EV, Strong WB, *et al.*: Longitudinal exercise hemodynamics in children with sickle cell anemia. *Am J Dis Child* 1984, 138:1021–1024.

24. Barret O, Saunders DE, McFarland DE, *et al.*: Myocardial infarction in sickle cell anemia. *Am J Hematol* 1984, 16:139–147.

25. Berezowski K, Mautner GC, Roberts WC: Scarring of the left ventricular papillary muscles in sickle-cell disease. *Am J Cardiol* 1992, 70:1368–1370.

26. Collins FS, Orringer EP: Pulmonary hypertension in the sickle hemoglobinopathies. *Am J Med* 1982, 73:814–821.

27. Norris SL, Johnson CS, Haywood LJ: Sickle cell anemia: does myocardial ischemia occur during crisis? *J Natl Med Assoc* 1991, 83:209–213.

28. Pearl W, Zeballos RJ, Gregory G, *et al.*: ECG in sickle cell trait at rest and during exercise and hypoxia. *J Electrocardiol* 1994, 27:215–219.

29. Lippman SM, Ginzton LE, Thigpen T, *et al.*: Mitral valve prolapse in sickle cell disease: presumptive evidence for a linked connective tissue disorder. *Arch Intern Med* 1985, 145:435–438.

30. Niederau C, Fischer R, Sonnenberg AM, *et al.*: Survival and causes of death in cirrhotic and in noncirrhotic patients with primary hemochromatosis. *N Engl J Med* 1985, 313:1256–1262.

31. Rahko PS, Salerni R, Uretsky BF, *et al.*: Successful reversal by chela-tion therapy of congestive cardiomyopathy due to iron overload. *J Am Coll Cardiol* 1986, 8:436–440.

32. James TN: Pathology of the cardiac conduction system in hemochromatosis. *N Engl J Med* 1964, 271:92–94.

33. Peeters S, Vandenplas Y, Jochmans K, *et al.*: Myocardial infarction in a neonate with hereditary antithrombin III deficiency. *Acta Paediatr* 1993, 82:610–613.

34. Carrie D, Beard T, Sie P, *et al.*: Simultaneous thrombosis of the left anterior, interventricular, and right coronary arteries in a 27-year-old patient with protein S deficiency. *Arch Mal Coeur Vaiss* 1993, 86:921–924.

35. Kam RM, Tan AT, Chee TS, *et al.*: Massive acute pulmonary embolism in protein S deficiency—a case report. *Ann Acad Med Singapore* 1994, 23:396–399.

36. De Stefano V, Leone G, Micalizzi P, *et al.*: Arterial thrombosis as a clinical manifestation of congenital protein C deficiency. *Ann Hematol* 1991, 62:180–183.

37. Kattwinkel N, Villanueva AG, Labib SB, *et al.*: Myocardial infarc-tion caused by cardiac microvasculopathy in a patient with the primary antiphospholipid syndrome. *Ann Intern Med* 1992, 116:974–976.

38. Asherson RA, Higenbottam TW, Dinh-Xuan AT, *et al.*: Pulmonary hypertension in a lupus clinic: experience with twenty-four patients. *J Rheumatol* 1990, 17:1298–1308.

39. Roberts WC, Brodey GP, Wertake PT: The heart in acute leukemia—a study of 420 cases. *Am J Cardiol* 1968, 21:388–412.

40. Terry LN, Kligerman MM: Pericardial and myocardial involvement by lymphomas and leukemias. *Cancer* 1970, 25:1003–1008.

41. Kosmo MA, Gale RP: Plasma cell leukemia with IgA paraproteinemia and hyperviscosity. *Am J Hematol* 1988, 28:113–115.

42. Escalante CP: Causes and management of superior vena cava syndrome. *Oncology* 1993, 7:61–77.

43. Tak T, Rashtian M, Detar M, *et al.*: Unusual case of metastatic intracardiac plasmacytoma. *Can J Cardiol* 1994, 10:857–860.

44. Devoy MA, Tomson CR: Fatal cardiac failure after a single dose of doxorubicin in myeloma-associated cardiac amyloid. *Postgrad Med J* 1992, 68:69.

45. McBride W, Jackman JD Jr, Grayburn PA: Prevalence and clinical characteristics of a high cardiac output state in patients with multiple myeloma. *Am J Med* 1990, 90:21–24.

46. Nand S, Orfei E: Pulmonary hypertension in polycythemia vera. *Am J Hematol* 1994, 47:242–244.

47. Pick RA, Glover MU, Nanfro JJ, *et al.*: Acute myocardial infarction with essential thrombocythemia in a young man. *Am Heart J* 1983, 106:406–407.

48. Isner JM, Ferrans VJ, Cohen SR, *et al.*: Clinical and morphologic cardiac findings after anthracycline chemotherapy: analysis of 64 patients studied at necropsy. *Am J Cardiol* 1983, 51:1167–1174.

49. O'Connell TX, Berenbaum MC: Cardiac and pulmonary effects of high doses of cyclophosphamide and osiphosphamide. *Cancer Res* 1974, 34:1586–1591.

50. Gradishar WJ, Vokes EE: 5-Fluorouracil cardiotoxicity: a critical review. *Ann Oncol* 1990, 1:409–414.

51. Baello EB, Ensberg ME, Ferguson DW, *et al.*: Effect of high-dose cyclophosphamide and total body irradiation on left ventricular function in adult patients with leukemia undergoing allogeneic bone marrow transplantation. *Cancer Treat Rep* 1986, 70:1187–1193.

52. Brosius FC, Waller BF, Roberts WC: Radiation heart disease. Analysis of 16 young (aged 15 to 33 years) necropsy patients who received over 3500 rads to the heart. *Am J Med* 1981, 70:519–530.

ANTICOAGULANT, ANTITHROMBOTIC, AND THROMBOLYTIC THERAPY

4

CHAPTER

Stephen M. Zaacks and Mihai Gheorghiade

Over the past two decades, the morbidity and mortality associated with thrombotic and embolic events in the cardiovascular system have been reduced significantly by antithrombotic therapy. Still, the incidence of serious thromboembolic events remains high. Thrombosis plays an important role in the pathophysiology of myocardial infarction (MI), unstable angina, sudden death, stroke, venous thrombosis, and pulmonary and systemic emboli. It may also be involved in the progression of coronary artery disease. At least 10 million people in the United States suffer from thromboembolic disease, and current anticoagulant, antithrombotic, and thrombolytic therapy is essential in the management of these conditions. As more is learned about the pathogenesis of thrombus formation, newer agents are being developed.

Thrombus formation is the result of three pathophysiologic steps. First, endothelial cells and subendothelial tissues, such as collagen and fibronectin, initiate the hemostatic process by activating platelets and the coagulation cascade by releasing substances that include tissue factor, von Willebrand factor, and platelet-activating factor. Second, platelets adhere to the vessel walls and secrete numerous granules as well as thromboxane, which in turn enhance platelet aggregation. Third, activation of the coagulation cascade leads to the formation of thrombin via a series of enzymatic conversions. Thrombin, a potent stimulator of platelet aggregation, stabilizes the hemostatic plug by converting fibrinogen to fibrin. In addition, the vascular system has an intrinsic, self-regulated thrombolytic system that prevents excessive thrombosis through the conversion of plasminogen into active plasmin.

Antithrombotic therapy has focused on blocking individual steps in this process. *Warfarin* prevents the formation of thrombin by interfering with vitamin K metabolism, thereby reducing the levels of activated factors II, VII, IX, and X. This anticoagulant has been shown to prevent embolic events in a variety of conditions, including atrial fibrillation, rheumatic heart disease, prosthetic heart valves, left ventricular thrombus, and venous thromboembolic disease. Warfarin's safety and efficacy have recently been improved by using the International Normalized Ratio (INR). Data now suggest that combining warfarin with aspirin is beneficial in patients with mechanical prosthetic valves, and trials are now under way to evaluate this combination in atrial fibrillation and in the period after MI.

Heparin, a complex linear polysaccharide, inhibits the action of thrombin indirectly by forming a complex with antithrombin III and also inhibits the activity of factor X in the coagulation cascade. Heparin appears to be an effective therapy for patients who present with unstable angina or pulmonary embolus. It is also being used in patients with MI, either alone or in combination with thrombolytic agents. Low-molecular-weight heparins (LMWH) can bind to thrombin directly, thus reducing its procoagulant effects, and may even be superior to standard heparin in certain clinical situations. Since LMWH do not require regular monitoring, they may be more useful in the outpatient setting.

The antiplatelet agents *aspirin* and *ticlopidine* partially inhibit platelet aggregation by their negative effects on thromboxane synthesis and ADP, respectively. Although aspirin is highly beneficial in patients with suspected MI, stable and unstable angina, and atrial fibrillation, doses of 75 to 325 mg appear to be beneficial. Since not all patients respond to aspirin, future research should seek to identify these unresponsive patients and to determine the correct dose for a particular patient. Ticlopidine appears to be an alternative to aspirin, and more studies are needed to establish its place in clinical practice. Despite the proven antiplatelet effects of dipyridamole, the clinical usefulness of this agent seems limited.

Thrombolytic drugs activate the body's own clot-destroying mechanisms by converting plasminogen to plasmin. They have become one of the most important interventions to limit infarct size and improve survival. A limitation of thrombolytic therapy is a small risk of hemorrhagic stroke.

Hirudins are proteins that are still under investigation as effective inhibitors of thrombus formation, although they may also increase the risk of bleeding. Other small peptides that bind to platelet GpIIb/IIIa receptor are also being evaluated.

HISTORY OF ANTITHROMBOTIC THERAPY

2400 years ago	Hippocrates reported therapeutic benefits of extracts of willow bark (source of salicylic acid)
1826–1829	Leroux (Paris), Buchner (Munich), and Fontana and Brugnatelli (Italy) isolated salicin
1861	Von Burke reported the proteolytic activity of human urine
1884	Haycraft discovered hirudins
1916	McLean isolated heparin from dog liver
Early 1930s	Discovery by Tillet of fibrinolysin, called streptokinase by Christensen and MacLeod
1935	Jorpes purified heparin and determined its chemical structure
1935	Quick developed the prothrombin time test
1939	Link found dicumarol to be the cause of sweet clover disease, a hemorrhagic disorder in cows
1942	Nichol and Wright first to treat MI with a warfarin derivative
1942	Warfarin identified by Link
1943	Link reports on the anticoagulant effects of aspirin
1947	Sherry first to administer streptokinase to humans
1957	Markwardt described the antithrombotic effects and structure of hirudins
1976	Chazov in the USSR is first to report intracoronary use of streptokinase in acute MI
1979	t-PA first isolated by Rijken

FIGURE 4-1. History of antithrombotic therapy [1]. The therapeutic effects of anticoagulant agents were first reported as far back as 2400 years ago, when Hippocrates described willow bark as a source of salicylic acid. It was not until the early 1800s, however, that salicin was isolated by researchers in Paris, Munich, and Italy; then, in 1943, Link published the first reports of the anticoagulant effects of aspirin. Vane received the Nobel Prize in 1971 for noting that aspirin exerts its effect by inhibiting prostaglandin synthetase. Another agent, heparin, was first isolated from dog liver in 1916 by a medical student named McLean; later, in the 1930s, its chemical structure was determined by Jorpes. Warfarin, first synthesized in 1942, was initially used as rat poison; it was not until 1978 that its actual mechanism as an anticoagulant was elucidated when Whitlon and Bell showed that warfarin inhibits the enzyme vitamin K epoxide reductase. Finally, the impact of thrombolytic therapy on the treatment of acute myocardial infarction (MI) did not become fully apparent until the 1980s, although streptokinase was discovered in the early 1930s by Christensen and MacLeod. Tissue-type plasminogen activator (t-PA) was first isolated by Rijken from uterine tissue in 1979 and then from human melanoma cell cultures.

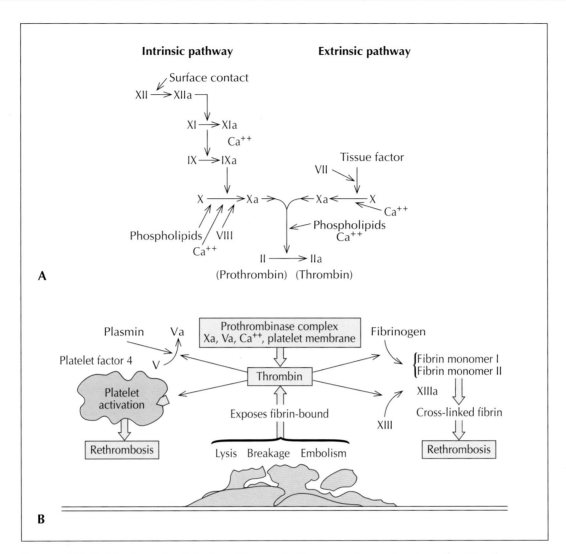

FIGURE 4-2. Intrinsic and extrinsic pathways in the cascade mechanisms for blood coagulation. Several triggers activate the coagulation cascade, including tumor necrosis factor, endotoxin, and endothelial injury. For example, in the development of the acute coronary syndromes, atherosclerotic plaque rupture results in the exposure of collagen and initiation of the coagulation cascade via the intrinsic pathway. The extrinsic pathway may be activated by tissue factor release from endothelial cells.

B, The important role of thrombin in thrombus formation. With a molecular weight of approximately 30,000 D, thrombin is a protein enzyme with proteolytic properties. It is a breakdown product of prothrombin, an α_2-globulin with a molecular weight of 68,700 D. Active thrombin will convert fibrinogen to fibrin and activate factor XIII, which accelerates fibrin cross-linking. In addition, thrombin enhances platelet aggregation by the upregulation of IIb/IIIa receptors on platelets and also activates factor V, thereby accelerating further thrombin formation. Platelet activation by thrombin leads to the production of platelet factor 4, a natural inhibitor of heparin [2,3]. (Part B *adapted from* Webster and coworkers [2]; with permission.)

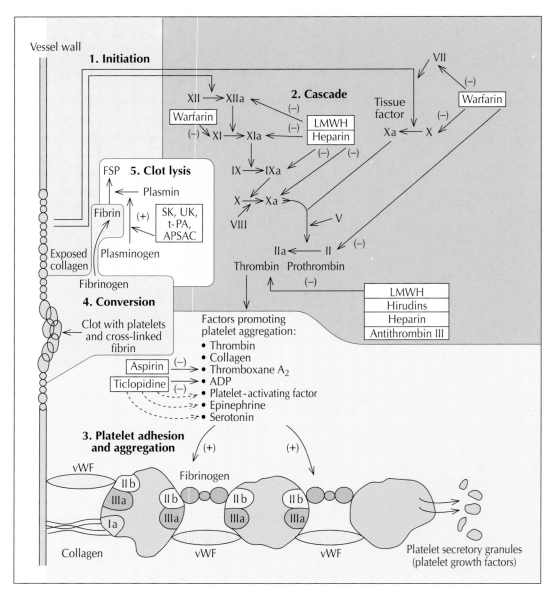

FIGURE 4-3. Five steps in thrombus formation in coronary arteries and the sites of action of anticoagulant, antithrombotic, and thrombolytic agents: (1) initiation, (2) the coagulation cascade, (3) platelet adhesion and aggregation, (4) conversion of fibrinogen to fibrin, and (5) clot lysis [4–6]. The mechanism of thrombus formation in arteries, veins, and cardiac chambers is similar, although the initiating factors in each setting may be different. A certain stimulus (tissue injury, exposed collagen) initiates the process by activating the coagulation cascade, enabling the production of thrombin, which acts along with several plasma, endothelial, and platelet-derived factors as a potent mediator of platelet aggregation. Thrombin is also responsible for the conversion of fibrinogen to fibrin, which stabilizes the hemostatic plug with the help of factor XIIIa, also activated by thrombin.

Warfarin inhibits the generation of thrombin, while heparins and hirudins inhibit thrombin's activity. The antiplatelet agents aspirin and ticlopidine inhibit platelet aggregation by preventing thromboxane and ADP formation, respectively. Current research is focused on small peptides that inhibit platelet receptors IIb/IIIa and Ia, preventing platelet binding mediated by fibrinogen and von Willebrand factor (vWF). The endogenous thrombolytic system, the body's natural defense against excess thrombosis, forms plasmin. Plasmin is an active enzyme capable of lysing clots and is regulated by α_2-anti-plasmin. The thrombolytic agents streptokinase (SK), urokinase (UK), tissue-type plasminogen activator (t-PA), and APSAC (anisoylated plasminogen-streptokinase activator complex) enhance the conversion of plasminogen produced in endothelial cells to plasmin, thereby destroying thrombi. FSP—fibrin split products; LMWH—low molecular weight heparin. (*Adapted from* Ellis and coworkers [4] and Fuster and coworkers [5]; with permission.)

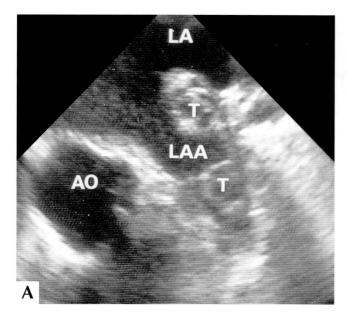

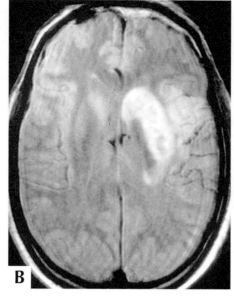

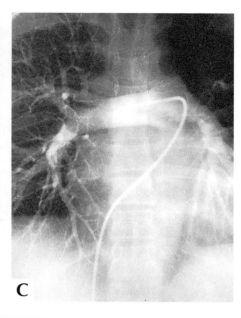

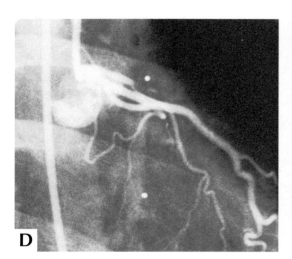

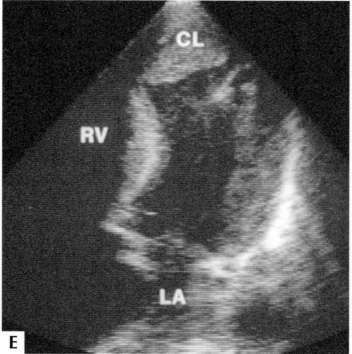

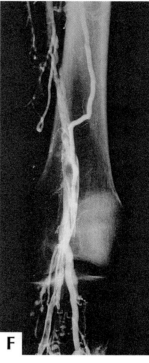

FIGURE 4-4. Spectrum of clinical conditions caused by thrombi and emboli in the cardiovascular system. **A,** Left atrial (LA) thrombus (T) is usually associated with atrial fibrillation and can be detected by transesophageal echocardiography. **B,** A cerebral infarction caused by emboli or thrombi is often seen on a computed tomographic scan of the brain and results in significant morbidity and mortality. **C,** Pulmonary embolus, which is diagnosed most effectively by angiography, is often the consequence of proximal deep venous thrombosis.

D, Coronary thrombosis causes a number of acute events, with myocardial infarction and sudden death being the most severe outcomes. **E,** Left ventricular thrombus detected by transthoracic echocardiography. **F,** Deep venous thrombosis of the lower extremities can be well visualized on a venogram. AO—aorta; CL—clot; LAA—left atrial appendage; RV—right ventricle. (Courtesy of the Department of Radiology, Division of Vascular Surgery, and Division of Cardiology, Northwestern Memorial Hospital, Chicago, IL.)

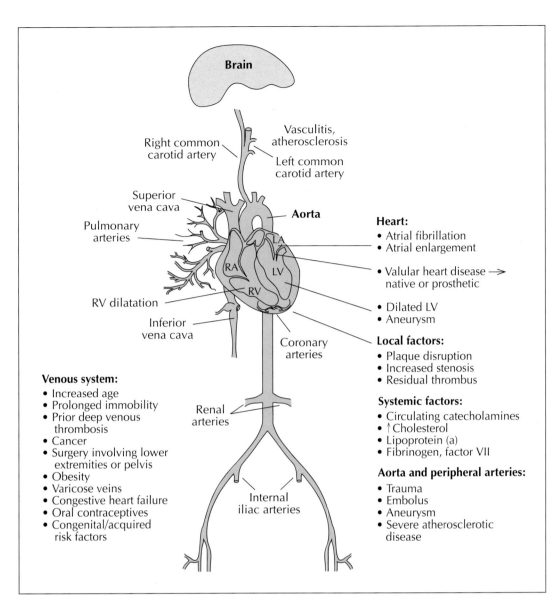

FIGURE 4-5. Factors predisposing to thrombus in the heart and arterial and venous systems are complex. In the coronary arteries and presumably the peripheral arteries, thrombus formation is triggered primarily by atherosclerotic plaque rupture, with the degree of rupture determining the acute coronary syndrome; deep ulceration likely results in the formation of an occlusive, persistent thrombus that leads to infarction, while a small fissure may cause small, labile thrombi to form transiently, resulting in unstable angina [7]. Thrombi in the cardiac chambers usually form when blood is static near a hypokinetic wall or aneurysm. In general, thrombi that form in the venous system are due to trauma or stasis and are composed mainly of red blood cells; arterial thrombi, on the other hand, form under conditions of high flow and are composed mainly of platelet aggregates bound together by thin fibrous strands. Finally, when evaluating other causes of arterial or venous thromboembolism, one should consider congenital disorders resulting in a hypercoagulable state such as antithrombin III deficiency, protein C and protein S deficiencies, disorders of plasminogen activation, the lupus anticoagulant, and polycythemia vera [5,8,9]. LA—left atrium; LV—left ventricle; RA—right atrium; RV—right ventricle.

Diagram labels:
Brain
Right common carotid artery
Vasculitis, atherosclerosis
Left common carotid artery
Superior vena cava
Aorta
Pulmonary arteries
RA, LA, LV, RV
RV dilatation
Inferior vena cava
Coronary arteries
Renal arteries
Internal iliac arteries

Heart:
- Atrial fibrillation
- Atrial enlargement
- Valvular heart disease → native or prosthetic
- Dilated LV
- Aneurysm

Local factors:
- Plaque disruption
- Increased stenosis
- Residual thrombus

Systemic factors:
- Circulating catecholamines
- ↑Cholesterol
- Lipoprotein (a)
- Fibrinogen, factor VII

Aorta and peripheral arteries:
- Trauma
- Embolus
- Aneurysm
- Severe atherosclerotic disease

Venous system:
- Increased age
- Prolonged immobility
- Prior deep venous thrombosis
- Cancer
- Surgery involving lower extremities or pelvis
- Obesity
- Varicose veins
- Congestive heart failure
- Oral contraceptives
- Congenital/acquired risk factors

WARFARIN

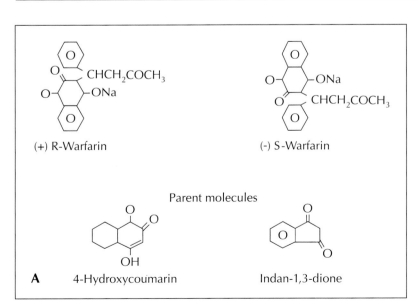

(+) R-Warfarin

(-) S-Warfarin

Parent molecules

4-Hydroxycoumarin

Indan-1,3-dione

A

FIGURE 4-6. A, Stereoisomers of warfarin and its parent compounds. The oral anticoagulants can be divided into two groups: those derived from 4-hydroxycoumarin and those derived from indan-1,3-dione. Only those compounds related to the former are frequently used in a clinical setting. Warfarin is the most commonly used agent, and commercial preparations consist of racemic mixtures of S-warfarin and R-warfarin. The S-warfarin isomer is more important clinically, since it is five times more potent as a vitamin K antagonist than is the R form [10]. (*continued*)

1924	Schofield described "sweet clover disease"
1929	Roderick determined that "sweet clover disease" was the result of decreased prothrombin levels
1935	Quick developed the one-stage prothrombin time test to monitor warfarin therapy
1939	Link identified dicumarol as the offending agent in sweet clover disease
1940s	Synthesis of warfarin
1950s	Warfarin used in medical practice

FIGURE 4-6. (*continued*) **B,** In 1924, Paul Schofield described "sweet clover disease" in cattle who bled to death 30 days after ingesting spoiled clover. Roderick attributed this phenomenon to a toxic reduction in plasma prothrombin; later, it was shown that the effects could be reversed if vitamin K was administered. In 1939, Link identified dicumarol as the agent causing the disease, and in the 1940s a more potent form of the agent was used as a rodenticide. Warfarin was synthesized in 1944 and was introduced into medical practice in the early 1950s [11].

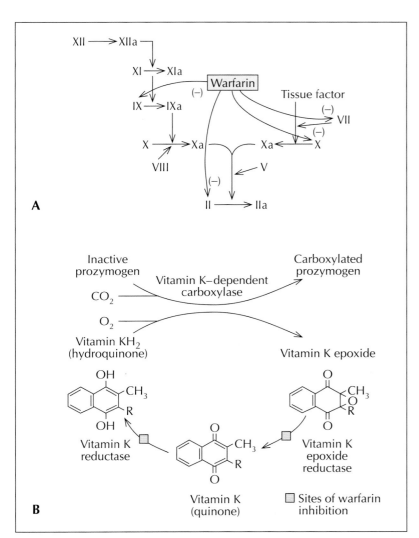

FIGURE 4-7. A, Inhibition of vitamin K–dependent clotting factors by warfarin. Factors II, VII, IX, and X are serine proteases that require the carboxylation of glutamate residues (usually 10 to 13 per factor) to γ-carboxyglutamic acid (Gla) in order to become active. The carboxylation process requires reduced vitamin K, oxygen, and carbon dioxide. In addition to its effects on these factors, warfarin also affects the formation of activated protein C, a proenzyme consisting of two identical polypeptide chains linked by disulfide bonds, and its cofactor, protein S. These two agents are at least partly responsible for regulation of the extrinsic coagulation system by inducing proteolysis of factors V and X and promoting fibrinolysis. **B,** By inhibiting vitamin K epoxide reductase and possibly vitamin K reductase, warfarin decreases the amount of reduced vitamin K available to form Gla residues and so prevents the formation of active enzymes (factors), impairing their biologic function. Glutamate residues must be carboxylated in order to bind, with the help of calcium, to phospholipid and become activated [12,13].

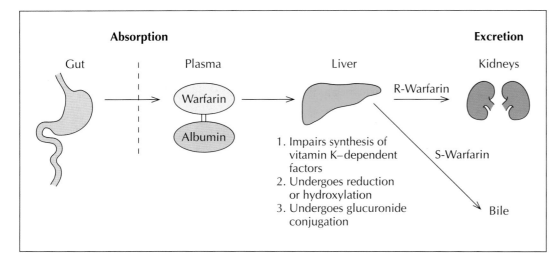

FIGURE 4-8. Absorption, metabolism, and excretion of warfarin. Warfarin is usually administered orally, although it can be injected. It is rapidly absorbed from the gastrointestinal tract and reaches maximal blood concentrations in 90 minutes. Warfarin circulates bound to plasma proteins, primarily albumin, and the racemic mixture has a half-life of 36 hours. It accumulates rapidly in the liver where it prevents synthesis of factors II, VII, IX, and X. The two isomers are metabolized by different pathways: S-warfarin is oxidized to 7-hydroxy-S-warfarin, which is eliminated in bile, and R-warfarin is reduced to warfarin alcohols, which are excreted in urine [12,14].

DRUGS AND CONDITIONS THAT INTERFERE WITH WARFARIN'S EFFECT

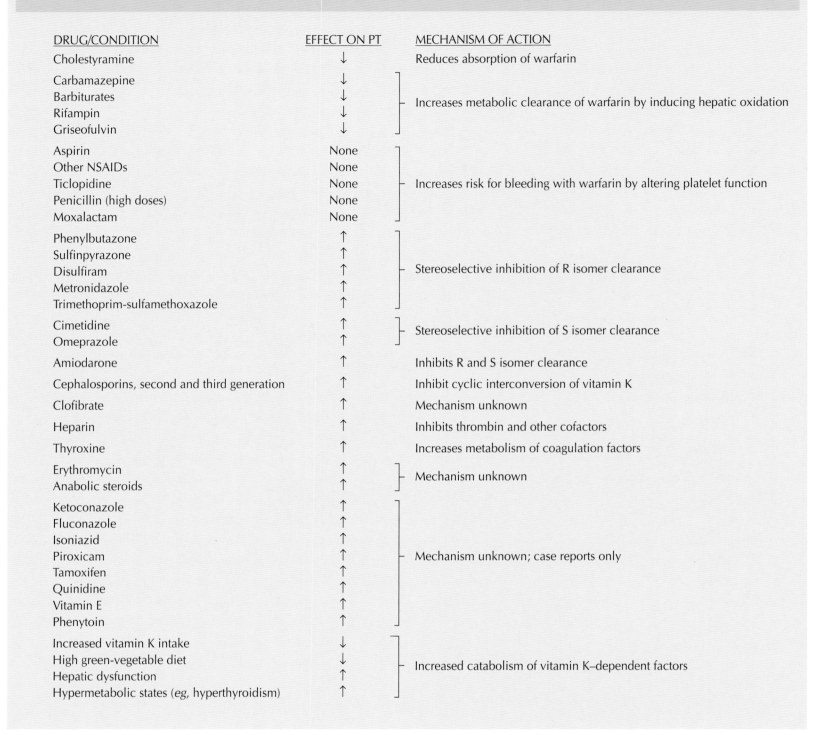

DRUG/CONDITION	EFFECT ON PT	MECHANISM OF ACTION
Cholestyramine	↓	Reduces absorption of warfarin
Carbamazepine	↓	
Barbiturates	↓	Increases metabolic clearance of warfarin by inducing hepatic oxidation
Rifampin	↓	
Griseofulvin	↓	
Aspirin	None	
Other NSAIDs	None	
Ticlopidine	None	Increases risk for bleeding with warfarin by altering platelet function
Penicillin (high doses)	None	
Moxalactam	None	
Phenylbutazone	↑	
Sulfinpyrazone	↑	
Disulfiram	↑	Stereoselective inhibition of R isomer clearance
Metronidazole	↑	
Trimethoprim-sulfamethoxazole	↑	
Cimetidine	↑	Stereoselective inhibition of S isomer clearance
Omeprazole	↑	
Amiodarone	↑	Inhibits R and S isomer clearance
Cephalosporins, second and third generation	↑	Inhibit cyclic interconversion of vitamin K
Clofibrate	↑	Mechanism unknown
Heparin	↑	Inhibits thrombin and other cofactors
Thyroxine	↑	Increases metabolism of coagulation factors
Erythromycin	↑	Mechanism unknown
Anabolic steroids	↑	
Ketoconazole	↑	
Fluconazole	↑	
Isoniazid	↑	
Piroxicam	↑	Mechanism unknown; case reports only
Tamoxifen	↑	
Quinidine	↑	
Vitamin E	↑	
Phenytoin	↑	
Increased vitamin K intake	↓	
High green-vegetable diet	↓	Increased catabolism of vitamin K–dependent factors
Hepatic dysfunction	↑	
Hypermetabolic states (eg, hyperthyroidism)	↑	

FIGURE 4-9. Drugs and conditions that interfere with warfarin's effect. Although none of these is a contraindication to warfarin prescription, prothrombin time (PT) should be followed carefully, at least during the initial period of combination therapy. Aspirin has no effect on the PT but may, at doses above 1 g/d, predispose patients on warfarin to gastrointestinal bleeding because of its potential to cause gastric erosions. Low doses of aspirin (eg, 100 mg) have minimal gastric side effects with similar antithrombotic efficacy and can be used with relative safety in combination with warfarin. Of note, several reports have described hereditary resistance to warfarin in humans and rats, thought to be due to decreased receptor affinity for this drug; such patients may therefore require doses 5 to 20 times the average [11,12,14]. NSAIDs—nonsteroidal anti-inflammatory agents.

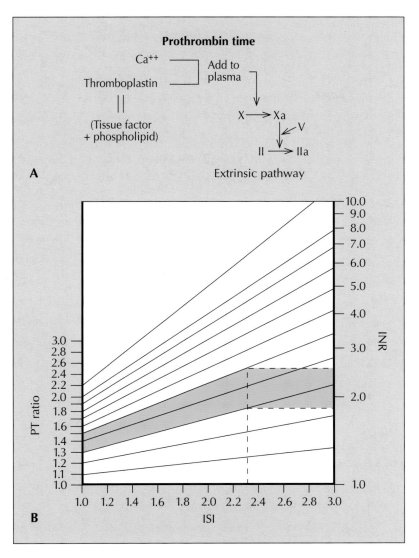

A

Prothrombin time

Ca++ → Add to plasma

Thromboplastin

||

(Tissue factor + phospholipid)

X → Xa
↙ V
II → IIa

Extrinsic pathway

B

PT ratio / INR / ISI

FIGURE 4-10. Warfarin therapy is monitored using the prothrombin time (PT) and the International Normalized Ratio (INR). **A,** The PT is a measure of the extrinsic pathway of coagulation. Initially, it reflects a reduction in factor VII levels, since this factor has the shortest half-life (6 hours); later, it reflects reduced levels of factors II and X. Of note, protein C activity actually declines within 6 hours after the administration of warfarin, and patients deficient in this proenzyme (about one in 16,000) are prone to warfarin-induced skin necrosis. Thromboplastin is a phospholipid-protein extract of lung, brain, or placental tissue that contains the tissue factor necessary to promote activation of factor X by factor VII. The various thromboplastins differ in their "responsiveness" (ie, ability to activate factor X) and significantly affect the PT for the same level of anticoagulation (ie, inactivation of clotting factors II, VII, X) by warfarin.

B, The INR and its relationship to the PT ratio over a range of International Sensitivity Index (ISI) values for thromboplastin reagents. The ISI is a measure of thromboplastin's ability to activate factor X; the lower the ISI, the more responsive the reagent. The Manchester reagent, a standardized human brain thromboplastic reagent, was introduced in 1962. In 1977, the World Health Organization designated this reagent as the first International Referent Preparation (IRP) for thromboplastin; subsequently, in 1982, a calibration system was adopted that allowed each preparation of thromboplastin to be standardized to the IRP by being assigned an ISI value. Each PT ratio could then be standardized by conversion to an INR. The ISI of the IRP is 1, while the ISI of most thromboplastins used in the United States ranges from 1.8 to 2.8 [10,12,14]. *Shaded area* indicates values for a PT ratio of 1.3 to 1.5 for a thromboplastin preparation of ISI 2.3; the $INR = PT^{ISI}$ ($1.3^{2.3}$ to $1.5^{2.3}$), or 1.83 to 2.54. (*Adapted from* Hirsh [12]; with permission.)

RATES OF BLEEDING DURING WARFARIN THERAPY

INDICATION FOR ANTICOAGULANT THERAPY	PATIENTS, n	MAJOR BLEED, n(%)	FATAL BLEED, n(%)
Ischemic cerebrovascular disease	588	41(7.0)	28(4.8)
Prosthetic mechanical heart valves	921	38(4.1)	11(1.2)
Atrial fibrillation	935	37(4.0)	3(0.3)
Ischemic heart disease	2497	101(4.0)	22(0.9)
Venous thromboembolism — More intense	112	13(8.1)	0
Venous thromboembolism — Less intense	361	6(1.7)	0

FIGURE 4-11. Pooled data from several trials indicate that bleeding is the major complication of warfarin therapy [12,15]. The risk for bleeding is increased by (1) concomitant use of other medications, especially high-dose aspirin; (2) the intensity of anticoagulation; and (3) additional factors, such as advanced age, history of stroke, gastrointestinal bleeding, atrial fibrillation, renal insufficiency, and anemia. (*Adapted from* Levine and coworkers [15]; with permission.)

TREATMENT TO REVERSE RISK OF WARFARIN-INDUCED HEMORRHAGE

INR	ACTIVE BLEEDING*	TREATMENT (VITAMIN K)
<6	No	Omit several doses
6–10	No	0.5 mg IV *or* subcutaneous
10–20	No	3–5 mg IV *or* subcutaneous
>20	No	10 mg IV *or* subcutaneous

*Factor concentrate or platelet transfusion should be given in addition to the recommended treatment.

FIGURE 4-12. Reversal of warfarin-induced bleeding. In cases of severe bleeding, intravenous vitamin K and replacement with factor concentrate are indicated. However, it may take 6 hours before vitamin K is effective, and patients usually do not respond to reinstituted warfarin therapy for 1 week after vitamin K has been administered. When treatment with warfarin is discontinued, the International Normalized Ratio (INR) may not change for 2 to 3 days because of the 36-hour half-life of the drug [14]. IV—intravenous.

UNCOMMON SIDE EFFECTS OF WARFARIN THERAPY

Warfarin-induced skin necrosis

"Purple toe" syndrome

Alopecia

Urticaria

Dermatitis

Fever

Nausea

Diarrhea

FIGURE 4-13. Uncommon side effects associated with warfarin therapy. All these reactions are rare, but the first two can cause considerable morbidity. Warfarin skin necrosis may occur 2 to 5 days after therapy is begun and usually affects women. Necrosis of skin, soft tissue, and muscle may require amputation of limbs. The underlying mechanism is thought to be a reduction in proteins C and S in patients with low levels of these factors that occurs more rapidly than a reduction in factors II and X, resulting in a hypercoagulable state and thrombus formation in the vasculature of affected tissue. Simultaneous therapy with heparin may prevent this hypercoagulable state. The "purple toe syndrome" usually occurs 3 to 8 weeks after warfarin is begun and is caused by bleeding into atheromatous plaques in the aorta, with subsequent cholesterol emboli to the extremities. Of note, warfarin is contraindicated in pregnancy, since numerous fetal abnormalities may result, such as warfarin-induced central nervous system and ocular abnormalities, fetal hemorrhage, and spontaneous abortion or stillbirth [16].

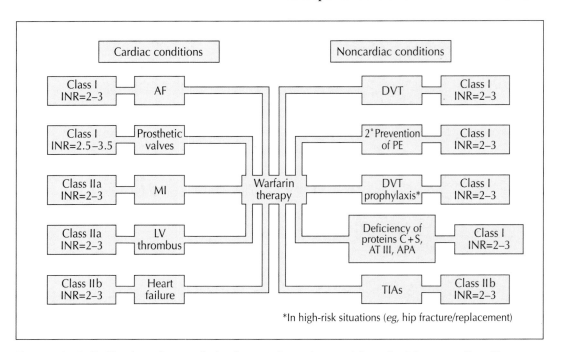

FIGURE 4-14. Indications for warfarin therapy in patients with and without cardiac disease [17]. For class I, warfarin is usually indicated, always acceptable, and considered useful or effective. For class II, warfarin is acceptable, of uncertain efficacy, and may be controversial; for class IIa, the weight of evidence is in favor of usefulness/efficacy, whereas for class IIb its use is not well established by evidence, although it can be helpful and is probably not harmful. For patients with cardiac disease, warfarin is indicated chronically for nonvalvular and valvular atrial fibrillation (AF) and for 3 weeks prior to elective cardioversion in patients with AF for at least 48 hours. However, it is not indicated for the "lone atrial fibrillator" under 60 years of age. In addition, it is indicated for lifetime use in patients with mechanical prosthetic mitral or aortic valves and for at least 3 to 6 months in patients with a large anterior wall infarction or documented left ventricular (LV) thrombus. Warfarin is effective for secondary prevention of reinfarction, stroke, and death after myocardial infarction (MI). The ongoing Coumadin-Aspirin Reinfarction Trial (CARS) has enrolled more than 7000 patients and will determine whether combination low-dose aspirin (80 mg) with 1 or 3 mg of warfarin is superior to aspirin alone for secondary prevention in patients recovering from acute MI.

Patients with proximal deep venous thrombosis (DVT), symptomatic calf-vein thrombosis, and pulmonary embolus (PE) should be treated with warfarin for 3 to 6 months. Those with hip fractures or those undergoing total hip replacement should receive warfarin with a targeted International Normalized Ratio (INR) of 2 to 3; the 1-mg dose is not effective, as was once believed. Warfarin therapy should be started prior to surgery or on the first postoperative day. Furthermore, patients with congenital deficiencies of antithrombin (AT) III, protein C or S, or antiphospholipid antibody (APA) require anticoagulation indefinitely. In the management of strokes, stable and unstable angina, and in patients who have undergone coronary angioplasty, the efficacy of warfarin is not clear [9,14,18]. TIAs—transient ischemic attacks. (*Adapted from* ACC/AHA Task Force [17]; with permission from the American College of Cardiology.)

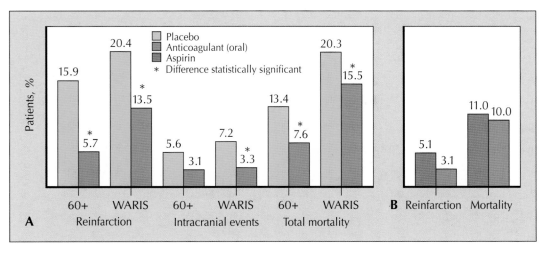

FIGURE 4-15. Results of the three large randomized studies comparing oral anticoagulant therapy with placebo and aspirin in patients who had had a myocardial infarction (MI). **A,** The 60+ Reinfarction Study was a randomized, double-blind, placebo-controlled, multicenter trial that enrolled 878 patients to placebo or warfarin for a mean follow-up of 2 years [19]. The Warfarin Reinfarction Trial (WARIS) was a placebo-controlled, randomized, double-blind trial in which 1214 patients recovering from acute MI were assigned to placebo or warfarin for a mean follow-up period of 37 months [20]. Both studies reported a statistically significant beneficial effect of warfarin therapy for long-term use after acute MI. However, higher International Normalized Ratios (INRs) were maintained and the incidence of bleeding from anticoagulants was increased.

B, The EPSIM (Enquete de Prevention Secondaire de L'Infarctus du Myocarde) multicenter clinical trial randomized 1303 patients to aspirin or oral anticoagulants for an average follow-up of 29 months [21]. The evidence suggests that warfarin and aspirin have similar effects on mortality and reinfarction. Although more patients experienced gastrointestinal bleeding in the aspirin-treated group, there were four times as many patients with severe bleeding complications in the anticoagulant group. (Part A *adapted from* Report of the 60+ Reinfarction Study Research Group [19] and Smith and coworkers [20]; part B *adapted from* The EPSIM Research Group [21]; with permission.)

WARFARIN THERAPY FOR PATIENTS WITH PROSTHETIC HEART VALVES

All patients with mechanical prosthetic valves should receive chronic warfarin therapy.

The INR should be kept between 2.5 and 3.5.

Patients who suffer embolic events on warfarin therapy should also receive aspirin or dipyridamole. Although there is some increased risk of bleeding, 100 mg of aspirin may offer additional protection.

For patients with bioprosthetic valves, warfarin is recommended for the first 3 months if there is no history of AF, left atrial thrombus, or systemic embolus; in such cases, patients should receive chronic warfarin therapy.

For patients undergoing elective noncardiac surgery, warfarin may be discontinued for a few days prior to surgery and then restarted. However, patients at higher risk, such as those with mitral valve prostheses and/or AF, should receive continuous intravenous heparin therapy during the perioperative period.

FIGURE 4-16. Warfarin therapy for patients with prosthetic heart valves. Long-term warfarin therapy is indicated for all patients with mechanical heart valves in the aortic or mitral position, since the benefits of anticoagulation outweigh the risks for bleeding. Warfarin doses that cause the International Normalized Ratio (INR) to exceed 4.5 are associated with an excessive bleeding risk. Conversely, when the INR drops below 1.8, the risk for thromboembolic events is high. Dipyridamole appears to offer some additional protection against thromboembolic events, although some studies have shown little or no benefit. In addition, Turpie *et al.* [22] recently found that the addition of aspirin to warfarin, with the INR maintained at 3 to 4.5, offered a significant benefit; although there was a higher incidence of bleeding events, the risks of combined treatment were more than offset by the considerable benefits [23]. AF—atrial fibrillation. (*Adapted from* Stein and coworkers [23]; with permission.)

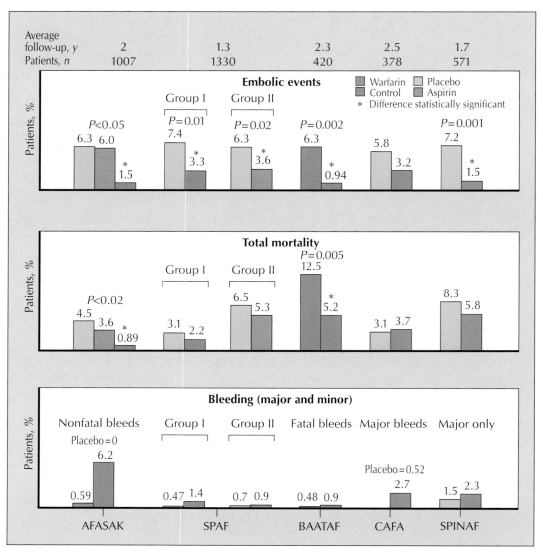

FIGURE 4-17. Results of five major clinical trials of warfarin for nonrheumatic atrial fibrillation (AF). All trials included patients with nonrheumatic AF as well as those with paroxysmal AF.

The AFASAK (Atrial Fibrillation, Aspirin, Anticoagulation) study randomized over 1000 patients to aspirin (75 mg/d), warfarin (Coumadin), or placebo for an average duration of 2 years and found that warfarin significantly reduced embolic events and vascular deaths compared with aspirin or placebo [24]. Target International Normalized Ratio (INR) = 2.8 to 4.2.

The SPAF (Stroke Prevention in Atrial Fibrillation) trial divided 1330 patients into two groups: Group I included patients assigned to warfarin, aspirin (325 mg), or placebo, and Group II included patients assigned to aspirin or placebo. Patients were followed on average for 1.3 years, and both aspirin and warfarin significantly reduced the incidence of embolic events, although the relative risk reduction was greater with warfarin (67%) than with aspirin (42%) [25]. Target INR = 2 to 3.5.

BAATAF (Boston Area Anticoagulation Trial for Atrial Fibrillation) randomized 420 patients to warfarin or control for 2.3 years and found a significant reduction in embolic events and total mortality [26]. Target INR = 1.5 to 2.7.

The CAFA (Canadian Atrial Fibrillation Anticoagulation) study randomized 378 patients to warfarin or placebo for 2.5 years and found no significant reduction in mortality or embolic events, although the trend favored warfarin [27]. Target INR = 2 to 3.

The SPINAF (Stroke Prevention in Nonrheumatic Atrial Fibrillation) study randomized 571 men to warfarin or placebo for 1.7 years and significantly reduced cerebral infarction without a significant increase in bleeding [28]. Based on these results and the recent SPAF II study, warfarin is recommended for all patients with chronic or paroxysmal AF except those under age 75 years who are free of clinical risk factors (history of congestive heart failure, hypertension, or stroke) and echocardiographic risk factors (left ventricular global dysfunction or left atrial enlargement); this latter group is at low risk for stroke development (approximately 1%/year), so aspirin may be used instead [11,29]. Target INR = 1.5 to 2.5.

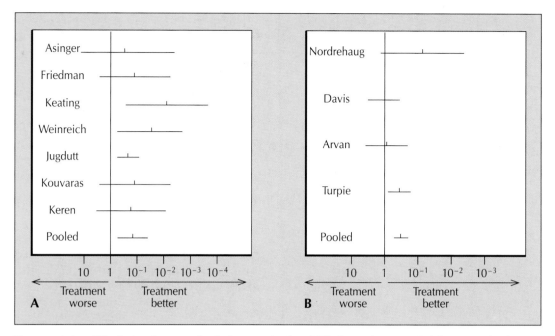

FIGURE 4-18. Warfarin therapy for left ventricular (LV) thrombus. **A,** Odds ratios (*ticks*) and 95% confidence intervals (*horizontal bars*) for seven studies showing the benefit of oral anticoagulants in reducing the embolic risk of mural thrombi in patients with an anterior myocardial infarction (MI). The trials enrolled a total of 270 patients with anterior MI who were found to have LV thrombus on two-dimensional echocardiography. Embolic complications occurred more frequently in the untreated patients, with a risk reduction of 33% in the treated group.

B, Odds ratios and 95% confidence intervals for four studies showing the advantage of anticoagulation in reducing the incidence of mural thrombi after anterior MI. This meta-analysis further suggests that reliance on echocardiographic studies alone to demonstrate mural thrombi is risky; therapy should be initiated rapidly after a large anterior MI, before thrombi are seen on echocardiography. Early therapy with heparin and warfarin is indicated, since warfarin alone may increase the incidence of thrombus formation. Overall, the risk for embolic complications is increased fivefold in patients who have an acute anterior wall MI with mural thrombi compared with those without [18,30]. Indications for warfarin therapy to prevent or treat LV thrombus along with overlapping heparin therapy for the first 5 days include (1) a large anterior wall MI, (2) a diffusely dilated and poorly contracting LV, (3) thrombus, and (4) a large akinetic region in the LV apex [17]. (*Adapted from* Vaitkus and Barnathan [18]; with permission from the American College of Cardiology.)

ANTIPLATELET AGENTS

ASPIRIN

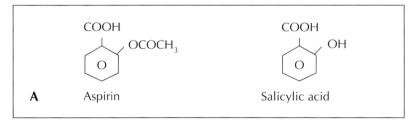

FIGURE 4-19. A, Structural formulas for aspirin and salicylic acid. (*continued*)

FIGURE 4-19. (*continued*) **B,** Historical perspective. The medicinal effect of willow bark had been recognized for centuries, but it was not until 1829 that Leroux (Paris), Buchner (Munich), and Fontana and Brugnatelli (Italy) isolated the active ingredient salicin, which can be converted into salicylic acid. Sodium salicylate was first used as an antipyretic and anti-inflammatory agent in 1876 to treat rheumatic fever. It was introduced into clinical medicine by Dreser in 1899 as "aspirin" derived from *Spiraea*, the plant species from which salicylic acid was once prepared. The antiplatelet effects of aspirin were not discovered until 1967, and in 1971 Vane found aspirin to be an inhibitor of prostaglandin synthesis [31,32].

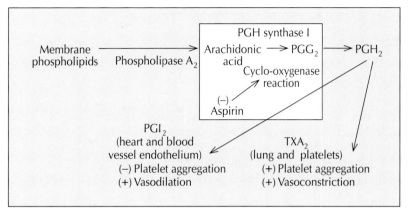

FIGURE 4-20. Aspirin acts by inhibiting the formation of thromboxane A$_2$ (TXA$_2$). Although some studies have suggested other mechanisms to explain the inhibition of platelet function by aspirin, most indicate that the major antithrombotic effect is exerted via the irreversible inhibition of cyclo-oxygenase, which normally converts arachidonic acid to prostaglandin G$_2$ (PGG$_2$). Within platelets, aspirin blocks the synthesis of TXA$_2$ by irreversible acetylation of a serine residue, interfering with cyclo-oxygenase function. PGG$_2$ is converted to prostaglandin H$_2$ (PGH$_2$), which may be converted to prostacyclin (PGI$_2$), an inhibitor of platelet aggregation; to TXA$_2$; or to other prostaglandins. The extent to which aspirin inhibits PGI$_2$ is controversial, and there is some suggestion that at low doses (75 mg) aspirin may selectively inhibit platelet cyclo-oxygenase (thromboxane) without inhibiting endothelial cyclo-oxygenase (PGI$_2$). However, in most clinical trials, the antithrombotic effects of aspirin predominate, regardless of dose, so the degree of prostacyclin inhibition remains unclear [32–35].

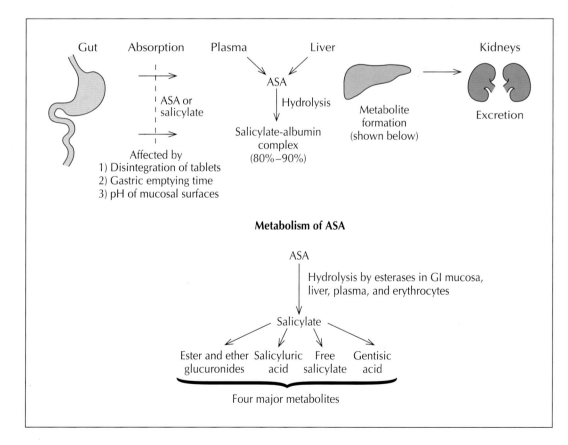

FIGURE 4-21. Absorption, fate, and excretion of aspirin (ASA). ASA is rapidly absorbed in the stomach and upper intestine and reaches peak plasma levels in 20 minutes, whereas rectal absorption is unreliable and much slower. By 1 hour, there is some inhibition of platelet aggregation, and peak blood concentration is reached after 2 hours and then gradually declines. The plasma half-life of ASA is 15 minutes, but alkalinization of the urine can dramatically increase this half-life and promote the elimination of salicylic acid. Absorption is enhanced if the particles are smaller; therefore, for a more rapid effect (*eg*, during an acute myocardial infarction), the tablet should be chewed before it is swallowed. Although ASA's solubility is increased in the ionized form, absorption is similar in either the ionized or nonionized form. However, mucosal damage may occur with nonionized salicylic acid, which is retained by the mucosal epithelial cells to a greater extent. Of note, buffered ASA is initially converted to salicylic acid, and at least four metabolites are produced in the liver and eventually excreted in the urine [30]. GI—gastrointestinal.

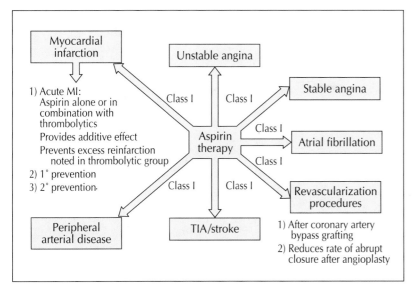

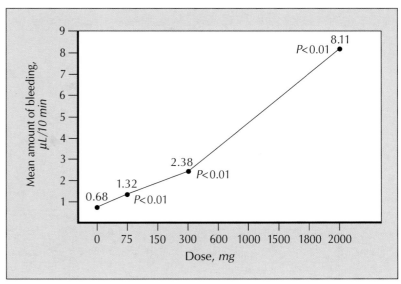

FIGURE 4-22. Although aspirin is clearly indicated for a number of cardiovascular conditions, the physician should be aware of the following special conditions. The effectiveness of aspirin in the prevention of venous thrombosis is still somewhat controversial. The addition of aspirin therapy is indicated for patients with prosthetic heart valves who develop systemic embolus while on warfarin. Aspirin may be used instead of warfarin in patients with atrial fibrillation who are 75 years of age or younger with no history of rheumatic heart disease, hypertension, congestive heart failure, or previous thromboembolic events. Aspirin is indicated for patients with atrial fibrillation for whom warfarin is contraindicated. Aspirin is not recommended for primary prevention of myocardial infarction (MI) except in patients 40 years of age and older who have significant risk factors for coronary artery disease [33].

FIGURE 4-23. Gastrointestinal bleeding (mean values) during aspirin therapy in 48 healthy volunteers over 5 days. Such bleeding has been observed to be dose-related, and several studies using aspirin at different doses have confirmed these findings [33,36]. The precise reason for aspirin-induced damage to the gastric mucosa is unclear, although one proposed mechanism is the inhibition of prostaglandin synthesis in this tissue. Gastrointestinal side effects of aspirin can be minimized by the concurrent use of antacids, H_2-receptor antagonists, or enteric-coated or buffered aspirin. Other side effects of aspirin given in high doses include convulsions, confusion, dizziness, tinnitus, psychosis, hearing loss, and nausea. In addition, IgE-mediated reactions to aspirin may also occur, including angioedema, asthma, and allergic interstitial nephritis (*Adapted from* Prichard and coworkers [36]; with permission.)

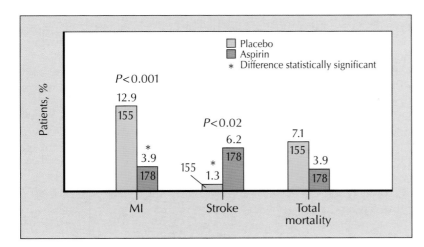

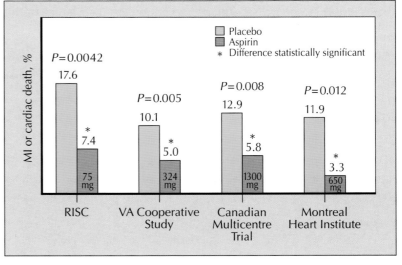

FIGURE 4-24. Results of a randomized, double-blind trial involving a subset of 333 male physicians from the Physicians' Health Study [37]. Patients with chronic stable angina and no history of a previous myocardial infarction (MI), stroke, or transient ischemic attack were followed for an average of 60.2 months while taking either aspirin (325 mg/d) or placebo. Aspirin plays a significant role in the prevention of MI in patients with chronic stable angina. The risk of first MI was significantly reduced in the aspirin-treated group. Although in this study the risk for stroke was higher among those who took aspirin, several other large trials have shown that the risk for developing cerebrovascular disease was reduced in patients assigned to aspirin therapy. The reason for aspirin's beneficial effect in stable angina is unclear, but some studies have suggested that aspirin's inhibition of platelet aggregation during certain high-risk periods of the day may be the mechanism. Numbers inside each bar represent the number of patients studied. (*Adapted from* Ridker and coworkers [37]; with permission.)

FIGURE 4-25. Results of four trials showing the significant reduction in the incidence of myocardial infarction (MI) and cardiac death with aspirin therapy in patients with unstable angina [34]. All four trials were placebo-controlled and double-blinded. The study by the European Research Group on Instability in Coronary Artery Disease (RISC) randomized 199 patients to placebo and 189 to aspirin (75 mg/d) for 3 months. The VA Cooperative Study randomized 641 patients to placebo and 625 patients to buffered aspirin (325 mg/d) for 3 months. The Canadian Multicentre Trial randomized 139 patients to placebo and 139 to aspirin (1300 mg/d) for 24 months. The Montreal Heart Institute Study randomized 118 patients to placebo and 121 to aspirin (650 mg/d) for an average of 6 days (range, 3 to 9 days). Overall, aspirin reduced the incidence of MI and death from cardiac causes by 50% to 70% in patients with unstable angina. (*Adapted from* Willard and coworkers [34]; with permission.)

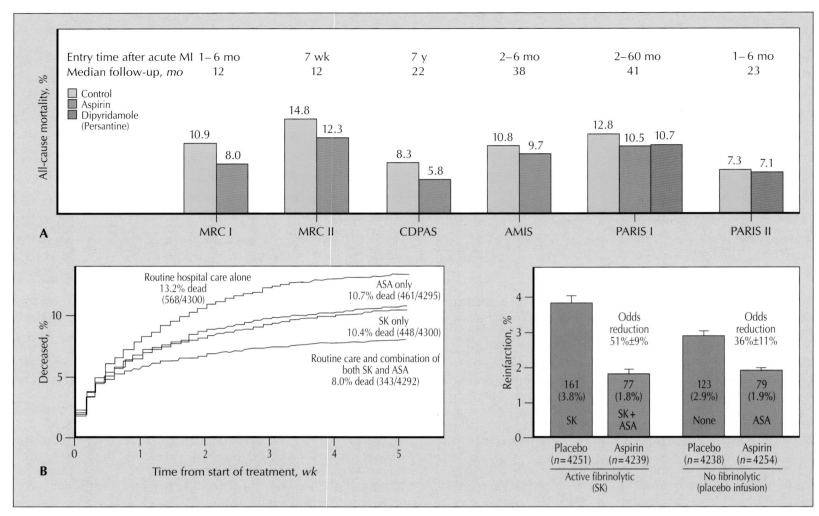

FIGURE 4-26. A, Results of six major trials comparing antiplatelet drugs with placebo for secondary prevention of all-cause mortality after myocardial infarction (MI): the Medical Research Council (MRC) Studies I and II, the Coronary Drug Project Aspirin Study (CDPAS), the Aspirin in Myocardial Infarction Study (AMIS), and the Persantine-Aspirin Reinfarction Studies (PARIS) I and II [37] (Persantine, Boehringer Ingelheim Ltd, Ridgefield, CT). The first three trials randomized over 1000 patients; AMIS included over 4500; and the last two included approximately 2000 and 3100 patients, respectively. None of the six trials showed a statistically significant decrease in all-cause mortality, although the trends appeared favorable; however, only the MRC II focused on early administration of aspirin (within 21 days of infarction), resulting in a significant reduction in cardiac death or nonfatal MI from 22% in the placebo-treated group to 16% in the aspirin-treated group. PARIS II also found a significant reduction in these endpoints.

In addition, two meta-analyses of pooled trials from 1980 and 1988 revealed a significant benefit with aspirin therapy to reduce recurrent MI and overall mortality. Aspirin therapy is therefore recommended as soon as possible during or following acute MI [38].

B, Results of the Second International Study of Infarct Survival (ISIS-2). In this study, 17,187 patients who presented within 24 hours of symptoms consistent with an acute evolving MI were randomized to one of four regimens: intravenous streptokinase (SK), 160 mg of oral aspirin (ASA) for 30 days, both drugs, or neither drug [39]. Three important conclusions emerged: (1) ASA alone is beneficial in reducing reinfarction and death compared with controls, (2) ASA in combination with SK produces an additive beneficial effect, and (3) ASA prevented the excess reinfarction rate noted in the SK-treated group when this group was compared with those given placebo. (Part A *adapted from* Jafri and coworkers [38]; part B *adapted from* ISIS-2 Collaborative Group [39]; with permission.)

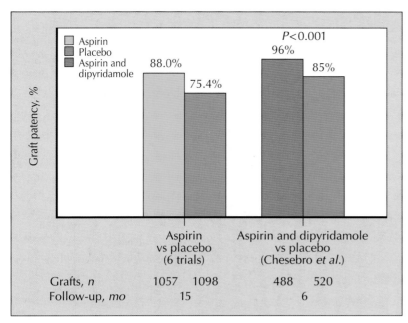

FIGURE 4-27. Effects of aspirin on patency rates of saphenous vein grafts following coronary artery bypass surgery. Six studies compared aspirin with placebo/control over a mean follow-up period of 15 months; the dose range for aspirin was 100 to 1200 mg. When the data are pooled, there is strong evidence to suggest that aspirin should be given perioperatively or within 6 to 12 hours after surgery and then indefinitely to all patients with saphenous vein grafts. When aspirin is started later, the effects may not be as pronounced [30]. Aspirin should be started on the day of surgery or 1 day prior to surgery. Aspirin may be less beneficial for internal mammary artery grafts, since the occlusion rate is low. A randomized, double-blind, placebo-controlled trial by Chesebro *et al.* showed a significant increase in patency rates at 6-month follow-up in patients treated early with a combination of dipyridamole and aspirin compared with placebo [40]. (*Adapted from* Fuster and coworkers [32] and Chesebro and coworkers [40]; with permission.)

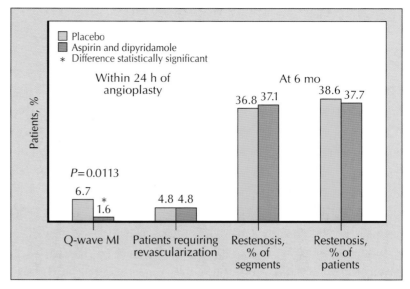

FIGURE 4-28. Role of aspirin in patients undergoing coronary angioplasty. Results of a prospective, multicenter, double-blind, placebo-controlled trial in which 376 patients were randomized to aspirin (330 mg) and dipyridamole (75 mg) three times a day beginning 24 hours before angioplasty [41]. These findings are similar to those of other prospective and retrospective studies showing that antiplatelet agents are effective in reducing periprocedural Q-wave myocardial infarction (MI) but have no effect on the rates of restenosis 6 months later. Coronary angioplasty disrupts atherosclerotic plaque, with subsequent thrombus formation, and aspirin probably has a role in preventing the aggregation and deposition of platelets at the site of rupture. Antiplatelet agents should therefore be started at least 24 hours before the procedure [32,34,42]. (*Adapted from* Schwartz and coworkers [41]; with permission.)

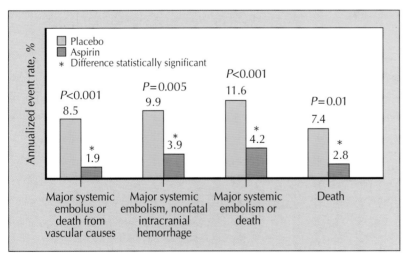

FIGURE 4-29. Effects of aspirin in patients with prosthetic valves who are receiving warfarin. Turpie *et al.* [22] randomized 370 patients who had mechanical heart valves, tissue valves with atrial fibrillation, or a history of thromboembolism to treatment with aspirin (100 mg/d) or placebo in addition to their usual warfarin dose (International Normalized Ratio 3 to 4.5). The patients were followed for an average of 2.5 years, and the rate of principal outcome events was found to be significantly reduced by the addition of aspirin. Of note, risk for minor bleeding (hematuria, epistaxis, bruising) was significantly increased in the aspirin-treated group, but even with these events, in combination with the other major endpoints, aspirin had a net beneficial effect. (*Adapted from* Turpie and coworkers [22]; with permission.)

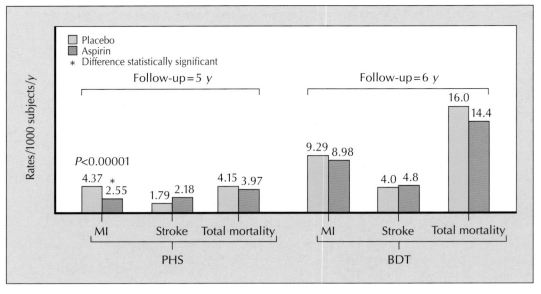

FIGURE 4-30. Primary prevention of cardiovascular events by aspirin in the Physicians' Health Study (PHS) and the British Doctors' Trial (BDT) [43]. The PHS was a double-

blind, placebo-controlled trial in which more than 22,000 US physicians (aged 40 to 80 years) were randomized to low-dose aspirin or placebo. Although there was a 44% reduction in the incidence of myocardial infarction (MI), a significant increase in gastrointestinal hemorrhage required transfusion in the aspirin-treated group. In the BDT, over 5000 male physicians (ages 50 to 70) were randomized to aspirin, 500 mg (two thirds of patients), or no medication. Over a total follow-up period of 6 years, there was no significant reduction in event rate or increase in side effects in the aspirin-treated group. Currently, the only recommendation for prophylactic aspirin is for men 40 years of age and older who are at risk for coronary artery disease and have no contraindications to the drug. (*Adapted from* Cairns and coworkers [43]; with permission.)

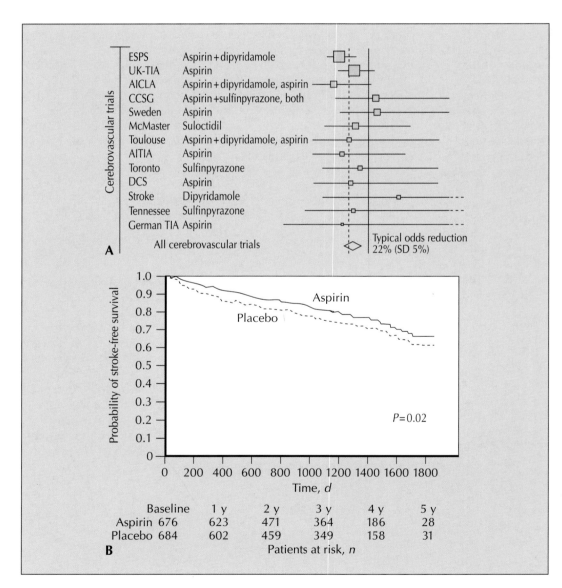

FIGURE 4-31. The benefit of aspirin therapy in reducing vascular and nonvascular mortality in patients with prior transient ischemic attacks (TIAs) or stroke. **A,** Cumulative results of 13 trials that enrolled patients with a history of TIA and/or stroke. The United Kingdom Transient Ischemic Attack Aspirin Trial (UK-TIA), which randomized patients to both high-dose (1200 mg) and low-dose (300 mg) aspirin, demonstrated a significant (18%) reduction in important vascular events [44].

B, The Swedish Aspirin Low-dose Trial (SALT) [45] was the first placebo-controlled study to show a benefit from low-dose aspirin (less than 300 mg/d). A total of 1360 patients with TIA, stroke, or retinal artery occlusion within the previous 3 months were enrolled for a median follow-up of 32 months. Only a mild increase in gastrointestinal side effects was noted in the aspirin-treated group. Overall, aspirin is strongly recommended for secondary prevention in patients with symptomatic cerebrovascular disease. AISLA—Accidents Ischémiques Cérébraux Liés à l'athérosclerose; AITIA—Aspirin and Transient Ischemic Attacks; CCSG—Canadian Cooperative Study Group; DCS—Danish Cooperative Study; ESPS—European Stroke Prevention Study. (Part A *adapted from* Antiplatelet Trialists' Collaboration [44]; part B *adapted from* The SALT Collaborative Group [45]; with permission.)

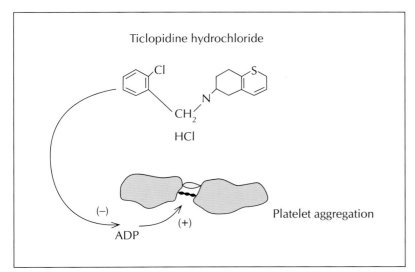

FIGURE 4-32. Structural formula and mechanism of action of ticlopidine [46]. Ticlopidine is structurally distinct from the other antiplatelet agents. It differs from aspirin in that its primary mechanism of action *in vivo* is inhibition of platelet aggregation induced by ADP, with variable effects on other platelet aggregation inducers such as adrenaline, thrombin, and serotonin. Since ticlopidine does not inhibit the cyclo-oxygenase pathway, it may thereby reduce the availability of the fibrinogen receptor on the platelet membrane and prevent binding of fibrinogen to the glycoprotein IIb/IIIa receptor on platelets. Ticlopidine is well absorbed orally, and the onset of its effect is 24 to 48 hours, with a maximal effect reached after 3 to 6 days of administration. It is metabolized extensively by the liver and excreted via the kidney or gastrointestinal tract; one of its metabolites may be more potent than ticlopidine. After discontinuation of the drug, ADP-induced aggregation returns to normal in approximately 4 to 8 days. The usual oral dose of ticlopidine is 250 mg twice daily. (*Adapted from* Saltiel and Ward [46]; with permission.)

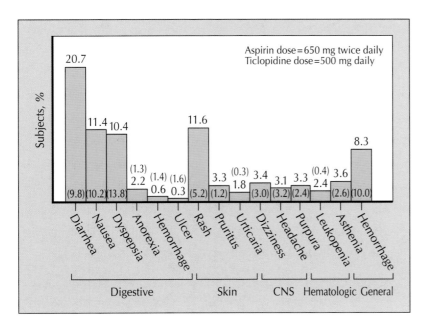

FIGURE 4-33. Side effects of ticlopidine as reported in the Canadian American Ticlopidine Study (CATS) (*N*=1072) [47] and the Ticlopidine Aspirin Stroke Study (TASS) (*N*=3069) [48]. Of note, treatment was terminated because of adverse effects in 20.9% of patients receiving ticlopidine in TASS compared with 14.5% of patients receiving aspirin over 3 years, although many patients with intolerance or contraindications to aspirin were excluded. Ticlopidine did appear to be safer than aspirin for patients with peptic ulcers or a history of gastrointestinal bleeding and could be a substitute for aspirin in such cases. The most significant side effect of the drug is reversible leukopenia, which is more severe earlier in the course of treatment (*ie*, within 3 months) but milder later; for this reason, complete blood counts should be obtained at least every 2 weeks for the first 3 months of therapy and every 3 months thereafter. *Numbers in parentheses* indicate the percentages of patients taking aspirin who developed side effects. CNS—central nervous system. (*Adapted from* Haynes and coworkers [49]; with permission.)

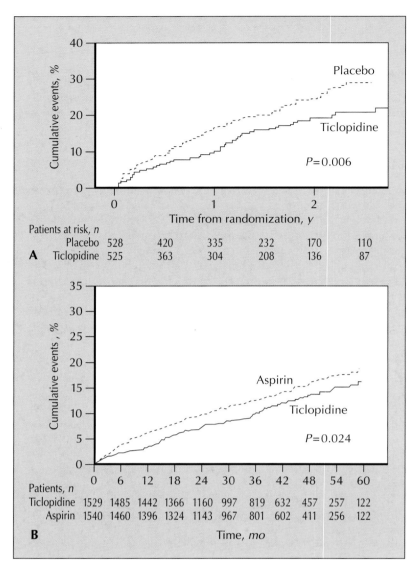

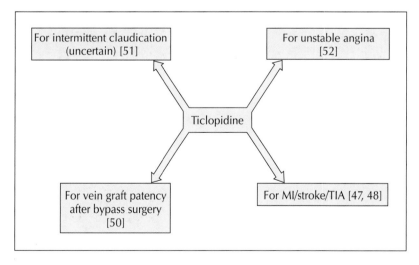

FIGURE 4-34. Results of two trials of ticlopidine therapy for patients with symptomatic cerebrovascular disease: the Canadian American Ticlopidine Study (CATS) [47] and the Ticlopidine Aspirin Stroke Study (TASS) [48]. **A,** CATS was a large double-blind, placebo-controlled trial that randomized over 1000 patients with recent strokes (within 4 months) to 500 mg ticlopidine or placebo for 3 years and found a 30.2% reduction in relative risk for significant events. **B,** TASS enrolled over 3069 patients with recent transient ischemic attacks or cerebrovascular accidents and randomized them to ticlopidine (500 mg/d) or aspirin (1300 mg/d) for 5 years. Although ticlopidine offered a small overall benefit compared with aspirin, adverse reactions were more prevalent with ticlopidine, especially diarrhea and severe neutropenia, while hemorrhage occurred less frequently. Currently, ticlopidine is recommended for patients with previous cerebrovascular events who suffer recurrent events while taking aspirin. (Part A *adapted from* Gent and coworkers [47]; part B *adapted from* Hass and coworkers [47]; with permission.)

FIGURE 4-35. Clinical applications of ticlopidine therapy [47,48,50–52]. To date, ticlopidine is not the agent of choice for these conditions because of its troublesome side effects, such as serious neutropenia and diarrhea; nevertheless, it is certainly indicated for patients who are allergic to aspirin or are at risk for significant gastrointestinal bleeding. The drug appears to be beneficial in preventing myocardial infarction (MI), stroke, or transient ischemic attack (TIA) in patients with peripheral vascular disease [47,48], while in patients with cerebrovascular disease ticlopidine may even be superior to aspirin in preventing major events. In a study of patients with coronary artery bypass vein grafts, ticlopidine increased patency significantly from 74% to 84% over controls [50]. However, several other studies have shown little or no benefit. Ticlopidine is being used with increasing frequency while still more trials are needed to compare it directly with the other commonly used agents [33,49].

DIPYRIDAMOLE

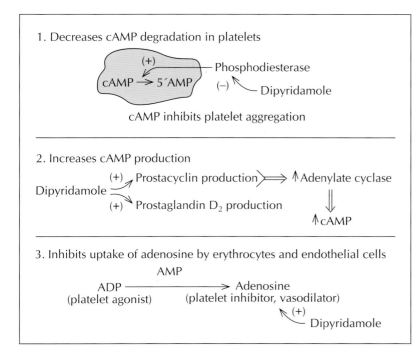

1. Decreases cAMP degradation in platelets

$$cAMP \xrightarrow{(+)} 5'AMP$$

Phosphodiesterase

(−) Dipyridamole

cAMP inhibits platelet aggregation

2. Increases cAMP production

Dipyridamole $\xrightarrow{(+)}$ Prostacyclin production $\Longrightarrow$ ↑ Adenylate cyclase

$\xrightarrow{(+)}$ Prostaglandin D_2 production

⇓

↑cAMP

3. Inhibits uptake of adenosine by erythrocytes and endothelial cells

AMP

ADP $\longrightarrow$ Adenosine
(platelet agonist)   (platelet inhibitor, vasodilator)

(+) Dipyridamole

FIGURE 4-36. Structure and possible mechanisms of action of dipyridamole [53]. The exact mechanism of action of dipyridamole is unclear, but possible actions include the following: (1) decreased degradation of cAMP by inhibition of the phosphodiesterase, which normally degrades cAMP to 5'AMP in platelets; cAMP is a potent inhibitor of platelet aggregation; (2) increased cAMP production, whereby dipyridamole increases the formation of prostaglandin D_2 and prostacyclin; these agents in turn promote the formation of adenylate cyclase, an enzyme that causes cAMP to accumulate; and (3) inhibition of adenosine uptake by endothelial cells and erythrocytes; adenosine is a platelet inhibitor and a vasodilator. Dipyridamole absorption is variable. In plasma, the drug becomes highly bound to albumin and α_1-acid glycoprotein. The agent is conjugated in the liver and then excreted, primarily via the biliary tract. There is no evidence to suggest that dipyridamole potentiates aspirin's antithrombotic effects *in vivo*, and this may reflect the results of clinical trials that show little advantage to using these drugs simultaneously. The actual effects of dipyridamole on platelet function *in vivo* suggest that it may modify the interaction of platelets with foreign surfaces and perhaps damaged blood vessels in humans; the effects on platelet survival are unclear. (*Adapted from* FitzGerald [53]; with permission.)

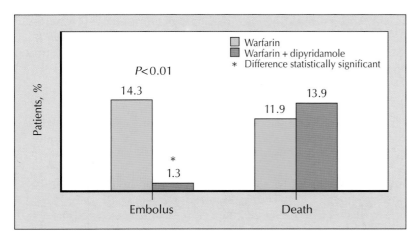

FIGURE 4-37. Results of dipyridamole therapy in patients with prosthetic heart valves. This study from 1971 involved 163 patients who survived prosthetic cardiac valve replacement [54]. Patients were randomized to treatment with warfarin, either alone or in combination with dipyridamole, on the 18th postoperative day and were then followed for 1 year. Cardioembolic events were significantly reduced with the drug combination, although there was no overall reduction in mortality. Since this report, subsequent studies have not shown that dipyridamole is superior to aspirin alone or in combination for the prevention of reinfarction, stroke, or reocclusion of coronary artery bypass vein grafts. In combination with aspirin, dipyridamole may prevent occlusion of arterial segments in patients with peripheral vascular disease. Overall, in patients with mechanical prosthetic heart valves, there is some benefit to adding dipyridamole to warfarin therapy in patients with or at high risk for systemic emboli, using it along with warfarin in patients unable to take aspirin, and adding it to aspirin when full-dose warfarin therapy is contraindicated. Patients with mechanical prosthetic valves in whom emboli develop despite warfarin therapy may benefit from aspirin administration [32,54]. (*Adapted from* Sullivan and coworkers [54]; with permission.)

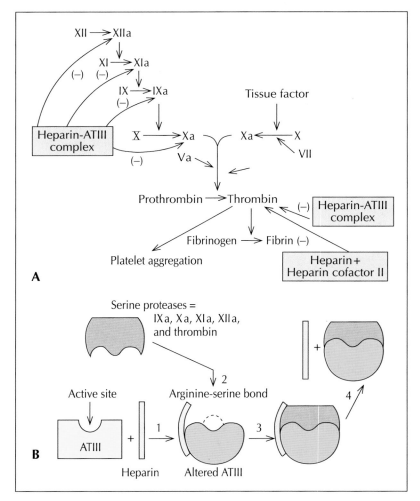

R' = -H or -SO3-
R'' = COCH3 or SO3-

A

1916	Medical student McLean discovered heparin
1922	Howell and Holt described it in detail and named it heparin because of its abundance in liver
1935	Jorpes purified heparin and determined its chemical structure
1939	Brinkhous found heparin cofactor necessary for heparin's anticoagulant activity
1968	Abildgaard found heparin cofactor, antithrombin III
1970s	Mechanism of interaction between heparin and antithrombin III identified

FIGURE 4-38. Structural formula (**A**) and historical perspective (**B**) of heparin. Heparin is a complex linear polysaccharide consisting of about 50 monosaccharide chains with a molecular weight of 5000 to 30,000 D (mean, 15,000 D). It is produced in large amounts by mast cells, basophils, and other cell lines and can be extracted from lung and intestinal mucosa for commercial preparation. Heparins are glycosaminoglycans composed of chains of alternating d-glycosamine and a uronic acid, and they contain several unique pentasaccharide sequences that are able to bind to antithrombin III. (*Arrows* indicate binding sites.)

Specifically, the third residue of the pentasaccharide consists of a 3-0-sulfated glucosamine that is essential for binding to that molecule. Other roles for heparin, in addition to its anticoagulant activity, include regulating angiogenesis, modulating lipoprotein lipase, and maintaining endothelial wall competence. Heparan sulfate is found primarily on the luminal surface of vascular endothelial cells and acts as a "natural" anticoagulant by binding to circulating antithrombin III [1,31,55,56]. (*Adapted from* Freedman [56]; with permission.)

FIGURE 4-39. Mechanism of action of heparin. **A,** When heparin is complexed to antithrombin III (ATIII), most of its antithrombotic action is directed against factor Xa and thrombin, although it also inhibits factors IXa, XIa, and XIIa. In addition, heparin binds to heparin cofactor II to catalyze the inactivation of thrombin and binds to platelets, inhibiting platelet aggregation. **B,** To exert its effect, the heparin molecule must contain at least 18 saccharides so it can bind to both ATIII and thrombin and form a complex; after heparin causes a conformational change in antithrombin (1), serine proteases are able to bind rapidly to ATIII by lysis of an arginine-serine bond (2), forming a complex (3). Heparin then dissociates, leaving ATIII with inhibitory power that is increased at least 1000-fold (4). Inhibition of factor Xa requires heparin binding of ATIII only and not the factor itself. The ATIII molecule is a glycosylated, single-chain polypeptide that rapidly inhibits thrombin only in the presence of heparin. Other actions of heparin include increased vessel wall permeability, platelet binding, and suppression of vascular smooth muscle proliferation [31,56,57].

CHARACTERISTICS OF STANDARD HEPARINS AND LMWH

	STANDARD HEPARINS	LMWH
Mean molecular weight, D	12,000–15,000	4000–6500
Saccharide units (mean)	40–50	13–22
Anti-Xa:anti-IIa activity	1:1	2:1 to 4:1
Inactivates factor Xa on platelet surface	Weak	Strong
Inhibitable by platelet factor 4	Yes	No
Dose-dependent clearance	Yes	No
Bioavailability at low doses	Poor	Good
Augments microvascular bleeding	++++	++
Main action through inhibition of factor IIa	Yes	Yes
Once-daily dosing without laboratory monitoring	No	Yes

FIGURE 4-40. Characteristics of low-molecular-weight heparins (LMWH) compared with standard heparin. LMWH are produced by chemical or enzymatic depolymerization of standard heparin and are approximately one third its size. Unlike standard heparin, LMWH do not bind to plasma proteins, so they have excellent bioavailability, even at low doses, and can be administered once daily without laboratory monitoring. Standard heparin, unlike LMWH, binds to platelet factor 4 and histidine-rich glycoprotein, which neutralizes some of its anticoagulant effects. The binding of standard heparin to von Willebrand factor, which reduces platelet function, may account for the increase in microvascular bleeding seen with standard heparin but not with LMWH. Although LMWH are not yet widely used in clinical practice, a number of trials have demonstrated that they are more effective than and as safe as low-dose heparin, dextran, or warfarin for prophylaxis of deep venous thrombosis in general surgical patients, orthopedic patients at high risk, and patients with paralytic stroke or spinal cord injury. Also, the risk for significant bleeding is much lower with LMWH. For treatment of venous thromboembolism, evidence suggests that some of the LMWH preparations administered by subcutaneous injection are at least as effective as standard heparin for secondary prevention [58,59]. (*Adapted from* Hirsh and Levine [58]; with permission.)

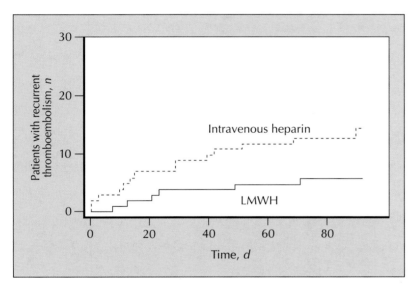

FIGURE 4-41. Results of a study in which low-molecular-weight heparin (LMWH) was used to treat deep venous thrombosis [60]. In this multicenter, double-blind trial, 432 patients with proximal deep venous thrombosis documented by venography were randomized to once-daily LMWH (Logiparin, Novo Nordisk, Denmark) (*n*=213) or continuous intravenous heparin (*n*=219) as initial treatment for 6 days, followed by warfarin therapy for 3 months. Compared with intravenous heparin therapy, Logiparin was as safe and at least as effective for preventing thrombus extension or pulmonary embolus in patients with acute proximal venous thrombosis. Logiparin can be given once daily without monitoring and may be an option in the outpatient setting. Of note, the protective effect of LMWH was lost during long-term therapy with warfarin. The majority of recurrent embolic events occurred within the first 6 weeks after diagnosis of the acute event. (*Adapted from* Hull and coworkers [61]; with permission.)

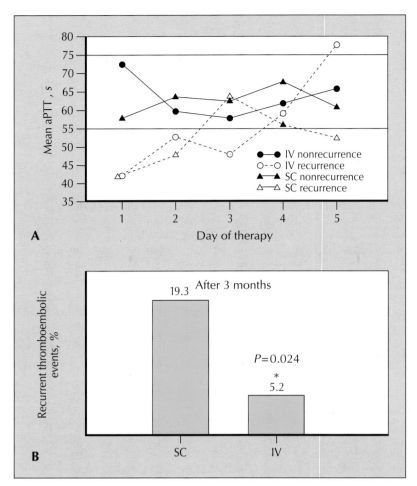

A

B

FIGURE 4-42. The importance of monitoring activated partial thromboplastin time (aPTT) during intravenous (IV) or subcutaneous (SC) heparin therapy. In this study by Hull *et al.* [61], mean values for aPTT were assessed during initial therapy with IV or SC heparin in patients with and without recurrent venous thromboembolism (**A**). The difference in mean aPTTs between patients with and without recurrent thromboembolism was significant (*P*=0.006); those patients who achieved an aPTT less than 50 were at increased risk for recurrent disease (**B**).

This study revealed the important difference in anticoagulant effect manifested by a reduced PTT when similar doses of IV or SC heparin are administered and therefore demonstrates the significance of maintaining adequately intense heparin therapy: patients who are inadequately anticoagulated are at increased risk for serious morbidity and mortality. After injection into the bloodstream, heparin is bound to several proteins, and its bioavailability and elimination cannot be predicted according to first-order kinetics; therefore, the anticoagulant response to a particular IV or SC dose of heparin is not linear and may not increase proportionately as the dose is increased. The average half-life of heparin is 60 minutes when the drug is given in therapeutic doses, and it is excreted primarily by the kidneys [55,59,61]. (*Adapted from* Hull and coworkers [61]; with permission.)

A. INTRAVENOUS HEPARIN: MONITORING AND ADJUSTING DOSAGE*

aPTT, s†	RATE CHANGE, mL/h	DOSE CHANGE, U/24 h	ADDITIONAL ACTION	NEXT aPTT
≤45	+6	+5760	Repeat bolus with 5000 U	4–6 h
46–54	+3	+2880	None	4–6 h
55–85‡	0	0	None	Next morning§
86–110	-3	-2880	Stop infusion 1 h	4–6 h after restart
>110	-6	-5760	Stop infusion 1 h	4–6 h after restart

*A starting bolus of 5000–10,000 U is given IV followed by IV infusion of 1300 U/h (heparin 20,000 U in 500 mL D₅W at approximately 33 mL/h). The concentration of heparin is 40 U/mL. When aPTT is checked at 6 h or longer, steady-state kinetics can be assumed. Dosage adjustments are made according to the protocol.

†Normal aPTT range with Dade-Actin FS reagent of 27 to 35 s.

‡This therapeutic range is roughly equivalent to plasma heparin concentration range of 0.2–0.4 U/mL by protamine titration or to 0.35–0.70 U/mL by inhibition of factor Xa. The therapeutic range will vary with different aPTT reagents and coagulation machines.

§During the first 24 h, repeat aPTT in 4 to 6 h. Thereafter, monitor aPTT daily unless it is subtherapeutic.

FIGURE 4-43. Heparin dosing and monitoring. Heparin therapy is followed by measuring the activated partial thromboplastin time (aPTT), a test sensitive to the inhibitory effects of heparin on thrombin factors Xa and IXa. **A,** Recommendations for dose adjustments based on the aPTT from a recent study by Hull *et al.* [61]. Considerable evidence indicates that an aPTT of 1.5 times control is the minimum therapeutic level for treatment of venous thromboembolism, unstable angina, and acute myocardial infarction (MI). The aPTT should be monitored every 6 to 8 hours during the first few days after an event and then daily thereafter. Of note, warfarin therapy should overlap heparin therapy by at least 5 days and may be started simultaneously. (*continued*)

B. FAILURE TO REACH LOWER LIMIT OF THERAPEUTIC RANGE OF aPTT RELATIVE TO THROMBOEMBOLIC EVENTS

STUDY	CONDITION	OUTCOME	RELATIVE RISK
Hull et al.	DVT	Recurrent venous thromboembolism	15.0
Basu et al.	DVT	Recurrent venous thromboembolism	10.7
Turpie et al.	Acute MI	LV mural thrombosis	22.2
Kaplan et al.	Acute MI	Recurrent MI/angina pectoris	6.0
Camilleri et al.	Acute MI	Recurrent MI/angina pectoris	13.3

FIGURE 4-43. (*continued*) **B,** Importance of maintaining the PTT in the therapeutic range to prevent thromboembolic events as shown in at least five studies, although higher doses of heparin may increase the risk for bleeding [57]. *Relative risk* refers to the relative increase in event rates when the rates in patients with subthera-peutic aPTT are compared with the rates in patients whose values are in the therapeutic range. (Part A *adapted from* Hyers and coworkers [62]; part B *adapted from* Hirsh and Fuster [57]; with permission from the American Heart Association, Inc.)

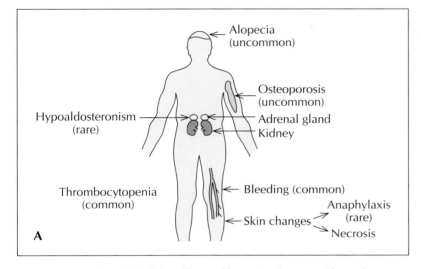

A

B. FACTORS INCREASING RISK OF BLEEDING

Aspirin use

Platelet count <100,000/mm^3

Heavy alcohol consumption

Serious concurrent illness

Renal failure

Concurrent gastrointestinal ulcers

Heparin dose

FIGURE 4-44. A and **B,** Side effects of heparin therapy. Thrombo-cytopenia is thought to be caused by an IgG-heparin immune complex binding to platelets. It usually occurs between 3 and 15 days after initiating therapy, but the platelet count returns to normal within 4 days of stopping therapy. Bleeding complications can occur with intravenous therapy or intermittent subcutaneous injection and may be exacerbated by the conditions listed in *panel A*. Osteoporosis associated with heparin therapy has been described in case reports, although the mechanism remains unclear. Skin necrosis has been reported at both the site of injection and other sites during intra-venous infusion. Hypoaldosteronism results from heparin inhibi-tion of aldosterone synthesis, possibly at the point of corticosterone conversion to 18-hydroxycorticosterone, but this condition is usually of little clinical significance [55,59].

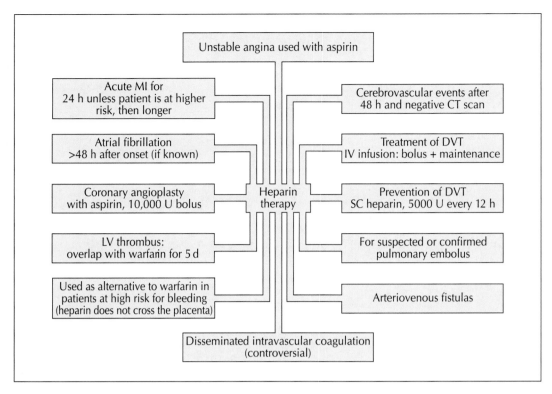

FIGURE 4-45. Role of heparin in cardiovascular disease. To prevent venous thromboembolic disease, subcutaneous heparin should be administered to bedridden patients and to general surgical patients at moderate to high risk. Treatment of symptomatic calf-vein thrombosis,

proximal deep venous thrombosis (DVT), or pulmonary embolus should be initiated upon presentation and continued for at least 5 days, overlapping with the initiation of warfarin therapy. For symptomatic cerebrovascular disease, heparin is recommended in progressing ischemic strokes and longer for small-to-moderate cardioembolic strokes in which computed tomographic scans have demonstrated no evidence of hemorrhage 48 hours after the onset of symptoms. Heparin is not recommended for completed thrombotic strokes. In cardiac disease, early heparin therapy is indicated for new-onset atrial fibrillation and after mechanical valve replacement until the INR is 2.5 to 3.5 on warfarin, as well as for unstable angina, although it may result in a reactivation of symptoms when discontinued if aspirin is not given concurrently. Heparin should be infused during angioplasty, with therapy continuing up to 24 hours after the procedure, depending upon the result obtained. In the setting of acute MI, heparin should be given with thrombolytic therapy and in its absence for at least 24 hours in patients at low risk and longer for patients at risk for LV thrombus.

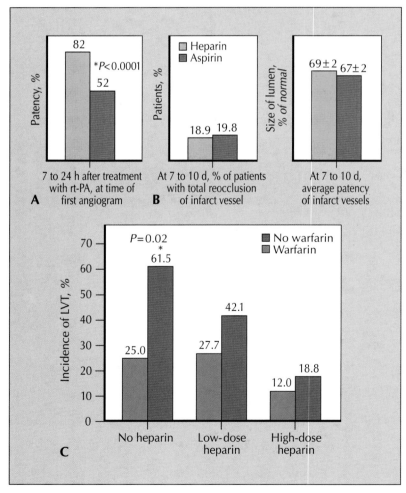

FIGURE 4-46. Heparin use in acute MI. **A,** The Heparin-Aspirin Reperfusion Trial (HART) [63] randomized 205 patients to immediate and continuous intravenous heparin following bolus, or immediate, daily aspirin after recombinant tissue-type plasminogen activator (rt-PA) therapy was initiated within the first 6

hours after presentation. Heparin was superior to aspirin in preserving early patency of the infarct vessel, but heparin and aspirin showed similar efficacy in preserving patency on days 1 to 7. Of note, the dose of aspirin taken was only 80 mg, so these results might have been different if higher doses had been administered. Side effects were similar with the two drugs.

B, The results of the Australia Coronary Thrombolysis Group study [64] complemented HART in that it concluded that heparin could be discontinued safely 24 hours after rt-PA therapy and could be replaced by aspirin. The study involved 241 patients with acute MI who were randomized to continuous heparin for 7 days or intravenous heparin for 24 hours followed by aspirin. Angiography at 7 to 10 days revealed no difference in patency rates between the two groups. In addition, LV function assessed at 2 days and at 1 month by cardiac catheterization did not differ significantly.

C, Finally, a prospective, randomized study by Koutny *et al.* [30] showed the importance of early heparin therapy in addition to warfarin therapy in patients at high risk with acute anterior wall infarctions (*n* = 229). Heparin was continued for several days in those randomized to heparin and warfarin therapy. When warfarin was given alone, the incidence of LV thrombi (LVT) formation was actually higher when compared with the group receiving no anticoagulation. However, when heparin was given with warfarin, the incidence of thrombus formation was lower when compared with both the control group and the group receiving warfarin alone. Several conclusions can be drawn about heparin therapy in acute MI: (1) Heparin should be given with or without thrombolytics in addition to aspirin. (2) Heparin may be used for only 24 hours in patients at lower risk. (3) Heparin should probably be administered for a longer time in patients at higher risk (*eg*, those with LV thrombus) and should overlap with warfarin therapy. (4) Patients who are also receiving intravenous nitroglycerin may be somewhat resistant to heparin. (Part A *adapted from* Hsia and coworkers [63]; part B *adapted from* Thompson and coworkers [64]; with permission from the American Heart Association, Inc.; part C *adapted from* Koutny and coworkers [30]; with permission.)

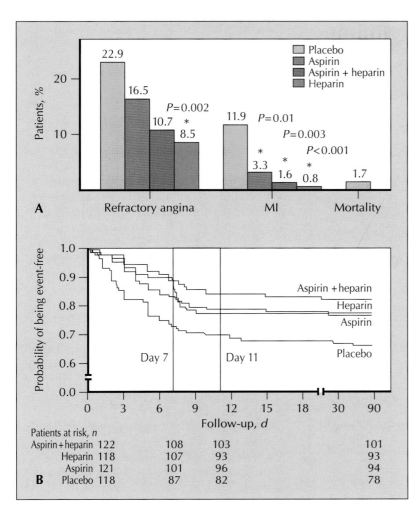

FIGURE 4-47. Heparin for unstable angina. **A,** In a double-blind, randomized, placebo-controlled trial, Theroux *et al.* compared early treatment with aspirin alone, heparin alone, or the combination for 6±3 days in 479 consecutive patients admitted with the diagnosis of unstable angina [65]. All three major endpoints— refractory angina, myocardial infarction (MI), and death—were significantly reduced with heparin therapy, although there was no increased benefit in giving aspirin and heparin together. All treatment except placebo reduced mortality to 0%. However, subsequent studies, ATACS (Antithrombotic Therapy in Acute Coronary Syndromes) and RISC (Research on Instability in Coronary Artery Disease), have shown a further reduction of recurrent ischemic events in the early phase of unstable angina when aspirin is added to heparin therapy.

B, In a later study by Theroux *et al.* [66], the discontinuation of therapy in patients treated with heparin alone resulted in more severe reactivation of unstable angina that required urgent intervention. However, patients treated with either aspirin alone or heparin and aspirin in combination in whom heparin therapy was discontinued after a mean of 6 days were not as likely to have recurrent events when compared with the control group. The earlier study (*A*) revealed the importance of heparin therapy in the management of unstable angina, while the later study (*B*) emphasizes the importance of combining aspirin with heparin to prevent reactivation of the disease process upon discontinuation of heparin. (Part A *adapted from* Theroux and coworkers [65]; part B *adapted from* Theroux and coworkers [66]; with permission.)

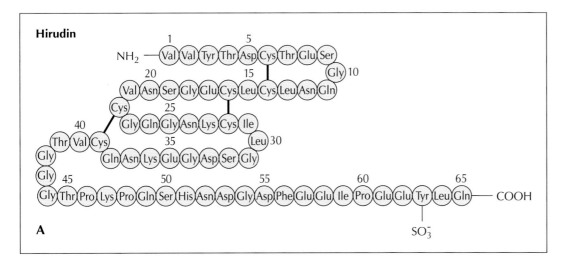

HIRUDINS AND HIRULOG

FIGURE 4-48. Hirudins and hirulog. **A,** Complete covalent structure of hirudin, variant 1 [67]. (*continued*)

B. COMPARISON OF HIRUDIN AND HEPARIN AS ANTICOAGULANTS

HIRUDIN	HEPARIN
Polypeptide (7000 D)	Heteropolysaccharide with various chain lengths (5000–25,000 D)
Direct interaction with thrombin	Needs antithrombin III as cofactor
Selective for thrombin	Heparin/antithrombin III complexes also react with various other factors of the coagulation/fibrinolysis cascades
Pharmacologically inert	High affinity for many other compounds (eg, platelets, endothelium)
No side effects observed	May cause thrombocytopenia, bleeding, etc.
Smaller synthetic hirudin derivatives (~2000 D) effectively inhibit thrombin	Low-molecular-weight heparins (~3000–5000 D) with special properties are available

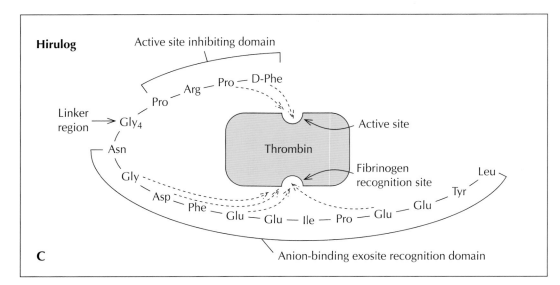

FIGURE 4-48. (*continued*) **B,** Comparison of the properties of hirudin and heparin. Hirudins are a family of natural isoproteins with molecular weights of about 7000 D that are structurally related and composed of 65 or 66 amino acid residues. They are isolated from the saliva of the medicinal leech and were first characterized in the 1950s by Markwardt. Hirudin is a bivalent inhibitor consisting of two functional domains; the C terminus induces a conformational change in thrombin, allowing the N terminus to inhibit the active site of thrombin. The bioavailability after subcutaneous injection is about 85%, and hirudin forms a noncovalent complex with thrombin [68].

C, The structure of hirulog and its interaction with thrombin. Hirulog is a 20–amino acid synthetic peptide derived from the natural hirudins. It selectively and reversibly binds to thrombin and appears to inhibit clot-bound thrombin more effectively than do natural hirudins. *In vitro*, both hirudin and hirulog appear superior to heparin as anticoagulants and are currently being investigated as possible substitutes. Potential advantages of hirulog compared with heparin are as follows: (1) Hirulog does not require antithrombin III as a cofactor. (2) Hirulog can almost equally inhibit both clot-bound and circulating thrombin. (3) Hirulog is not inhibited by activated platelets. Two recent studies in patients with coronary artery disease undergoing diagnostic cardiac catheterization revealed that hirulog can produce dose-dependent prolongation of the partial thromboplastin time (PTT), which can be reversed rapidly if necessary because of hirulog's 40-minute half-life [69]. Furthermore, in patients with unstable angina, hirulog infusions quickly and reproducibly yield stable, dose-dependent anticoagulant and antithrombotic effects with a favorable clinical efficacy profile [70]. (Part A *adapted from* Mao and coworkers [68]; part B *adapted from* Bichler and coworkers [67]; part C *adapted from* Cannon and coworkers [69]; with permission.)

THERAPEUTIC CONSIDERATIONS FOR HIRUDINS

Prevention of venous thrombosis and treatment

Patients with antithrombin III deficiency

Prevention of reocclusion after angioplasty

Prevention of reocclusion after thrombolysis

Extracorporeal circulation

Disseminated intravascular coagulation

Patients with thrombocytopenia or osteoporosis

FIGURE 4-49. Therapeutic considerations of hirudins [67]. Hirudins have been under careful investigation in both *in vitro* and *in vivo* animal studies. In rabbits, hirudin was found to be twice as effective as standard heparin in preventing pulmonary embolus and venous thrombosis. Furthermore, in pigs, hirudin significantly reduced platelet and fibrin deposition in coronary arteries opened by angioplasty and was five times more effective than standard heparins. Particularly encouraging are *in vitro* studies showing hirudin's superiority in preventing reocclusion after coronary thrombolysis; because hirudin has equal affinities for fibrin-bound thrombin and circulating thrombin, it may be more effective than heparin in lysing residual thrombus. Other potential uses may be in extracorporeal circulations, such as heart-lung machines and arteriovenous fistulas, as well as in patients with the syndrome of disseminated intravascular coagulation [67]. (*Adapted from* Bichler and Fritz [67]; with permission.)

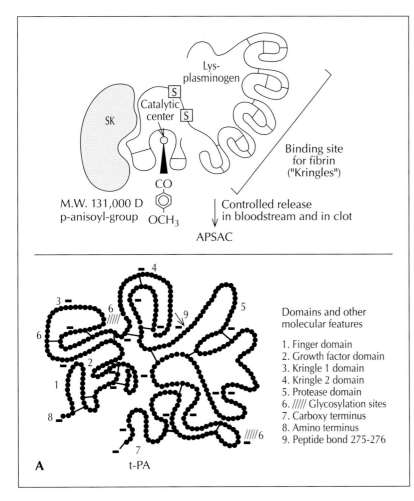

A   t-PA

Domains and other molecular features

1. Finger domain
2. Growth factor domain
3. Kringle 1 domain
4. Kringle 2 domain
5. Protease domain
6. ///// Glycosylation sites
7. Carboxy terminus
8. Amino terminus
9. Peptide bond 275-276

B. HISTORICAL LANDMARKS

1912   Herrick noted that acute myocardial infarction is caused by thrombus

1930s   Discovery by William Tillet of fibrinolysin, renamed SK by Christensen and MacLeod in 1944

1947   Sol Sherry and his team are the first to administer SK to humans

1959   First published trial of thrombolytic therapy

1976   Intracoronary SK used in a small study

1979   Fully purified t-PA prepared by Rijken *et al.*, first from uterine tissue and then, in 1981, from human melanoma cell cultures

FIGURE 4-50. Thrombolytic agents (**A**) and historical perspective (**B**) [1]. Streptokinase (SK) is a single-chain polypeptide, the complete structure of which has not been fully determined. It is secreted by group C α-hemolytic streptococci and does not possess protease activity. SK must first form a complex with plasminogen in order to activate other plasminogen molecules. APSAC (anisoylated plasminogen-streptokinase activator complex) is a synthesized molecule consisting of streptokinase and lys-plasminogen held together and inactivated by acylation of the enzymatically active center of the plasminogen molecule. Spontaneous deacylation occurs in plasma, forming a streptokinase-plasminogen activator complex. Urokinase, an enzyme that was first isolated from urine and later from renal parenchymal cultures, exists in single- and double-chain forms. The single-chain form is produced by recombinant DNA techniques. Urokinase is able to directly cleave the arginine-valine bond in plasminogen and convert it to active plasmin. Tissue-type plasminogen activator (t-PA) is a naturally occurring protease that consists of 527 amino acids synthesized by a variety of tissues, including vascular endothelial cells. Recombinant tissue-type plasminogen activator (rt-PA) is produced for therapeutic use by recombinant DNA techniques and has a high affinity for fibrin, which allows it to act preferentially at the site of a thrombus, converting plasminogen to plasmin [1,71].

PROFILES OF AVAILABLE THROMBOLYTIC AGENTS

	SK	APSAC	UROKINASE	rt-PA
Molecular weight, *D*	47,000	131,000	31,000–55,000	70,000
Half-life, *min*	23	90	16	4–8
Transient hypotension	Yes	Yes	No	No
Potential allergic reaction	Yes	Yes	No	No
Duration of infusion	1 h	2–5 min	5–15 min	10 mg IV bolus and 90-min infusion
Average dose	1.5 million U	30 U	2 million U	100 mg
Bleeding complications	Yes	Yes	Yes	Yes
Approximate charges to patient in 1993	$532/1.5 million U	—	$840/250,000 U	$6000/100 mg

FIGURE 4-51. Profiles of available thrombolytic agents. The Thrombolysis in Myocardial Infarction (TIMI-1) trial [72] and the recent Global Utilization of Streptokinase and Tissue Plasminogen Activator for Occluded Arteries (GUSTO) trial [73] have shown recombinant tissue-type plasminogen activator (rt-PA) to be superior to the other thrombolytic agents in achieving vessel patency 90 minutes after the onset of therapy. A longer plasma half-life allows APSAC (anisoylated plasminogen-streptokinase activator complex) one advantage in that its required duration of infusion is only 2 to 5 minutes. While all four agents are associated with bleeding compli-

cations, APSAC and streptokinase (SK) are antigenic and may cause allergic reactions such as cutaneous rash, nausea, fever, or a rare anaphylactic reaction (0.1% incidence); rapid infusion may cause hypotension. Another difference between the agents is cost, with rt-PA being the most expensive and SK the least expensive per dose. The GUSTO trial has also shown that it is safe to use front-loaded rt-PA with heparin. Of note, except with rt-PA, heparin may be started 6 hours after infusion of the thrombolytic agent [1,74–76]. (*Adapted from* Mueller and Scheidt [1], Alpert [74], and Marder and Sherry [75]; with permission.)

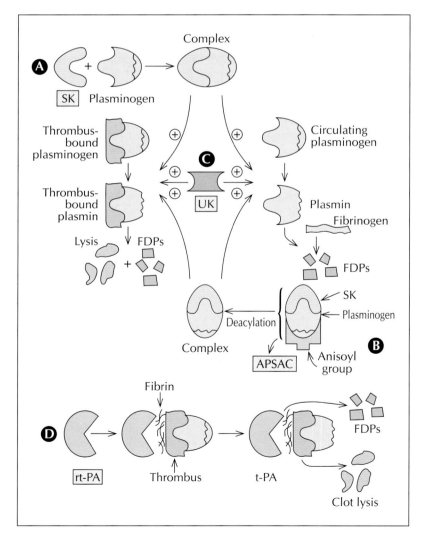

FIGURE 4-52. Mechanisms of action of thrombolytic agents. **A,** Streptokinase (SK) molecules form 1:1 complexes with circulating plasminogen, which then convert both thrombus-bound and circulating plasminogen to active plasmin by cleavage of an arginine-valine bond that splits the molecule into a heavy chain and a light chain capable of proteolytic activity. Plasmin causes clot lysis and reduces fibrinogen to fibrin degradation products (FDPs). Formation of the complex opens up an enzymatic center in plasminogen capable of activating other plasminogen molecules. **B,** APSAC (anisoylated plasminogen-streptokinase activator complex) undergoes deacylation when it is introduced into plasma to form the same SK-plasminogen complex and similarly converts plasminogen to plasmin. **C,** Urokinase (UK), in contrast, does not need to form complexes with plasminogen to become active; it directly cleaves clot-bound and circulating plasminogen into plasmin. **D,** Recombinant tissue-type plasminogen activator (rt-PA) is unique compared with the other agents in that it has a special affinity for fibrin. When bound to fibrin as part of a thrombus, rt-PA undergoes a conformational change that makes it 1000 times more active and thereby able to cleave thrombus-bound plasminogen to plasmin to achieve clot lysis [1,74,75].

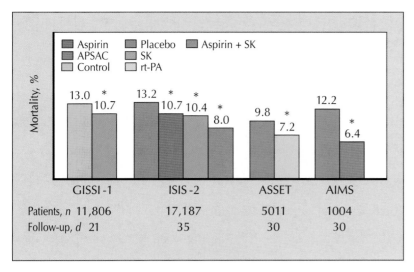

Figure 4-53. Four large trials demonstrating the reduction in mortality with thrombolytic therapy soon after acute myocardial infarction (MI). Gruppo Italiano per lo Studio della Streptochinasi nell'Infarto Miocardico (GISSI-1) [77] was the first large trial to show a reduction in mortality with intravenous streptokinase (IV SK). It randomized 11,806 patients presenting less than 12 hours after onset of symptoms to IV SK, 1.5 million units over 1 hour, or placebo with or without additional anticoagulation. Mortality was significantly reduced during the 21-day follow-up in those patients who received treatment early (between 0 and 6 hours).

The Second International Study of Infarct Survival (ISIS-2) [39] included over 17,000 patients randomized to one of four groups when presenting within 24 hours (median, 5 hours) of a suspected acute MI: SK alone, aspirin alone, the two drugs in combination, or placebo. The results at 5 weeks (35 days) and up to 2 years show a significant reduction in mortality, especially in those patients who received both SK and aspirin, and there was also benefit to treating patients who were older than 65 years, presented after 6 hours, or suffered an acute inferior wall MI. Aspirin prevented the excess reinfarction rate that was noted in the group receiving SK alone compared with placebo.

The Anglo-Scandinavian Study of Early Thrombolysis (ASSET) [78] randomized over 5000 patients under age 75 years who presented within 5 hours of onset of a suspected acute MI to recombinant tissue-type plasminogen activator (rt-PA) and heparin or heparin alone (no aspirin was used) and followed them for 30 days. Mortality was significantly improved in those receiving rt-PA regardless of age, time to treatment, previous MI, or site of infarction.

The APSAC Intervention Mortality Study (AIMS) [79] enrolled 1004 patients to anisoylated plasminogen-streptokinase activator complex (APSAC) or placebo followed by heparin within 6 hours of presentation with electrocardiographic evidence of infarction (ST-segment elevation > 0.1 mV in two leads) and followed them for 30 days. As in the first three trials with SK and rt-PA, APSAC also led to a significant reduction in mortality. *Asterisks* indicate statistically significant differences.

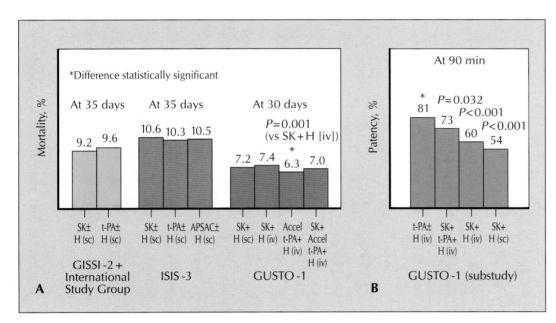

Figure 4-54. Trials comparing thrombolytic agents in acute myocardial infarction (MI) [80]. **A,** GISSI-2 [81] and the International Study Group [82] enrolled over 20,000 patients admitted to the critical care unit within 6 hours of onset of symptoms and randomized them to streptokinase (SK) or tissue-type plasminogen activator (t-PA). At 35 days, there was no significant difference in mortality or major side effects. The Third International Study of Infarct Survival (ISIS-3) compared SK, t-PA, and APSAC (anisoylated plasminogen-streptokinase activator complex) by randomizing over 41,000 patients to one agent within 24 hours of presentation [83]. As in GISSI-2, there was no difference in overall mortality.

The GUSTO trial [76] randomized over 41,000 patients presenting within 6 hours of acute MI to one of four treatments: SK with subcutaneous (sc) heparin, SK and intravenous (iv) heparin, accelerated (Accel) t-PA with heparin, and accelerated t-PA combined with SK and heparin. Mortality was significantly reduced in the accelerated t-PA group by 0.9% over the SK and subcutaneous heparin group and over the SK and intravenous heparin group. When considering the group consisting of mortality and nonfatal strokes, there was actually an absolute reduction of 0.7% with t-PA compared with the other two groups. Interestingly, there was no survival advantage in those who received the combination of SK and recombinant tissue-type plasminogen activator (rt-PA) compared with those who received t-PA only [76,81,83]. **B,** A GUSTO substudy [73] also assessed coronary artery patency, reocclusion, and left ventricular function. As shown, rt-PA with heparin produced a significantly higher patency rate at 90 minutes after institution of thrombolytic therapy, which resulted in lower mortality. At 180 minutes, the patency rates were similar.

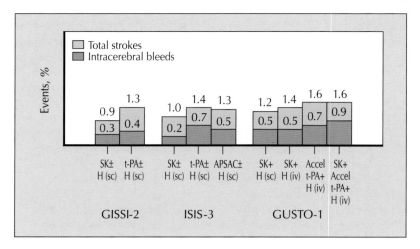

FIGURE 4-55. Bleeding and stroke complications associated with thrombolytic therapy. Although the three agents APSAC (anisoylated plasminogen-streptokinase activator complex), streptokinase (SK), and accelerated-dose tissue-type plasminogen activator (Accel t-PA) are associated with a low risk for stroke or hemorrhagic stroke, accelerated t-PA appeared to be associated with a higher incidence of stroke compared with SK in all three trials. The excess in total strokes per 1000 patients treated was four in ISIS-3 [83] and GISSI-2 [81] and two in the GUSTO trial [76], with the majority of events occurring on day 1 after thrombolytic therapy was instituted [76,84]. iv—intravenous; sc—subcutaneous. (*Adapted from* the GUSTO Investigators [76] and Collins and coworkers [84]; with permission.)

THROMBOLYTIC THERAPY IN ACUTE MI

INDICATIONS

1. Patients presenting with ischemic chest pain and ST-segment elevation in two contiguous leads or bundle branch block up to a least 12 h from symptom onset
2. Concomitant administration of aspirin reduces risks of reinfarction and stroke, especially when it is continued daily following the MI
3. Further evidence is needed to show that thrombolytics are beneficial in patients in cardiogenic shock and those with ischemic chest pain who have electrocardiographic changes but no ST-segment elevation or bundle branch block

CONTRAINDICATIONS

Absolute:
1. Active internal bleeding
2. Suspected aortic dissection
3. Prolonged or traumatic cardiopulmonary resuscitation
4. Recent head trauma or known intracranial neoplasm
5. Diabetic hemorrhagic retinopathy or other hemorrhagic ophthalmic condition
6. Pregnancy
7. Previous allergic reaction to the thrombolytic agent (SK or APSAC)
8. Recorded blood pressure above 200/120 mm Hg
9. History of cerebrovascular accident known to be hemorrhagic
10. Underlying bleeding disorder
11. Trauma or surgery more than 2 wk earlier; trauma or surgery more recent than 2 wk, which could be a source of rebleeding

Relative:
1. Trauma or surgery more than 2 wk earlier (trauma or surgery more recent than 2 wk, which could be a source of rebleeding, is an absolute contraindication)
2. History of chronic severe hypertension with or without drug therapy
3. Active peptic ulcer
4. History of cerebrovascular accident
5. Known bleeding diathesis or current use of anticoagulants
6. Significant liver dysfunction
7. Prior exposure to SK or APSAC (particularly important in the initial 6- to 9-mo period after SK or APSAC administration; applies to reuse of any SK-containing agent but does *not* apply to rt-PA or urokinase)
8. Puncture of a noncompressible artery

FIGURE 4-56. Indications and contraindications for thrombolytic therapy in acute myocardial infarction (MI). In addition, the following correlates are important: (1) Time from onset of symptoms to treatment and patency rate correlate with survival. (2) In younger patients ages 55 to 75 years with early presentation, front-loaded tissue-type plasminogen activator (t-PA) with heparin is superior to streptokinase (SK). (3) Aspirin alone or in combination with t-PA is highly beneficial. (4) Routine catheterization followed by immediate percutaneous transluminal coronary angioplasty is not necessary after thrombolytic therapy. (5) Although the rate of stroke is low with thrombolytic agents, the rate with t-PA is higher than with SK [17, 85]. (*Adapted from* Fibrinolytic Therapy Trialists' Collaborative Group [17,85]; with permission.)

INCIDENCE OF CARDIOVASCULAR EVENTS WITHIN 42 DAYS OF THERAPY WITH t-PA OR PLACEBO FOR UNSTABLE ANGINA*

EVENT (ALL PATIENTS)	t-PA	PLACEBO	P VALUE
Death	2.3	2.0	0.67
MI (fatal and nonfatal)	7.4	4.9	0.04
Death or MI	8.8	6.2	0.05
Stroke	1.6	0.8	0.14

*Numbers are % of total patients in each group (placebo or t-PA).

FIGURE 4-57. Role of thrombolytics in the treatment of unstable angina [86,87]. The Thrombolysis in Myocardial Infarction Trial IIIB (TIMI-IIIB) evaluated 1473 patients with unstable angina or non–Q-wave myocardial infarction (MI) who were seen within 24 hours of ischemic chest discomfort at rest and were randomized to accelerated-dose tissue-type plasminogen activator (t-PA) or placebo as initial therapy. All patients were treated with aspirin, β-blockers, calcium antagonists, long-acting nitrates, and intravenous heparin. At 6 weeks, the overall infarction rate was 6.3% and mortality was 2.4%. MI and intracerebral bleeds were more frequent in the t-PA–treated group. Based on this study and others, thrombolytic agents are not beneficial—and may be detrimental—in patients with unstable angina. Current research is focused on combining thrombolytics, the use of prostaglandins, monoclonal antibodies against platelet receptors, and serotonin-thromboxane receptor blockers for use in treating unstable angina and MI [86,87]. (*Adapted from* The TIMI-IIIB investigators [87]; with permission from the American Heart Association, Inc.)

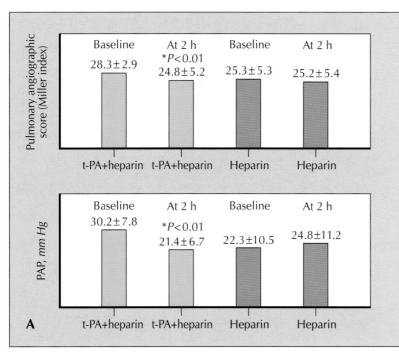

B. THROMBOLYTIC AGENTS IN VENOUS THROMBOEMBOLISM

STOP HEPARIN INFUSION: START THROMBOLYTIC INFUSION WHEN αPTT OR TT IS ≤1.5 × CONTROL

SK*	250,000 IU loading dose
	100,000 IU/h maintenance dose
UK†	4400 IU/lb loading dose
	4400 IU/lb/h maintenance dose
t-PA‡	100 mg (56 million IU) over 2 h

After terminating thrombolytic infusion, restart heparin infusion without a loading dose or with a small loading dose when aPTT or TT ≤ 1.5 × control.

*Recommended for 24-h infusion in PE and for 48–72 h in DVT.
†Recommended for 12-h infusion in PE and for 24–48 h in DVT.
‡Recommended for 2-h infusion in PE to a total dose of 100 mg.

FIGURE 4-58. Thrombolytic agents for venous thromboembolic disease. **A,** In this Italian multicenter trial [88], 20 patients with angiographically documented pulmonary embolus were given a 2-hour infusion of recombinant tissue-type plasminogen activator (rt-PA; 10-mg bolus, then 90 mg over 2 hours), followed by heparin; 16 patients were given only an intravenous heparin infusion. (The Miller index is a measure of the number of patent pulmonary arterial segments prior to thrombolytic therapy.) As shown, rt-PA significantly improved both perfusion and mean pulmonary artery pressure (PAP) at 2 hours. However, there were three major bleeding episodes in the rt-PA–treated group, resulting in two deaths, and two bleeds in the heparin group, resulting in one death. Overall, thrombolytic therapy is indicated only for patients with massive pulmonary embolus who are hemodynami-cally unstable. There have been no studies to date demonstrating reductions in short- or long-term mortality with thrombolytic agents for pulmonary embolus.

B, Dosing recommendations for treatment of venous thromboembolic disease [62]. In deep venous thrombosis (DVT), the indications for thrombolytic therapy are unclear. It appears that in venous disease, thrombolytic therapy may cause only partial dissolution of a thrombus, because these thrombi are older and more organized than coronary thrombi. There may be some easing of symptoms in these patients. PE—pulmonary embolism; SK—streptokinase; TT—thrombin time; UK—urokinase. (Part A *adapted from* Dalla-Volta and coworkers [88]; part B *adapted from* Hyers and coworkers [62]; with permission.)

REFERENCES

1. Mueller RL, Scheidt S: History of drugs for thrombotic disease. *Circulation* 1994, 89:432–449.

2. Webster MWI, Chesebro JH, Fuster V: Antithrombotic therapy in acute myocardial infarction: enhancement of thrombolysis, reduction of reocclusion, and prevention of thromboembolism. In *Acute Myocardial Infarction*. Edited by Gersch BG, Rahimtoola S. New York: Elsevier; 1990:333–348.

3. Fuster V, Stein B, Ambrose JA, *et al.*: Atherosclerotic plaque rupture and thrombosis: evolving concepts. *Circulation* 1990, 82(suppl II):II-47–II-59.

4. Ellis SG, Bates ER, Schaible T, *et al.*: Prospects for the use of antagonists to the platelet glycoprotein IIb/IIIa receptor to prevent postangioplasty restenosis and thrombosis. *J Am Coll Cardiol* 1991, 17:89B–95B.

5. Fuster V, Badimon L, Badimon JJ, *et al.*: The pathogenesis of coronary artery disease and the acute coronary syndromes (first of two parts). *N Engl J Med* 1992, 326:242–317.

6. Anderson HV, Willerson JT: Current concepts: thrombolysis in acute myocardial infarction. *N Engl J Med* 1993, 329:703–709.

7. Shah PK, Forrester JS: Pathophysiology of acute coronary syndromes. *Am J Cardiol* 1991, 68:16C–23C.

8. Clagett GP, Graor RA, Salzman EW: Antithrombotic therapy in peripheral arterial occlusive disease. *Chest* 1992, 102(suppl):516S–528S.

9. Clagett GP, Anderson FA, Levine MN, *et al.*: Prevention of venous thromboembolism. *Chest* 1992, 102(suppl):391S–407S.

10. Freedman MD: Oral anticoagulants: pharmacodynamics, clinical indications and adverse effects. *J Clin Pharmacol* 1992, 32:196–209.

11. Hirsh J, Fuster V: Guide to anticoagulant therapy. Part 2: Oral anticoagulants. *Circulation* 1994, 89:1469–1480.

12. Hirsh J: Oral anticoagulant drugs. *N Engl J Med* 1991, 324:1865–1873.

13. Furie B, Furie BC: Molecular basis of vitamin K–dependent gamma-carboxylation. *Blood* 1990, 75:1753–1762.

14. Hirsh J, Dalen JE, Deykin D, *et al.*: Oral anticoagulants: mechanism of action, clinical effectiveness, and optimal therapeutic range. *Chest* 1992, 102(suppl):312S–326S.

15. Levine MN, Hirsh J, Landefeld S, *et al.*: Hemorrhagic complications of anticoagulant treatment. *Chest* 1992, 102(suppl):352S–363S.

16. Peterson CE, Kwaan HC: Current concepts of warfarin therapy. *Arch Intern Med* 1986, 146:581–584.

17. ACC/AHA Task Force: Guidelines for the early management of patients with acute myocardial infarction. A report of the American College of Cardiology/American Heart Association Task Force on assessment of diagnostic and therapeutic cardiovascular procedures. (Subcommittee to Develop Guidelines for the Early Management of Patients with Acute Myocardial Infarction.) *J Am Coll Cardiol* 1990, 16:249–292.

18. Vaitkus PT, Barnathan ES: Embolic potential, prevention and management of mural thrombus complicating anterior myocardial infarction: a meta-analysis. *J Am Coll Cardiol* 1993, 22:1004–1009.

19. Report of the 60+ Reinfarction Study Research Group: a double-blind trial to assess long-term anticoagulant therapy in elderly patients after myocardial infarction. *Lancet* 1980, 2:989–994.

20. Smith P, Arnesen H, Holme I: The effect of warfarin on mortality and reinfarction after myocardial infarction. *N Engl J Med* 1990, 323:147–152.

21. The EPSIM Research Group: A controlled comparison of aspirin and oral anticoagulants in prevention of death after myocardial infarction. *N Engl J Med* 1982, 307:701–708.

22. Turpie AGG, Gent M, Laupacis A, *et al.*: A comparison of aspirin with placebo in patients treated with warfarin after heart valve replacement. *N Engl J Med* 1993, 329:524–529.

23. Stein PD, Alpert JS, Copeland J, *et al.*: Antithrombotic therapy in patients with mechanical and biological prosthetic heart valves. *Chest* 1992, 102(suppl):445S–455S.

24. Petersen P, Boysen G, Godtfredsen J, *et al.*: Placebo-controlled, randomized trial of warfarin and aspirin for prevention of thromboembolic complications in chronic atrial fibrillation: the Copenhagen AFASAK study. *Lancet* 1989, 1:175–179.

25. The Stroke Prevention in Atrial Fibrillation Investigators: The Stroke Prevention in Atrial Fibrillation trial: final results. *Circulation* 1991, 84:527–539.

26. The Boston Area Anticoagulation Trial for Atrial Fibrillation Investigators: The effect of low-dose warfarin on the risk of stroke in patients with nonrheumatic atrial fibrillation. *N Engl J Med* 1990, 323:1505–1511.

27. Connolly SJ, Laupacis A, Gent M, *et al.*: Canadian Atrial Fibrillation Anticoagulation (CAFA) Study. *J Am Coll Cardiol* 1991, 18:349–355.

28. Ezekowitz MD, Bridgers SL, James KE, *et al.*: VA cooperative study of warfarin in the prevention of stroke associated with nonrheumatic atrial fibrillation. *N Engl J Med* 1992, 327:1406–1412.

29. Stroke Prevention in Atrial Fibrillation Investigators: Warfarin versus aspirin for prevention of thromboembolism in atrial fibrillation: Stroke Prevention in Atrial Fibrillation II Study. *Lancet* 1994, 343:687–691.

30. Koutny F, Dale J, Abildgaard U, *et al.*: Adverse effect of warfarin in acute myocardial infarction: increased left ventricular thrombus formation in patients not treated with high-dose heparin. *Eur Heart J* 1993, 14:1040–1043.

31. Gilman AG, Rall TW, Nies AS, Taylor P, eds. *Goodman and Gilman's The Pharmacological Basis of Therapeutics*, ed 8. New York: Pergamon Press; 1990.

32. Fuster V, Dyken ML, Vokonas PS, *et al.*: Aspirin as a therapeutic agent in cardiovascular disease. *Circulation* 1993, 87:659–675.

33. Hirsh J, Dalen JE, Fuster V, *et al.*: Aspirin and other platelet-active drugs: the relationship between dose, effectiveness, and side effects. *Chest* 1992, 102(suppl):327S–336S.

34. Willard JE, Lange RA, Hillis LD: Current concepts: the use of aspirin in ischemic heart disease. *N Engl J Med* 1992, 327:175–181.

35. Patrono C: Aspirin as an antiplatelet drug. *N Engl J Med* 1994, 330:1287–1294.

36. Prichard PJ, Kitchingman GK, Hawkey CJ: Gastric mucosal bleeding: what dose of aspirin is safe? *Gut* 1987, 28:A1401.

37. Ridker PM, Manson JE, Gaziano M, *et al.*: Low-dose aspirin therapy for chronic stable angina: a randomized, placebo-controlled clinical trial. *Ann Intern Med* 1991, 114:835–839.

38. Jafri SM, Zarowitz B, Goldstein S, *et al.*: The role of antiplatelet therapy in acute coronary syndromes and for secondary prevention following a myocardial infarction. *Progr Cardiovasc Dis* 1993, 36:75–84.

39. ISIS-2 Collaborative Group: Randomized trial of intravenous streptokinase, oral aspirin, both, or neither during 17,187 cases of suspected acute myocardial infarction. *Lancet* 1988, 2:349–360.

40. Chesebro JH, Clements IF, Fuster V, *et al.*: A platelet inhibitor trial in coronary-artery bypass operations: benefit of perioperative dipyridamole and aspirin therapy on early vein-graft patency. *N Engl J Med* 1982, 307:73–78.

41. Schwartz L, Bourassa MG, Lesperance J, *et al.*: Aspirin and dipyridamole in the prevention of restenosis after percutaneous transluminal coronary angioplasty *N Engl J Med* 1988, 318:1714–1719.

42. Stein PD, Dalen JE, Goldman S, *et al.*: Antithrombotic therapy in patients with saphenous vein and internal mammary artery bypass grafts following percutaneous transluminal coronary angioplasty. *Chest* 1992, 102(suppl):508S–515S.

43. Cairns JA, Hirsh J, Lewis HD, *et al.*: Antithrombotic agents in coronary artery disease. *Chest* 1992, 102(suppl):456S–481S.

44. Antiplatelet Trialists' Collaboration: Secondary prevention of vascular disease by prolonged antiplatelet treatment. *Br Med J* 1988, 296:320–331.

45. The SALT Collaborative Group: Swedish Aspirin Low-dose Trial (SALT) of 75 mg as secondary prophylaxis after cerebrovascular ischaemic events. *Lancet* 1991, 338:1345–1349.

46. Saltiel E, Ward A: Ticlopidine: a review of its pharmacodynamic and pharmacokinetic properties, and therapeutic efficacy in platelet-dependent disease states. *Drugs* 1987, 34:222–262.

47. Gent M, Blakeley JA, Easton JD, *et al.*: The Canadian American Ticlopidine Study (CATS) in thromboembolic stroke. *Lancet* 1989, 1:1215–1220.

48. Hass WK, Easton JD, Adams HP, *et al.*: A randomized trial comparing ticlopidine hydrochloride with aspirin for the prevention of stroke in high-risk patients. *N Engl J Med* 1989, 321:501–507.

49. Haynes RB, Sandler RS, Larson EB, *et al.*: A critical appraisal of ticlopidine, a new antiplatelet agent: effectiveness and clinical indications for prophylaxis of atherosclerotic events. *Arch Intern Med* 1992, 152:1376–1380.

50. Limet R, David JL, Magotteaux P, *et al.*: Prevention of aorto-coronary bypass graft occlusion. *J Thorac Cardiovasc Surg* 1987, 94:773–783.

51. Janzon J, Bergqvist D, Boberg J, *et al.*: Prevention of myocardial infarction and stroke in patients with intermittent claudication: effects of ticlopidine. *J Intern Med* 1990, 227:301–308.

52. Balasano F, Rizzon P, Violi F, and the Studio della Ticlopidina nell'Angina Instabile Group: Antiplatelet treatment with ticlopidine in unstable angina: a controlled multicenter clinical trial. *Circulation* 1990, 82:17–26.

53. FitzGerald GA: Dipyridamole. *N Engl J Med* 1987, 316:1247–1257.

54. Sullivan JM, Harken DE, Gorlin R: Pharmacologic control of thromboembolic complications of cardiac-valve replacement. *N Engl J Med* 1971, 284:1391–1394.

55. Hirsh J: Heparin. *N Engl J Med* 1991, 324:1565–1574.

56. Freedman MD: Pharmacodynamics, clinical indications, and adverse effects of heparin. *J Clin Pharmacol* 1992, 32:584–596.

57. Hirsh J, Fuster V: Guide to anticoagulant therapy. Part 1: Heparin. *Circulation* 1994, 89:1449–1468.

58. Hirsh J, Levine MN: Low molecular weight heparin. *Blood* 1992, 79:1–17.

59. Hirsh J, Dalen JE, Deykin D, *et al.*: Heparin: mechanism of action, pharmacokinetics, dosing considerations, monitoring, efficacy, and safety. *Chest* 1992, 102(suppl):337S–351S.

60. Hull RD, Rakob GE, Pineo GF, *et al.*: Subcutaneous low-molecular-weight heparin compared with continuous intravenous heparin in the treatment of proximal-vein thrombosis. *N Engl J Med* 1992, 326:975–982.

61. Hull RD, Raskob GE, Hirsh J, *et al.*: Continuous intravenous heparin compared with intermittent subcutaneous heparin in the initial treatment of proximal-vein thrombosis. *N Engl J Med* 1986, 315:1109–1114.

62. Hyers TM, Hull RD, Weg JG: Antithrombotic therapy for venous thromboembolic disease. *Chest* 1992, 102(suppl):408S–425S.

63. Hsia J, Hamilton WP, Kleiman N, *et al.*: A comparison between heparin and low-dose aspirin as adjunctive therapy with tissue plasminogen activator for acute myocardial infarction. *N Engl J Med* 1990, 323:1433–1437.

64. Thompson PL, Aylward PE, Federman J, *et al.*: A randomized comparison of intravenous heparin with oral aspirin and dipyridamole 24 hours after recombinant tissue-type plasminogen activator for acute myocardial infarction. *Circulation* 1991, 83:1534–1542.

65. Theroux P, Ouimet H, McCans J, *et al.*: Aspirin, heparin, or both to treat acute unstable angina. *N Engl J Med* 1988, 319:1105–1111.

66. Theroux P, Waters D, Lam J, *et al.*: Reactivation of unstable angina after discontinuation of heparin. *N Engl J Med* 1992, 327:141–145.

67. Bichler J, Fritz H: Hirudin, a new therapeutic tool? *Ann Hematol* 1991, 63:67–76.

68. Mao SJT, Yates MT, Owen JT, *et al.*: Interaction of hirudin with thrombin: identification of a minimal binding domain of hirudin that inhibits clotting activity. *Biochemistry* 1988, 27:8170–8173.

69. Cannon CP, Maraganore JM, Loscalzo J, *et al.*: Anticoagulant effects of hirulog, a novel thrombin inhibitor, in patients with coronary artery disease. *Am J Cardiol* 1993, 71:778–782.

70. Lidon RM, Theroux P, Juneau M, *et al.*: Initial experience with a direct antithrombin, hirulog, in unstable angina (Part I). *Circulation* 1993, 88:1495–1501.

71. Cairns JA, Fuster V, Kennedy JW: Coronary thrombolysis. *Chest* 1992, 102(suppl):482S–507S.

72. Chesebro JH, Knatterud G, Roberts R, *et al.*: Thrombolysis in Myocardial Infarction (TIMI) Trial. Phase I: a comparison between intravenous tissue plasminogen activator and intravenous streptokinase: clinical findings through hospital discharge. *Circulation* 1987, 76:142–154.

73. The GUSTO Angiographic Investigators: The effects of tissue plasminogen activator, streptokinase, or both on coronary artery patency, ventricular function, and survival after acute myocardial infarction. *N Engl J Med* 1993, 329:1615–1622.

74. Alpert JS: Importance of the pharmacological profile of thrombolytic agents in clinical practice. *Am J Cardiol* 1991, 67:3E–7E.

75. Marder VJ, Sherry S: Thrombolytic therapy: current status (first of two parts). *N Engl J Med* 1988, 318:1512–1520.

76. The GUSTO Investigators: An international randomized trial comparing four thrombolytic strategies for acute myocardial infarction. *N Engl J Med* 1993, 329:673–682.

77. Gruppo Italiano per lo Studio della Streptochinasi nell'Infarto Miocardico (GISSI): Effectiveness of intravenous thrombolytic treatment in acute myocardial infarction. *Lancet* 1986, 1:397–402.

78. Wilcox RG, Van der Lippe G, Olsson CG, *et al.*: Trial of tissue plasminogen activator for mortality reduction in acute myocardial infarction: Anglo-Scandinavian Study of Early Thrombolysis (ASSET). *Lancet* 1988, 2:525–530.

79. AIMS Trial Study Group: Effect of intravenous APSAC on mortality after acute myocardial infarction: preliminary report of a placebo-controlled clinical trial. *Lancet* 1988, 1:545–549.

80. Ridker PM, Marder VJ, Hennekens CH, *et al.*: Large-scale trials of thrombolytic therapy for acute myocardial infarction: GISSI-2, ISIS-3, GUSTO-1. *Ann Intern Med* 1993, 119:530–532.

81. Gruppo Italiano per lo Studio dell Streptochinasi nell'Infarto Miocardico (GISSI). GISSI-2: A factorial randomised trial of alteplase versus streptokinase and heparin versus no heparin among 12,490 patients with acute myocardial infarction. *Lancet* 1990, 336:65–71.

82. The International Study Group: In-hospital mortality and clinical course of 20,891 patients with suspected acute MI randomised between alteplase and streptokinase with or without heparin. *Lancet* 1990, 336:71–75.

83. ISIS-3 (Third International Study of Infarct Survival Collaborative Group): ISIS-3: a randomised comparison of streptokinase vs. tissue plasminogen activator vs. anistreplase and of aspirin and heparin vs. heparin alone among 41,299 cases of suspected myocardial infarction. *Lancet* 1992, 339:765–770.

84. Collins R, Peto R, Parish S, *et al.*: ISIS-3 and GISSI-2: no survival advantage with tissue plasminogen activator over streptokinase, but a significant excess of strokes with tissue plasminogen activator in both trials. *Am J Cardiol* 1993, 71:1127–1128.

85. Fibrinolytic Therapy Trialists' (FTT) Collaborative Group: Indications for fibrinolytic therapy in suspected acute myocardial infarction: collaborative overview of early mortality and major morbidity results from all randomised trials of more than 1,000 patients. *Lancet* 1994, 343:311–322.

86. Shammas NW, Zeitler R, Fitzpatrick P: Intravenous thrombolytic therapy in myocardial infarction: an analytical review. *Clin Cardiol* 1993, 16:283–292.

87. The TIMI-IIIB investigators: Effects of t-PA and a comparison of early invasive and conservative strategies in unstable angina and non-Q-wave myocardial infarction: results of the TIMI-IIIB trial. *Circulation* 1994, 89:1545–1556.

88. Dalla-Volta S, Palla A, Santolicandro AM, *et al.*: PAIMS 2: alteplase combined with heparin versus heparin in the treatment of acute pulmonary embolism. *J Am Coll Cardiol* 1992, 20:520–526.

PREGNANCY AND THE HEART

Carole A. Warnes

Women with heart disease may present for the first time during pregnancy, and the physiologic effects of a normal pregnancy may mimic the signs and symptoms of cardiac disease. With the declining incidence of rheumatic heart disease, most maternal cardiac disease is now congenital in origin, particularly since more women with congenital heart disease are surviving to childbearing age. Among several physiologic changes that take place throughout pregnancy are significant changes in maternal hemodynamics, including increases in volume load and cardiac output along with a relative anemia. In addition, both systemic and pulmonary vascular resistances fall, so that stenotic lesions are less well tolerated than are regurgitant ones. Echocardiography is useful for evaluating these hemodynamics noninvasively before pregnancy is considered.

Assessment of women before pregnancy includes consideration of the cardiac lesion, functional class, ventricular function, and pulmonary artery pressure. Each patient should be managed individually, with the approach coordinated among the cardiologist, obstetrician, and anesthesiologist. Some women should be advised not to become pregnant; these include patients with primary pulmonary hypertension, Eisenmenger syndrome, symptomatic obstructive lesions (aortic stenosis, pulmonic stenosis, and coarctation), Marfan syndrome with a dilated aortic root, and patients with impaired ventricular function who are in New York Heart Association functional class III or IV. Other women may be managed safely through a pregnancy but are at increased risk; these include patients with a mechanical cardiac prosthetic valve who are on warfarin. All medications need to be reviewed prior to the pregnancy to ensure that any potentially teratogenic drug is discontinued and that only those drugs that are essential are continued through the pregnancy.

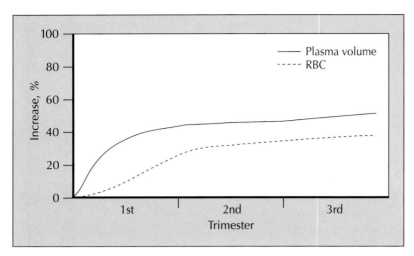

FIGURE 5-1. Early in pregnancy, the plasma volume begins to increase, peaking at almost 50% above baseline during the second trimester. This rise is followed by a lesser rise in red blood cell (RBC) mass, which produces the relative anemia of pregnancy [1–3]. Because anemia adds to the cardiac demands of pregnancy, it is important to ensure that pregnant women take iron and vitamin supplements to minimize this problem as much as possible.

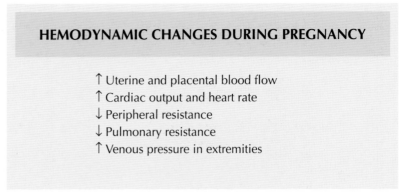

HEMODYNAMIC CHANGES DURING PREGNANCY

↑ Uterine and placental blood flow
↑ Cardiac output and heart rate
↓ Peripheral resistance
↓ Pulmonary resistance
↑ Venous pressure in extremities

FIGURE 5-2. During pregnancy, several hemodynamic changes take place. Uterine and placental blood flow increase, and cardiac output and heart rate increase to cope with the increased flow [4–6]. Owing to hormonal changes, peripheral resistance falls and pulmonary resistance may also fall slightly [7,8]. Venous pressure in the extremities rises, which is why approximately 80% of healthy women have pedal edema during pregnancy. Because of these hemodynamic changes, cardiovascular disease may be exacerbated by pregnancy or pregnancy may cause cardiac disease to become manifest for the first time.

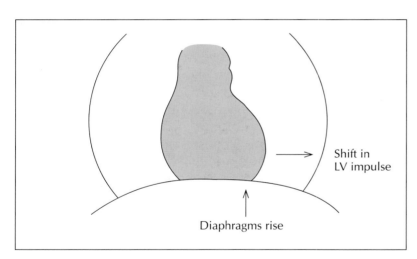

FIGURE 5-3. Left ventricular (LV) end-diastolic and end-systolic volumes increase during pregnancy. As pregnancy advances, the diaphragms are displaced upward, and the LV impulse may be shifted laterally, becoming displaced, forceful, and sustained [9]. Because of the increased cardiac output and fall in peripheral resistance, the carotid pulse may become brisk and full. Jugular venous pressure is normal or slightly elevated.

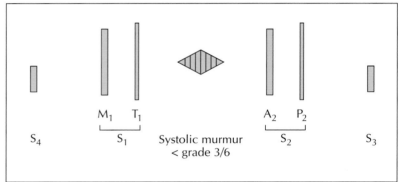

FIGURE 5-4. Because of the hemodynamic changes, physical examination of the heart in a pregnant woman will be altered beginning in the first trimester. The heart sounds become accentuated and, for the unwary physician, may mimic pulmonary hypertension. A systolic murmur at the upper left sternal edge is almost invariable [10]. It is less than grade 3/6 and arises from either the left and/or the right ventricular outflow tract. Although such a murmur may superficially suggest an atrial septal defect, the second heart sound (S_2) in a normal pregnant woman does not exhibit fixed splitting. A third sound (S_3) is also common and reflects the increased cardiac output. A_2—aortic second sound; M_1—first mitral sound; P_2—pulmonic second sound; S_4—fourth heart sound; T_1—tricuspid first sound.

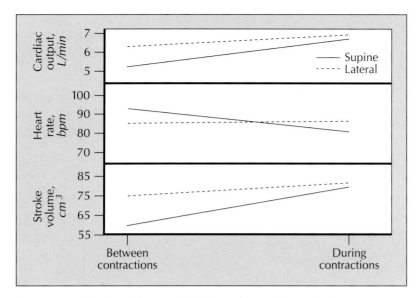

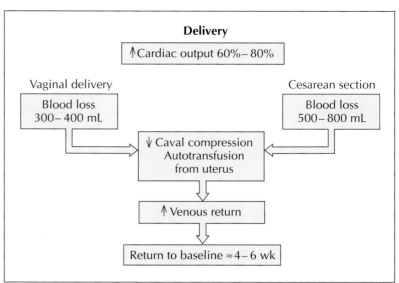

FIGURE 5-5. During labor and delivery, hemodynamic changes occur rapidly. With each uterine contraction, up to 500 mL of blood is squeezed out of the uterus and into the circulation, causing an increase in stroke volume and cardiac output and often a reflex fall in heart rate [11,12]. These changes are more marked in the supine than in the lateral (side-lying) position. When delivery is in the supine position, the fetus will be lying upon (and thus compressing) the inferior vena cava, so venous return will be reduced [13,14]. (*Adapted from* Metcalfe and Ueland [15]; with permission.)

FIGURE 5-6. Delivery is a time of sudden hemodynamic changes, which are also influenced by the method of anesthesia used [12–17]. Because blood loss associated with cesarean section is higher, a vaginal delivery is the preferred route for the vast majority of women with cardiac disease, unless obstetric indications dictate otherwise [14,17,18].

PRENATAL COUNSELING

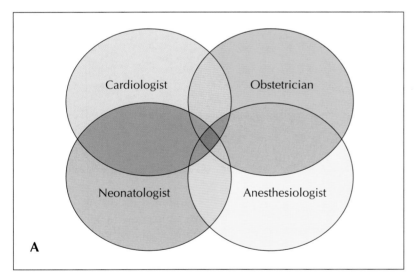

A

FIGURE 5-7. A, Planning among physicians and comprehensive patient counseling comprises a multidisciplinary approach involving cardiologists, obstetricians, anesthesiologists, and neonatologists. Labor and delivery can therefore be planned and coordinated.

B, When one is counseling a woman with heart disease about the risks posed by pregnancy, each patient must be considered individ-

B. CONSIDERATIONS IN PRENATAL COUNSELING

Maternal functional class
Ventricular function, hemodynamics
Genetic counseling
Avoidance of potential teratogens
Antepartum care: cardiovascular and obstetric
Labor: hemodynamic and obstetric considerations
Antibiotic prophylaxis
Postpartum care

ually. She should undergo a clinical examination and, if necessary, an exercise test to assess functional capacity. An ejection fraction of 35% or lower may pose significant risks, since the volume load of pregnancy may precipitate heart failure. If the patient has congenital heart disease, a careful family history must be taken, because the presence of a familial syndrome or a congenital anomaly in a sibling increases the chance that the child will have a congenital heart defect. Furthermore, any drugs that might be teratogenic or potentially harmful to the fetus (*eg,* warfarin or angiotensin-converting enzyme inhibitors) should be avoided (*see* Fig. 5-35).

FUNCTIONAL CLASS AND MATERNAL OUTCOME

NYHA FUNCTIONAL CLASS	MATERNAL MORTALITY, %	INTERVENTION
I or II	0.4	Rest, left lateral position
		Prenatal iron, vitamins
		Low-salt diet
		Limit strenuous activity
III or IV	6.8	Bed rest
		Hospitalization
		Operative intervention if decompensation

FIGURE 5-8. One determinant of maternal outcome is the mother's functional class [19], which must be assessed and reviewed when counseling patients who are considering pregnancy. Some simple interventions may help reduce the hemodynamic burden imposed by pregnancy. If cardiac status may be compromised, complete bed rest may be necessary; if the cardiac problem can be repaired surgically, operative intervention (ideally between the 25th and 28th weeks of pregnancy) may be necessary to save the mother. NYHA— New York Heart Association.

ROLE OF ECHOCARDIOGRAPHY IN RISK ASSESSMENT

Is pregnancy possible?
? LV function
? RV function
? Obstructive lesions
   Aortic stenosis ———
   Pulmonic stenosis ——————————————— Doppler gradient
   Coarctation ———
? Volume lesions
   Mitral regurgitation, tricuspid regurgitation —
   Aortic regurgitation, pulmonic regurgitation —————— Color Doppler
   VSD, ASD
   Shunts ———
? PA pressure

FIGURE 5-9. Echocardiography is particularly useful when assessing a potential mother's risk during pregnancy. A detailed noninvasive evaluation of hemodynamics and ventricular function can be performed. ASD—atrial septal defect; LV—left ventricular; PA—pulmonary artery; RV—right ventricular; VSD—ventricular septal defect.

MANAGING THE HIGH-RISK PREGNANCY

INTRAPARTUM MANAGEMENT OF HIGH-RISK PREGNANCY

Intravenous line, arterial line, Swan-Ganz catheter
Blood available
Analgesia/anesthesia
Delivery in left lateral position
Fetal/maternal electrocardiographic monitoring
Short second stage–facilitated delivery
Antibiotic prophylaxis

FIGURE 5-10. For women at high risk, labor should be planned and coordinated. Once the fetus is mature, labor may be induced, with a Swan-Ganz catheter inserted to optimize hemodynamic management. Pulmonary capillary wedge pressure should be maintained at 12 to 15 mm Hg. Particular attention should be paid to analgesia; epidural anesthesia with fentanyl can usually be employed safely, thus avoiding significant hypotension. Delivery in the left lateral position will avoid compression of the inferior vena cava by the fetus and thus help maintain venous return. Prolonged labor should be avoided; if labor is not progressing smoothly, the second stage should be facilitated with forceps or vacuum extraction.

INDICATIONS FOR INVASIVE HEMODYNAMIC MONITORING DURING LABOR AND DELIVERY

Aortic stenosis, moderate to severe
Coarctation of aorta, moderate to severe
Mitral stenosis, functional class III or IV
Impaired LV function, EF<40%
Pulmonary hypertension, PAP>50% systemic
Ischemic heart disease

FIGURE 5-11. Indications for invasive hemodynamic monitoring during labor and delivery. Patients at risk for compromised hemodynamic function should be considered for such monitoring and include those who are dependent on an adequate preload (in aortic stenosis and coarctation) and those at risk for pulmonary edema (in mitral stenosis and impaired left ventricular [LV] function). Therapeutic manipulation of the pulmonary capillary wedge pressure and systemic vascular resistance will permit rapid correction of the hemodynamic abnormality. EF—ejection fraction; PAP—pulmonary artery pressure.

AVOIDANCE/INTERRUPTION OF PREGNANCY: HIGH-RISK LESIONS AND CONDITIONS

CONDITIONS POSING HIGH RISK IN PREGNANCY

Pulmonary hypertension (PAP>75% of systemic)
Dilated cardiomyopathy with congestive heart failure
Symptomatic obstructive lesions
Marfan syndrome with dilated aortic root

FIGURE 5-12. For patients with the conditions listed here, pregnancy poses a significant risk. Patients with pulmonary hypertension include those with primary or thromboembolic pulmonary hypertension or Eisenmenger syndrome. Symptomatic obstructive lesions include aortic stenosis, pulmonic stenosis, and coarctation. Patients with Marfan syndrome are always at risk for dissection and rupture during pregnancy, even with a normal-sized aortic root; if the aortic root diameter exceeds 40 mm, this risk appears to be increased. PAP—pulmonary artery pressure.

EISENMENGER SYNDROME

EISENMENGER SYNDROME

44 cases firmly documented with 70 pregnancies
30% of pregnancies associated with maternal death
Overall maternal mortality=48%

FIGURE 5-13. Gleicher *et al.* [20] reviewed 44 patients with Eisenmenger syndrome who had 70 pregnancies. Maternal mortality approached 50%, and only 26% of the 70 pregnancies reached term. Even after a successful delivery, maternal death post partum as a result of either pulmonary infarction or progressive hemodynamic deterioration associated with hypotension is not uncommon. If a patient with Eisenmenger syndrome becomes pregnant against advice, interruption of pregnancy is less dangerous than continuing the pregnancy, although anesthesia itself also poses a risk for these patients.

AORTIC STENOSIS AND COARCTATION

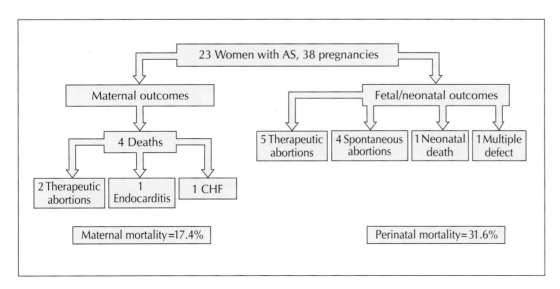

FIGURE 5-14. Symptomatic aortic valve stenosis (AS) poses both maternal and perinatal risks. In a review of the literature, Arias and Pineda [21] reported 38 pregnancies in 23 women with AS, the severity of which was not stated. Maternal mortality was 17.4%. Four pregnancies ended in spontaneous abortion and five in therapeutic abortion. Perinatal mortality was 31.6%. Although recent reports suggest a more favorable outcome for mothers with severe AS [22], this condition remains a significant threat to both mother and fetus. Ideally, patients should be evaluated before pregnancy; Doppler echocardiography greatly assists this evaluation [23]. CHF—congestive heart failure.

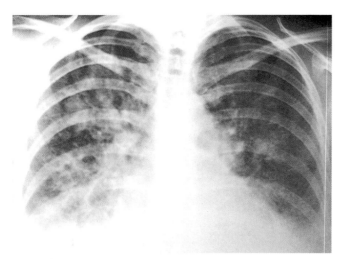

FIGURE 5-15. Chest radiograph of a 32-year-old woman with severe aortic valve stenosis (AS) and a left ventricular ejection fraction of 30% who presented *in extremis* at 30 weeks of pregnancy. Because of fetal distress, the baby was delivered by cesarean section followed immediately by emergency aortic valve replacement. AS in women of childbearing age is usually congenital, and most commonly the valve is bicuspid [24]. Although aortic balloon valvotomy has been used safely in pregnancy [25], it was not an option in this case because of grade 2/4 aortic valve regurgitation.

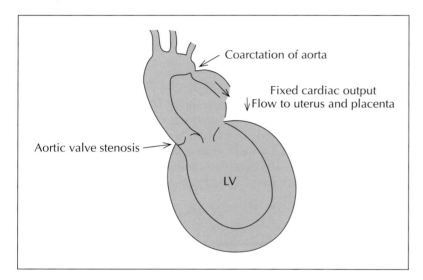

FIGURE 5-16. Both aortic valve stenosis and coarctation of the aorta prevent a normal increase in cardiac output during pregnancy, so the flow of blood to the uterus—and thus to the fetus— is restricted, increasing the likelihood of fetal loss. Following repair of coarctation, the chances of a successful pregnancy are much improved. LV—left ventricle.

AORTIC COARCTATION DURING PREGNANCY

COARCTATION	RESULTS
Uncorrected	
Nine women, 32 pregnancies	<10% of pregnancies uncomplicated
Cardiovascular or renal complications in 50% of pregnancies	40% of pregnancies → living child
Corrected	
Eight women, 21 pregnancies	85% of pregnancies uncomplicated
Cardiovascular or renal complications in <5% of pregnancies	90% of pregnancies → living child

FIGURE 5-17. In a study by Mortensen and Ellsworth [26] of nine women with uncorrected coarctation who had 32 pregnancies, less than 10% of the pregnancies were uncomplicated and only 40% resulted in a living child. Miscarriages occurred in 53% of the pregnancies. Maternal complications included systemic hypertension, dyspnea, albuminuria, and frank cardiac decompensation. Outcomes were considerably better in eight women with repaired coarctation; however, since the aorta in these patients is not normal, they are still at risk for aortic dissection and rupture during pregnancy. With modern medical management and good control of systemic hypertension, the outcome has almost certainly improved [27]. Maternal blood pressure should be meticulously controlled throughout pregnancy, preferably with β-blockers.

MARFAN SYNDROME

MARFAN SYNDROME

Fetal risk
   Spontaneous abortion
   Inheritance 50%
Maternal risk
   ? Pre-existing cardiovascular disease
   Hemodynamically significant MR, AR
   Aortic root diameter > 40 mm
   Advise against pregnancy
   Aortic root diameter < 40 mm—small risk
      for dissection and rupture, but unpredictable

FIGURE 5-18. Marfan syndrome poses risks to both the fetus and the mother. When the mother has Marfan syndrome, the risk for spontaneous abortion is increased and the chance that the fetus will inherit the disorder is 50% (since it is an autosomal dominant trait). Maternal risk is related to the congenital anomaly present, *ie*, whether the mother has mitral valve prolapse with mitral (MR) or aortic (AR) regurgitation. Dilation of the aortic root is a major concern because of the risk for dissection and rupture as the vessels soften during pregnancy. Pyeritz has recommended that women whose aortic root diameter exceeds 40 mm be counseled against childbearing [28]; however, even patients with a normal aortic root dimension are at risk for dissection and rupture [29]. If the patient is already on β-blockers, she should continue such therapy throughout pregnancy.

PROSTHETIC VALVES AND ANTICOAGULATION

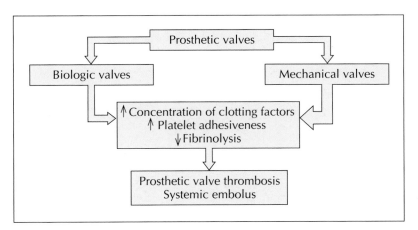

FIGURE 5-19. Because of the clotting tendency associated with pregnancy, the risk for valve thrombosis and emboli is increased in women with prosthetic heart valves. This risk is greater for those with a mechanical valve.

FETAL COMPLICATIONS OF WARFARIN THERAPY

Spontaneous abortion
Stillbirth
Premature delivery
Warfarin embryopathy

FIGURE 5-20. Fetal exposure to warfarin during the first trimester may cause serious central nervous system abnormalities that can result in neonatal optic atrophy, deafness, and mental retardation as well as nasal hypoplasia and stippling of the bony epiphysis [30–32]. In addition, the baby is at risk for intracranial hemorrhage, especially around the time of delivery.

FETAL COMPLICATIONS OF WARFARIN THERAPY

STUDY	PREGNANCIES, *n*	FETAL WASTAGE, %
Harrison and Roschke [33]	55	29
Bonnar [34]	216	15
Ibarra-Perez *et al.* [35]	25	36
Lutz *et al.* [36]	40	56
Ben Ismail *et al.* [37]	133	30
Salazar *et al.* [38]	223	28
	Total=692	Average=32

FIGURE 5-21. Fetal complications of warfarin therapy. Many reports confirm that warfarin is deleterious to the fetus. In various series, the rate of spontaneous abortion ranges from 15% to 56%, with an average of approximately 30% [33–38].

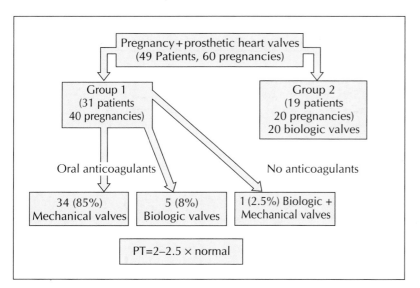

FIGURE 5-22. A recent study examined 60 pregnancies in 50 women who had prosthetic heart valves [39]. Group 1 patients were taking oral anticoagulants, and most of them (85%) had a mechanical valve prosthesis. Group 2 patients were not taking anticoagulants. The prothrombin time (PT) of each patient on anticoagulants was kept at 2 to 2.5 times normal.

A. MATERNAL MORBIDITY RELATED TO PROSTHETIC VALVES

MATERNAL COMPLICATIONS	GROUP 1 PREGNANCIES (n=40), n(%)	GROUP 2 PREGNANCIES (n=20), n(%)
Death	3(7.5)	1(5)
Heart failure	11(27.5)	7(35)
Supraventricular tachycardia	7(17.5)	2(10)
Valve thrombosis/embolus	4(10.0)	1(5)
Bleeding	1(2.5)	—
Endocarditis/prosthesis rupture	2(5.0)	—
Bioprosthesis stenosis	—	3(15)
Total	28(70)	14(70)

FIGURE 5-23. Morbidity related to prosthetic heart valves during pregnancy in the study described in Fig. 5-22 [39]. **A,** Maternal complications were similar in the two groups, occurring in 70% of pregnancies in those women taking anticoagulants (group 1) and

B. FETAL/NEONATAL MORBIDITY RELATED TO PROSTHETIC VALVES

FETAL/NEONATAL COMPLICATIONS	GROUP 1 PREGNANCIES (n=40), n(%)	GROUP 2 PREGNANCIES (n=20), n(%)
Spontaneous abortion	7(17.5)	—
Prematurity	14(46.5)	2(10.5)*
Low birthweight	15(50.0)	2(10.5)*
Stillbirth	1(3.2)	—
Neonatal mortality	5(16.2)	—
Birth defects	4(12.1)	—

*$P<0.05$.

in 70% of pregnancies in those not taking anticoagulants (group 2). **B,** The number of fetal/neonatal complications was significantly higher when the women were taking oral anticoagulants (group 1). In that group, 46.5% of the babies were born prematurely versus 10.5% in the group not taking anticoagulants (group 2). Neonatal mortality was also higher in group 1.

ORAL ANTICOAGULANTS AND FETAL/NEONATAL LOSS

Fetal loss (9/60 pregnancies)

  Spontaneous abortion (7)

  Stillbirth (1)

  Hydatidiform mole (1)

Neonatal death (5/60 pregnancies)

  Premature with RDS (3)

  Cerebral hemorrhage (1)

  Hypoplastic left heart (1)

All in mothers treated with anticoagulants

  Warfarin embryopathy (3)

FIGURE 5-24. Out of 60 pregnancies in the study described in Fig. 5-22, nine resulted in loss of the fetus (15%). Five resulted in neonatal death (16%): three babies were premature and had respiratory distress syndrome (RDS), one had a cerebral hemorrhage, and one had hypoplastic left heart syndrome. All these complications occurred in the group in which the mothers were taking oral anticoagulants. Three infants were born with warfarin embryopathy; two had only mild nasal hypoplasia and stippled epiphyses, but the third had severe embryopathy with respiratory distress from upper airway obstruction.

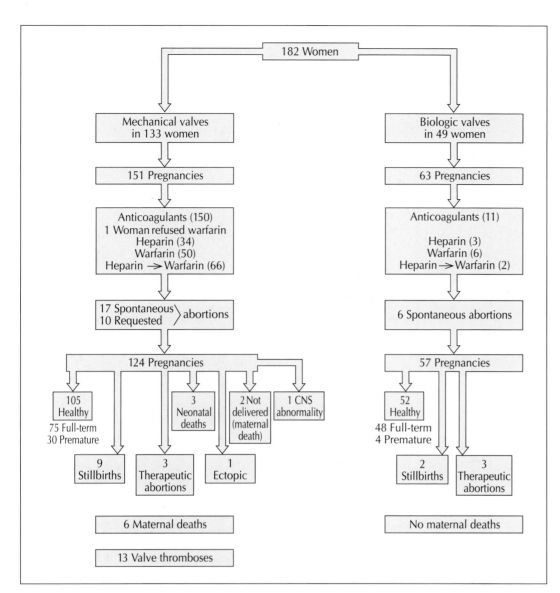

FIGURE 5-25. In a more recent study from Europe [40], Sbarouni and Oakley suggested that the risks of warfarin during pregnancy have been overstated and that its use is not as commonly associated with embryopathy as had been reported. Furthermore, these investigators found that treatment with heparin was associated with more thromboembolic complications and more bleeding complications than was warfarin. One hundred fifty-one pregnancies occurred in 133 women with mechanical valves and 63 pregnancies occurred in 49 women with biologic valves. The anticoagulant regimens for the two groups are shown as well as the incidence of stillbirths and spontaneous abortions. Although these events occurred with similar frequency in both groups, the incidence of prematurity was significantly lower among the women with the bioprostheses. CNS—central nervous system.

PREGNANCY OUTCOME BY ANTICOAGULANT REGIMEN

	NO ANTICOAGULANT (B=49), n(%)	HEPARIN FOR FIRST TRIMESTER, THEN WARFARIN (n=64, B=2), n(%)	WARFARIN THROUGHOUT (n=31, B=5), n(%)	HEPARIN THROUGHOUT (n=29, B=1), n(%)
Healthy babies	44(91)	61(92)[†]	30(83)	22(73)[†]
Full term	41(84)	42(64)	23(64)	17(57)
Premature	3(6)*	19(29)*	7(19)	5(17)
Stillbirths	2(4)	1(1.5)[‡]	4(11)[‡]	4(13)[‡]
Neonatal deaths	0(0)	1(1.5)	2(3)	0(0)
Therapeutic abortion	3(6)	0(0)	1(3)	2(7)

*†‡ $P<0.05$.

FIGURE 5-26. Pregnancy outcomes in the study described in Fig. 5-25 according to the different anticoagulant regimens [40]. Only one stillbirth occurred in the group taking heparin followed by warfarin (66 women), but four stillbirths occurred among those taking warfarin throughout the pregnancy (36 women). These stillbirths were associated with prematurity, but no fetal abnormality was detected. Four stillbirths occurred in the group taking heparin throughout gestation, and these were all associated with fatal valve thromboses. B—bioprostheses.

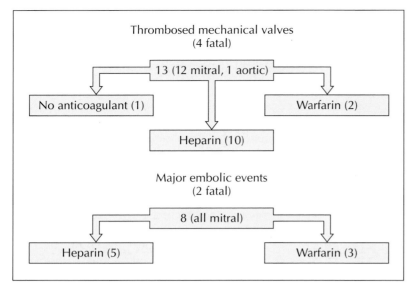

FIGURE 5-27. Anticoagulant regimens used in the group of women with mechanical prosthetic valves in the study described in Figs. 5-25 and 5-26 [40]. Valve thromboses occurred in 13 of the 133 women. One notable concern to these investigators was that the function of more than 17 (35%) of the 49 bioprostheses deteriorated markedly either during pregnancy or shortly thereafter. This finding suggests that pregnancy accelerates the degenerative process, perhaps in relation to the increased turnover of calcium. Such deterioration has also been reported by others [38,41].

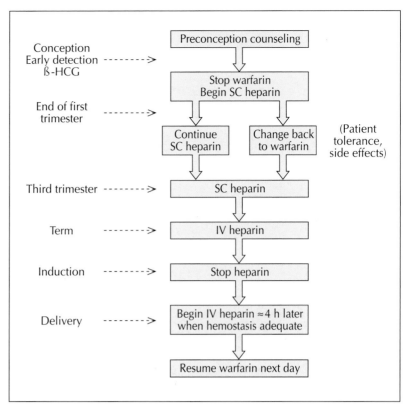

FIGURE 5-28. Proposed algorithm for anticoagulation for women with mechanical prosthetic valves. Since warfarin appears to pose the greatest risk during the first trimester, it is reasonable to switch to heparin as soon as pregnancy is confirmed. Meticulous control of the activated partial thromboplastin time must be established, after which the physician and the patient must choose between continuing heparin throughout the pregnancy and switching back to warfarin. This decision is based on the physician's preference and patient's tolerance of subcutaneous injections. If the patient returns to warfarin therapy, the regimen should be changed back to heparin again in the third trimester to avoid potential bleeding complications with a premature delivery. HCG—human chorionic gonadotropin; IV—intravenous; SC—subcutaneous.

MITRAL STENOSIS

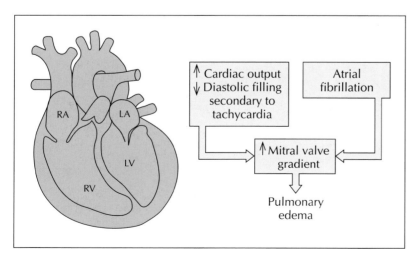

FIGURE 5-29. Hemodynamic changes with mitral stenosis during pregnancy. Pregnancy may pose significant risks for patients with mitral stenosis. The tachycardia of pregnancy exacerbates the transvalvular gradient and may lead to pulmonary edema, especially after the volume load peaks at the end of the second trimester. Pulmonary congestion develops in approximately 18% to 30% of these patients, more commonly in older patients and those in atrial fibrillation [42]. Atrial fibrillation may also cause acute hemodynamic embarrassment, sometimes necessitating cardioversion. Patients with mild mitral stenosis who are in functional class I or II, however, may tolerate pregnancy without difficulty [4]. LA—left atrium; LV—left ventricle; RA—right atrium; RV—right ventricle.

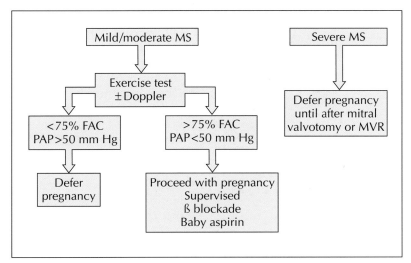

FIGURE 5-30. Proposed management strategy for patients with mitral stenosis (MS) in sinus rhythm. For women with mild or moderate MS, an exercise test, preferably with Doppler echocardiography, may help determine whether or not pregnancy is appropriate. For women who cannot achieve 75% of their functional aerobic capacity (FAC) or in whom pulmonary artery systolic pressure (PAP) exceeds 50 mm Hg, pregnancy should probably be deferred until the MS is corrected with valvotomy or mitral valve replacement (MVR). For women who can achieve 75% of their FAC and whose systolic PAP is less than 50 mm Hg, pregnancy can proceed with supervision. Therapy with β-blockers will slow the heart rate and reduce the diastolic gradient. The use of baby aspirin after the first trimester may help reduce the risk for thromboembolic complications. For women whose condition deteriorates during pregnancy or for those who present already pregnant with significant MS, bed rest and, if necessary, hospitalization must be instituted. Heart rate must be adequately controlled with β-blockers. If atrial fibrillation develops, sinus rhythm must be restored promptly, either pharmacologically or electrically. If atrial fibrillation has been present for more than 48 hours, heparin should be utilized first. Diuretics should be reserved for those women with pulmonary edema.

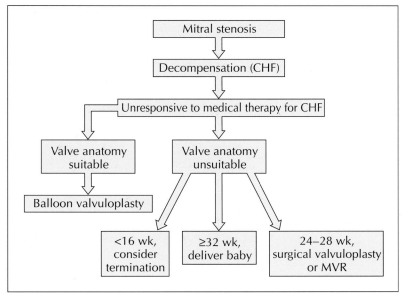

FIGURE 5-31. For women with mitral stenosis who decompensate during pregnancy, balloon valvuloplasty may be performed safely, provided that valve anatomy is deemed ideal based on two-dimensional echocardiography. During imaging, lead shielding must be used to protect the fetus from radiation. For women with calcified, thickened, immobile valves or chordal fusion, surgical commissurotomy should be considered. Ideally, this procedure should be performed between the 24th and 28th weeks of pregnancy, since it is preferable to delay open-heart surgery until organogenesis is complete; after 28 weeks, the risk for premature labor increases. Fetal monitoring should be performed throughout surgery, and flow through the extracorporeal circulation should be maintained at a high level. Even under ideal circumstances, however, the chance of fetal loss is increased, but survival of the mother should be the prime consideration. CHF—congestive heart failure; MVR—mitral valve replacement.

AORTIC AND MITRAL REGURGITATION

MEDICAL MANAGEMENT OF CHF

Bed rest (sitting or semi-recumbent)
   to decrease venous return

Oxygen

Morphine

Digoxin

Dopamine

Hydralazine

Operative intervention

FIGURE 5-32. Medical management of congestive heart failure (CHF) in aortic or mitral regurgitation during pregnancy. In contrast to the obstructive lesions of aortic and mitral valve stenosis, regurgitant valve lesions are usually well tolerated during pregnancy, provided the patient is in functional class I or II. This is because the fall in peripheral resistance during gestation helps to reduce left ventricular afterload. Left ventricular function and exercise capacity should be assessed at the time of preconception counseling. Even patients with severe regurgitation, if asymptomatic, will usually tolerate pregnancy if properly managed. In severe regurgitation with signs of left ventricular decompensation, valve surgery should be performed before conception. If the patient is already pregnant and CHF supervenes, medical management may be helpful.

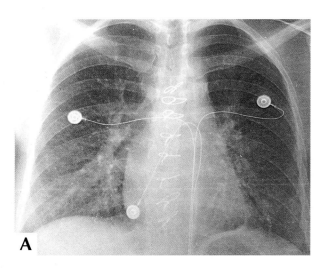 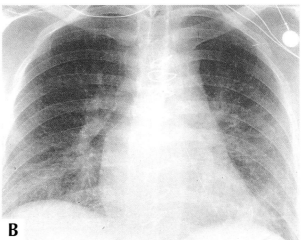

FIGURE 5-33. Chest radiographs of a patient with severe mitral regurgitation at the beginning of pregnancy (**A**) and at 32 weeks (**B**), when congestive heart failure developed and premature labor ensued. Following treatment with oxygen, diuretics, and morphine, a premature but healthy infant was delivered under epidural anesthesia. Three months later, the patient underwent successful mitral valve repair.

PHARMACOLOGIC THERAPY

TERATOGENIC AGENTS

LABELING OF TERATOGENIC DRUGS

FDA CATEGORY	TERATOGENICITY
A	Well-controlled human studies have not disclosed any fetal risk
B	Animal studies have disclosed no fetal risk or have suggested some risk not confirmed in controlled studies in women; or there are no adequate studies in women
C	Animal studies have revealed adverse fetal effects; there are no adequate controlled studies in women
D	Some fetal risk, but benefits may outweigh risk
X	Fetal abnormalities; contraindicated in pregnancy

FIGURE 5-34. Food and Drug Administration labeling for teratogenicity of drugs in general. (*Adapted from* Ferris [43]; with permission.)

FDA CATEGORIES OF TERATOGENICITY FOR CARDIAC DRUGS

B	C	D	X
Digoxin	Furosemide	Angiotensin-converting enzyme inhibitors	Warfarin
Dipyridamole	Heparin	Phenytoin	
Methyldopa	Hydralazine		
Thiazides	Procainamide		
	Propranolol		
	Quinidine		
	Verapamil		

FIGURE 5-35. Even though most cardiac drugs needed for pregnant patients have been assigned to category B or C by the Food and Drug Administration (FDA), many can be used safely.

POTENTIAL ADVERSE EFFECTS OF CARDIAC DRUGS

		ADVERSE EFFECTS	
CARDIAC DRUG	FDA CATEGORY*	MATERNAL	FETAL
Amiodarone [44]	C	Skin discoloration Liver and thyroid dysfunction Pulmonary fibrosis	Thyroid abnormalities
Atenolol [45]	B	Bronchospasm Hypotension Bradycardia CHF	Growth retardation Bradycardia Hypoglycemia
Digoxin [46]	A	Bradycardia Nausea	?
Disopyramide [47]	C	Dry mouth Urine retention Uterine contractility	?
Lidocaine [48]	B	Seizure	Bradycardia
Phenytoin [49]	X	Fatigue Rash Gingival hyperplasia	Teratogenicity (hydantoin syndrome)
Procainamide [50]	C	Lupus syndrome	?
Propranolol [51]	C	Bronchospasm Bradycardia Hypotension CHF	Growth retardation Bradycardia Hypoglycemia
Quinidine [50]	C	Diarrhea Thrombocytopenia	Thrombocytopenia
Verapamil [50]	C	Bradycardia Hypotension Uterine relaxation	AV block CHF

*See Fig. 5-34.

FIGURE 5-36. Some commonly used cardiac drugs and their potential adverse effects on the mother and fetus [44–51]. All 10 drugs cross the placenta. AV—atrioventricular; CHF—congestive heart failure.

ENDOCARDITIS PROPHYLAXIS

AHA RECOMMENDATIONS FOR ENDOCARDITIS PROPHYLAXIS DURING DELIVERY

NOT RECOMMENDED

Cesarean section

In the absence of infection for urethral catheterization, D & C, **uncomplicated** vaginal delivery, therapeutic abortion, sterilization procedures, or insertion/removal of IUDs

RECOMMENDED

Vaginal delivery in the presence of infection

In addition to prophylactic regimen for genitourinary procedures, antibiotic therapy should be directed against the most likely bacterial pathogen

FIGURE 5-37. The most recent American Heart Association (AHA) recommendations for endocarditis prophylaxis suggest that antibiotic prophylaxis is not necessary for "uncomplicated" vaginal delivery [52]. However, since the majority of deliveries are accompanied by an episiotomy, they are technically considered "complicated." Furthermore, many women have pyrexia after delivery, presumed to be secondary to endometritis. While the risk for endocarditis around the time of delivery is low, it is the author's preference to administer antibiotic prophylaxis as described here. In patients with prosthetic heart valves, a history of bacterial endocarditis, or surgical shunts, physicians may administer prophylactic antibiotics even for low-risk procedures involving the lower respiratory, gastrointestinal, or genitourinary tracts.

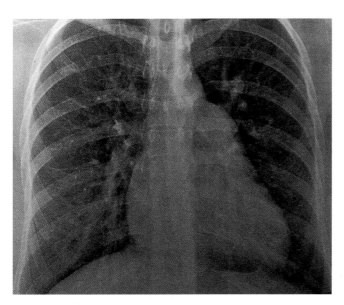

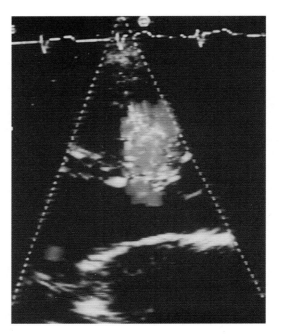

FIGURE 5-38. Chest radiograph of a woman who presented with a secundum atrial septal defect who tolerated one pregnancy without complication. With the declining incidence of rheumatic heart disease and increasing numbers of adults with congenital heart disease, most maternal cardiac disease is now congenital in origin. Atrial septal defect is one of the most common malformations to remain undetected until adulthood. This patient had a sizable shunt and right ventricular volume overload. Note the enlarged pulmonary artery, pulmonary plethora, and enlarged right ventricle.

During pregnancy, the major concern is the risk for paradoxical emboli arising from the leg veins, since phlebitis and phlebothromboses are common complications of pregnancy. Meticulous attention to leg care is therefore necessary, particularly peripartum, when venous stasis is common. For older women with atrial septal defect, atrial fibrillation is another possible complication. Ideally, the defect should be closed before pregnancy is contemplated. If a patient with an atrial septal defect presents already pregnant, daily baby aspirin is recommended after the first trimester to try to reduce the incidence of thrombosis.

FIGURE 5-39. Two-dimensional echocardiogram (long-axis view) showing a small, hemodynamically insignificant paramembranous ventricular septal defect. Women with a restrictive ventricular septal defect, normal ventricular function, and a normal pulmonary artery pressure should tolerate pregnancy without difficulty. This can usually be assessed noninvasively by two-dimensional echocardiography. The velocity across the defect was 5 m/s, predicting normal right ventricular systolic pressure. This patient tolerated the pregnancy without complication. In patients with larger ventricular septal defects, the risk during pregnancy increases if ventricular function is impaired and pulmonary artery pressure is elevated [53]. The added volume load of pregnancy may cause ventricular failure [54].

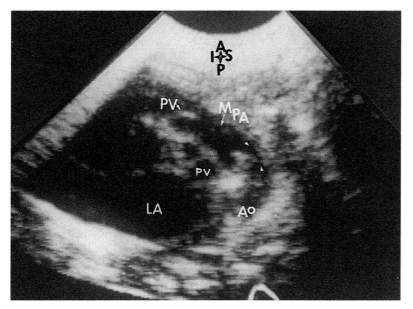

FIGURE 5-40. Two-dimensional echocardiogram showing a small patent ductus arteriosus. A small or moderate-sized ductus is not an impediment to pregnancy provided that ventricular function and pulmonary artery (PA) pressure are normal and the woman is asymptomatic [55]. If the ductus is large enough to produce left ventricular volume overload, it should be closed before pregnancy is contemplated. Ductal size, ventricular function, and PA pressure can usually be determined noninvasively by two-dimensional and Doppler echocardiography. For women with any kind of shunt, with a PA pressure that is 75% or more of systemic pressure, pregnancy poses a significant risk (*see* Fig. 5-13, Eisenmenger syndrome). Ao—aorta; LA—left atrium; MPA—main pulmonary artery; PV—pulmonic valve.

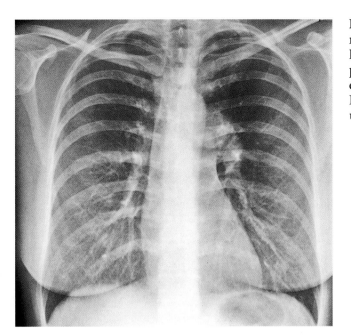

FIGURE 5-41. Chest radiograph of a patient with severe pulmonic stenosis and right ventricular pressure at the systemic level. Note the enlarged main and left pulmonary arteries, representing poststenotic dilatation. Mild or moderate pulmonic stenosis is usually well tolerated during pregnancy [56,57], and even patients with severe pulmonic stenosis may get through pregnancy safely. Ideally, however, this defect should be dealt with before pregnancy. This patient underwent successful balloon valvotomy prior to pregnancy.

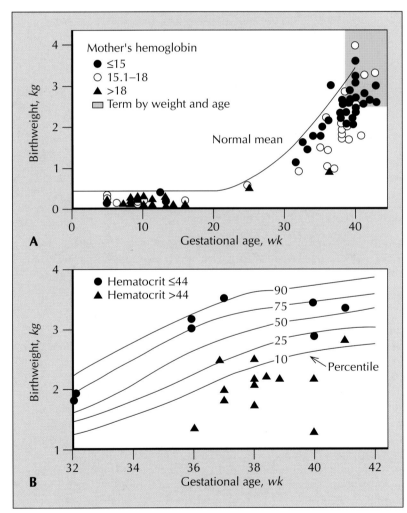

FIGURE 5-42. Maternal cyanosis poses a significant risk to fetal growth and survival. **A,** As cyanosis worsens (as reflected by an increasing maternal hemoglobin concentration), the incidence of spontaneous abortion increases and the impediment to fetal growth becomes more pronounced. In this study, no infant survived if the maternal hemoglobin exceeded 18 g [58]. **B,** In a study by Whittemore [59], the degree of cyanosis was assessed by examining the maternal hematocrit. For all infants born to mothers with an increased hematocrit, birthweight was below the 50th percentile for gestational age. (Part A *adapted from* Burwell and Metcalfe [60]; part B *adapted from* Whittemore [59]; with permission.)

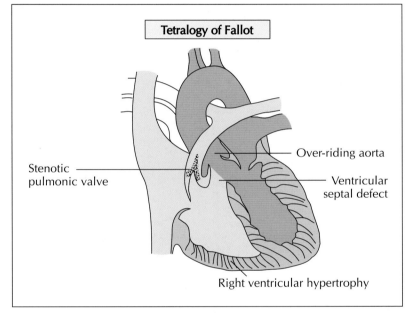

FIGURE 5-43. Tetralogy of Fallot consists of obstruction to right ventricular outflow, right ventricular hypertrophy, a large subaortic ventricular septal defect, and an over-riding aorta. Since blue blood cannot easily exit the obstructed pulmonary outflow tract, it enters the aorta. For women with unrepaired tetralogy of Fallot, pregnancy poses significant risks. The fall in peripheral resistance permits increased right-to-left shunting and worsening of cyanosis. In addition, the volume load of pregnancy and increased venous return may cause heart failure, so maternal mortality and morbidity are increased [61]. The peripartum period is an especially precarious time, when blood loss may cause hypotension, right-to-left shunting, and circulatory collapse. Following surgery, the prognosis is much improved. (*Adapted from* the American Heart Association [62]; with permission.)

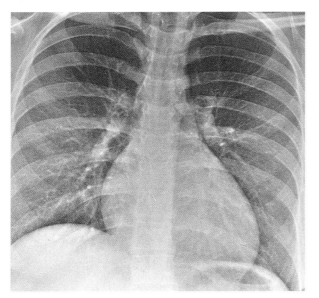

FIGURE 5-44. Chest radiograph of a patient with mild Ebstein anomaly showing right atrial enlargement and mild cardiomegaly. The major feature of this anomaly is inferior displacement of the tricuspid valve, which is abnormally formed and variably regurgitant. The right atrium is usually enlarged and incorporates the "atrialized" portion of the right ventricle. Fifty percent of patients have an atrial septal defect or patent foramen ovale through which blood may be shunted from right to left and cause cyanosis. Up to 25% of patients may have one or more accessory conduction pathways. Pregnancy is often well tolerated in women with Ebstein anomaly provided that the right-sided chambers are only moderately enlarged and ventricular function is not significantly impaired [63,64]. Patients with cyanosis, however, are at increased risk for fetal loss and paradoxical embolus. This woman with a small patent foramen ovale but no cyanosis was counseled that she can proceed with pregnancy with appropriate care.

RISK FOR RECURRENCE (%) IF ONE PARENT HAS CONGENITAL HEART DISEASE

CONGENITAL ANOMALY	NORA *et al.* [65]	WHITTEMORE *et al.* [54]	ROSE *et al.* [66]	MORRIS AND MENASHE [67]	CONNOLLY AND WARNES [64]
Aortic valve stenosis	4	—	12	—	—
Coarctation of aorta	—	—	8	—	—
Pulmonic stenosis	3.5	19	—	—	—
Atrial septal defect	3	11	11	5	—
Ventricular septal defect	4	22	—	8	—
Patent ductus arteriosus	4	11	—	—	—
Tetralogy of Fallot	4	13	—	2	—
Ebstein anomaly	—	—	—	—	6

FIGURE 5-45. Risk for recurrence of some common congenital cardiac anomalies [54,64–68]. If one parent has congenital heart disease, an appropriate question is "What are the chances my child will have congenital heart disease?" The considerable variation among these results can be attributed to ascertainment bias and level of expertise in examining the infant. Some studies suggest that the child's risk for inheriting congenital heart disease is greater if the mother is affected rather than the father [66,69].

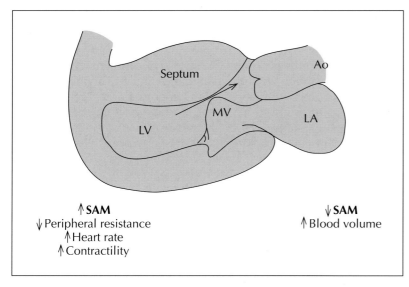

FIGURE 5-46. Hemodynamic changes in hypertrophic cardiomyopathy (HC) during pregnancy. Some of these changes make it possible for women with HC to tolerate pregnancy in most cases. For example, although there is a fall in systemic vascular resistance, and heart rate and contractility increase, these changes are partly offset by the increase in blood volume. In some patients dyspnea may develop during pregnancy because of worsening mitral regurgitation, increased filling pressure, or increasing left ventricular (LV) outflow tract obstruction. Acute atrial fibrillation is a possible cause of abrupt deterioration in hemodynamic status. Patients who have few or no symptoms and are not receiving any treatment usually do not need medical therapy and will tolerate pregnancy well. Hemodynamic status, including the presence or absence of LV outflow tract obstruction, mitral regurgitation, and diastolic dysfunction, should be assessed by two-dimensional and Doppler echocardiography prior to conception. If the patient is already taking β-blockers, such therapy should be continued throughout the pregnancy; if there is evidence of increasing LV outflow tract obstruction, the dosage may be increased. Fetal growth should be monitored, and if the patient is on large doses of β-blockers, the neonatologist should be alerted to the possibility of bradycardia and hypoglycemia.

Patients with significant hemodynamic abnormalities should be delivered according to the recommendations presented in Fig. 5-10, although the incidence of significant complications is low [70,71]. Because HC is transmitted in an autosomal dominant fashion, potential mothers should be warned about the risks of the child inheriting the disease. Ao—aorta; LA—left atrium; MV—mitral valve; SAM—systolic anterior motion.

REFERENCES

1. Metcalfe J, Ueland K: Maternal cardiovascular adjustments to pregnancy. *Progr Cardiovasc Dis* 1974, 16:363–374.

2. Lund CJ, Donovan JC: Blood volume during pregnancy. Significance of plasma and red cell volumes. *Am J Obstet Gynecol* 1967, 98:393–403.

3. Pritchard JA: Hematologic aspects of pregnancy. *Clin Obstet Gynecol* 1960, 3:378–385.

4. Elkayam U, Gleicher N: Cardiac problems in pregnancy. I. Maternal aspects: the approach to the pregnant patient with heart disease. *JAMA* 1984, 251:2838–2839.

5. Sullivan JM, Ramanathan KB: Management of medical problems in pregnancy: severe cardiac disease. *N Engl J Med* 1985, 313:304–309.

6. Lees MM, Taylor SH, Scott DB, *et al.*: A study of cardiac output at rest throughout pregnancy. *J Obstet Gynecol Br Commonw* 1967, 74:319–328.

7. Greiss FC Jr, Anderson SG: Effect of ovarian hormones on the uterine vascular bed. *Am J Obstet Gynecol* 1970, 107:829–836.

8. Ginsburg J, Duncan SLB: Peripheral blood flow in normal pregnancy. *Cardiovasc Res* 1967, 1:132–137.

9. Harvey WP: Alterations of the cardiac physical examination in normal pregnancy. *Clin Obstet Gynecol* 1975, 18:51–63.

10. Cutforth R, MacDonald CB: Heart sounds and murmurs in pregnancy. *Am Heart J* 1966, 71:741–747.

11. Hendricks CH, Quilligan EJ: Cardiac output during labor. *Am J Obstet Gynecol* 1956, 71:953–972.

12. Adams JQ, Alexander AM Jr: Alterations in cardiovascular physiology during labor. *Obstet Gynecol* 1958, 12:542–549.

13. Kerr MG, Scott DB, Samuel E: Studies of the inferior vena cava in late pregnancy. *BMJ* 1964, 1:532–533.

14. Bieniarz J, Crottogini JJ, Cururchet E, *et al.*: Aorto-caval compression by the uterus in late human pregnancy. II. An arteriographic study. *Am J Obstet Gynecol* 1968, 100:203–217.

15. Metcalfe J, Ueland K: Maternal cardiovascular adjustments to pregnancy. *Progr Cardiovasc Dis* 1974, 16:363–374.

16. Ueland K, Hanson JM: Maternal cardiovascular hemodynamics. III. Labor and delivery under local and caudal analgesia. *Am J Obstet Gynecol* 1969, 103:8–18.

17. Ueland K, Gills RE, Hanson JM: Maternal cardiovascular dynamics. I. Cesarean section under subarachnoid block anesthesia. *Am J Obstet Gynecol* 1968, 100:42–54.

18. Pritchard JA, Roland RC: Blood volume changes in pregnancy in the puerperium. III. Whole body and large vessel hematocrits in pregnant and nonpregnant women. *Am J Obstet Gynecol* 1964, 88:391–395.

19. Wood P: An appreciation of mitral stenosis. *BMJ* 1954, 1:1051–1063.

20. Gleicher N, Midwall J, Hochberger D, *et al.*: Eisenmenger's syndrome and pregnancy. *Obstet Gynecol Surv* 1979, 34:721–741.

21. Arias F, Pineda J: Aortic stenosis in pregnancy. *J Reprod Med* 1978, 20:229–232.

22. Easterling TR, Chadwick HS, Otto CM, *et al.*: Aortic stenosis in pregnancy. *Obstet Gynecol* 1988, 72:113–118.

23. Rose BI, Holbrook RH Jr, Wyner J, *et al.*: Efficacy of Doppler echocardiography in the evaluation of aortic stenosis during pregnancy. *Obstet Gynecol* 1987, 69:431–432.

24. Roberts WC: Valvular, subvalvular, and supravalvular aortic stenosis: morphologic features. *Cardiovasc Clin* 1973, 1:97–126.

25. Angel JL, Chapman C, Knuppel RA, *et al.*: Percutaneous balloon aortic valvuloplasty in pregnancy. *Obstet Gynecol* 1988, 72:438–440.

26. Mortensen JD, Ellsworth HS: Coarctation of the aorta in pregnancy: obstetric and cardiovascular complications before and after surgical correction. *JAMA* 1965, 191:596–598.

27. Barash PG, Hobbins JC, Hook R, *et al.*: Management of coarctation of the aorta during pregnancy. *J Thorac Cardiovasc Surg* 1975, 69:781–784.

28. Pyeritz RE: Maternal and fetal complications of pregnancy in the Marfan syndrome. *Am J Med* 1981, 71:784–790.

29. Rosenblum NG, Grossman AR, Gabbe SG, *et al.*: Failure of serial echocardiographic studies to predict aortic dissection in a pregnant woman with Marfan's syndrome. *Am J Obstet Gynecol* 1983, 146:470–471.

30. Hall JG, Pauli RM, Wilson KM: Maternal and fetal sequelae of anticoagulation during pregnancy. *Am J Med* 1980, 68:122–140.

31. Holzgreve W, Carey JC, Hall BD: Warfarin-induced fetal abnormalities. *Lancet* 1976, 2:914–915.

32. Pauli RM, Madden JD, Kranzler JK, *et al.*: Warfarin therapy initiated during pregnancy and phenotypic chondrodysplasia punctata. *J Pediatr* 1976, 88:506–508.

33. Harrison EC, Roschke EJ: Pregnancy in patients with cardiac valve prostheses. *Clin Obstet Gynecol* 1975, 18:107–123.

34. Bonnar J: Long-term self-administered heparin therapy for prevention and treatment of thromboembolic complications in pregnancy. In: *Heparin: Chemistry and Clinical Usage*. Edited by Kakkar VV, Thomas DP. London: Academic Press; 1976:247–260.

35. Ibarra-Perez C, Arevalo-Toledo N, Alvarez-de la Cadena O, *et al.*: The course of pregnancy in patients with artificial heart valves. *Am J Med* 1976, 61:504–512.

36. Lutz DJ, Noller KL, Spittell JA, *et al.*: Pregnancy and its complications following cardiac valve prostheses. *Am J Obstet Gynecol* 1978, 131:460–466.

37. Ben Ismail M, Fekih M, Taktak M, *et al.*: Prosthèses valvulaires cardiaques et grossesse. *Arch Mal Coeur* 1979, 77:192–199.

38. Salazar E, Zajarias A, Gutierrez N, *et al.*: The problem of cardiac valve prostheses, anticoagulants, and pregnancy. *Circulation* 1984, 70(suppl I):I-169–I-177.

39. Born D, Martinez EE, Almeida PAM, *et al.*: Pregnancy in patients with prosthetic heart valves: the effects of anticoagulation on mother, fetus, and neonate. *Am Heart J* 1992, 124:413–417.

40. Sbarouni E, Oakley CM: Outcome of pregnancy in women with valve prostheses. *Br Heart J* 1994, 71:196–201.

41. Bortolloti U, Milano A, Mazzucco A, *et al.*: Pregnancy in patients with a porcine valve prosthesis. *Am J Cardiol* 1982, 50:1051–1054.

42. Szekely P, Turner R, Snaith L: Pregnancy and the changing pattern of rheumatic heart disease. *Br Heart J* 1973, 35:1293–1303.

43. Ferris TF: Toxemia and hypertension. In: *Medical Complications During Pregnancy*, ed 2. Edited by Burro GN, Ferris TF. Philadelphia: WB Saunders Co; 1982:1–35.

44. Foster CJ, Love HG: Amiodarone in pregnancy: case report and review of the literature. *Int J Cardiol* 1988, 20:307–316.

45. Rubin PC, Butters L, Klark D, *et al.*: Obstetric aspects of the use in pregnancy-associated hypertension of the beta-adrenoceptor antagonist atenolol. *Am J Obstet Gynecol* 1984, 150:389–392.

46. Roger MC, Willerson JT, Goldblatt A, *et al.*: Serum digoxin concentrations in the human fetus, neonate and infant. *N Engl J Med* 1972, 287:1010–1013.

47. Tamari I, Eldar M, Robinowitz B, *et al.*: Medical treatment of cardiovascular disorders during pregnancy. *Am Heart J* 1982, 104:1357–1363.

48. Rotmensch HH, Rotmensch S, Elkayam U: Management of cardiac arrhythmias during pregnancy: current concepts. *Drugs* 1987, 33:623–633.

49. Alen RW Jr, Augden B, Bentley FL, *et al.*: Fetal hydantoin syndrome, neuroblastoma, and hemorrhagic disease in a neonate. *JAMA* 1980, 244:1464–1465.

50. Rotmensch HH, Elkayam U, Frishman WH: Antiarrhythmic drug therapy during pregnancy. *Ann Intern Med* 1983, 98:487–497.

51. Frishman WH, Chestnar M: Beta-adrenergic blockers in pregnancy. *Am Heart J* 1988, 115:147–152.

52. Dajani AS, Bisno AL, Chung KJ: Prevention of bacterial endo-carditis: recommendations by the American Heart Association. *JAMA* 1990; 264:2919–2922.

53. Schaefer G, Arditi LI, Solomon HA, *et al.*: Congenital heart disease and pregnancy. *Clin Obstet Gynecol* 1968, 11:1048–1063.

54. Whittemore R, Hobbins JC, Engle MA: Pregnancy and its outcome in women with and without surgical treatment of congenital heart disease. *Am J Cardiol* 1982, 50:641–651.

55. Metcalfe J, McAnulty JH, Ueland K: *Heart Disease and Pregnancy: Physiology and Management*. Boston: Little, Brown; 1986:223–264.

56. Neilson G, Galea EG, Blent A: Congenital heart disease and pregnancy. *Med J Aust* 1970, 1:1086–1088.

57. Mendelson CL: *Cardiac Disease in Pregnancy*. Philadelphia: FA Davis; 1960.

58. Neill CA, Swanson S: Outcome of pregnancy in congenital heart disease. *Circulation* 1961, 24:1003.

59. Whittemore R: Congenital heart disease: its impact on pregnancy. *Hosp Pract* 1983, 18:65–74.

60. Burwell CS, Metcalfe J: *Heart Disease and Pregnancy*, ed 2. Edited by Metcalfe J, McAnulty JH, Ueland K. Boston: Little, Brown; 1986.

61. Higgins CB, Mulder DG: Tetralogy of Fallot in the adult. *Am J Cardiol* 1972, 29:837–846.

62. American Heart Association Committee on Congenital Cardiac Defects of the AHA's Council on Cardiovascular Disease in the Young: *If Your Child Has a Congenital Heart Defect: A Guide for Parents*. Dallas: American Heart Association; 1991:34.

63. Donnelly JE, Brown JM, Radford DJ: Pregnancy outcome and Ebstein's anomaly. *Br Heart J* 1991, 66:368–371.

64. Connolly HM, Warnes CA: Ebstein's anomaly: outcome of pregnancy. *J Am Coll Cardiol* 1994, 23:1194–1198.

65. Nora JJ, Nora AH, Wexler P: Hereditary and environmental aspects as they affect the fetus and newborn. *Clin Obstet Gynecol* 1981, 2:851–861.

66. Rose V, Gold RJM, Lindsay G, *et al.*: Possible increase in the inci-dence of congenital heart defects among the offspring of affected parents. *J Am Coll Cardiol* 1985, 6:376–382.

67. Morris CD, Menashe VD: Recurrence of congenital heart disease in offspring of parents with surgical correction. *Clin Res* 1985, 33:68A.

68. Zellers TM, Driscoll DJ, Michels VV: Prevalence of significant congenital heart defects in children of parents with Fallot's tetralogy. *Am J Cardiol* 1990, 65:523–526.

69. Czeizel A, Pornoi A, Peterffy E, *et al.*: Study of children of parents operated on for congenital cardiovascular malformations. *Br Heart J* 1982, 47:290–293.

70. Oakley GDG, McGarry K, Limb DG, *et al.*: Management of preg-nancy in patients with hypertrophic cardiomyopathy. *BMJ* 1979, 1:1749–1750.

71. Shah DM, Sunderji SG: Hypertrophic cardiomyopathy in preg-nancy: report of maternal mortality and review of the literature. *Obstet Gynecol Surv* 1985, 40:444–448.

HEART DISEASE IN THE PRESENCE OF NEUROLOGIC DISEASE

6

CHAPTER

Ileana L. Piña
and Ross R. Zimmer

Neurologic disorders associated with heart disease can be either acquired (*eg*, subarachnoid hemorrhage) or inherited (*eg*, muscular dystrophy). The cardiac manifestations have been described extensively and can range from incidental electrocardiographic (ECG) findings to overt cardiac dysfunction, including sudden death. In addition, since primary cardiac disease can present as a neurologic event or can coexist independently, much time has been devoted to searching for a direct cause-and-effect relationship between disorders of the two systems. This is particularly true in the case of the inherited neuromuscular disorders. However, the astute clinician must not forget that neurologic and cardiovascular diseases can coexist but be unrelated.

In this chapter, the term "acute cerebral events" will be used to encompass the group of acquired neurologic disorders that includes subdural and subarachnoid hemorrhage, stroke, and head trauma. The classic ECG manifestations of an acute cerebral event have long been known to clinicians and can resemble those of ischemic heart disease. These abnormalities include deep and symmetric (neurogenic) T-wave inversion and Q-T prolongation. Both bradyarrhythmias and tachyarrhythmias have been described as well [1–10]. Although the ECG changes associated with acute cerebral events are well known, the initiating mechanism(s) remain unclear. As one possible mechanism, the role of the sympathetic nervous system has been studied extensively both in animal models and *in vivo*, and the role of catecholamines has been well established [11]. Supporting this theory are the autopsy findings in patients who have succumbed to an acute cerebral event in which the cardiac histopathologic changes are consistent with catecholamine excess [12]. In contrast, the echocardiographic and thallium perfusion abnormalities found in association with acute cerebral events have been less well recognized. An emerging body of echocardiographic data demonstrates that although significant wall motion abnormalities can exist in a patient with an acute cerebral event, the changes can be transient and inconsequential [13]. In addition, efforts to link thallium perfusion defects to specific ECG changes have failed [14].

The inherited neuromuscular disorders discussed in this chapter are primarily those having the strongest associations with cardiac pathology and those in which the heart is an integral part of the disease process. Charcot-Marie-Tooth disease has been included, although the heart is not consistently affected in this disorder. The *nonmyotonic dystrophies* include the sex-linked progressive Duchenne and Becker dystrophies, the facioscapulohumeral dystrophy of Landouzy- Déjèrine, and the limb-girdle dystrophy of Erb. The cardiac manifestations associated with these disorders range from minor ECG changes to severe heart failure. For example, Duchenne muscular dystrophy, perhaps the most extensively studied of all the dystrophies, is associated with a severe, insidious, and often fatal cardiomyopathy at an early age [15]. In contrast, patients with the less aggressive Becker's muscular dystrophy survive into adulthood, and although the cardiomyopathy is as severe as in Duchenne

dystrophy, cardiac transplantation is a viable option for these patients [16].

Cardiac involvement, specifically of the conduction system, is an integral part of *myotonic dystrophy*, also known as Steinert disease [15]. In a few cases, however, structural abnormalities have also been described (*eg*, mitral valve prolapse) [17]. Finally, in *Friedreich's ataxia*, the most common neurologic inherited disorder, the heart may manifest either a myopathic or a hypertrophic process (unlike that of genetic hypertrophic cardiomyopathy), which may be the cause of death. Research is now being directed toward the genetic mapping and early identification of the neuromuscular diseases. This chapter highlights the salient features of the cardiac manifestations of both acquired and inherited neurologic disorders.

ACQUIRED NEUROLOGIC DISORDERS

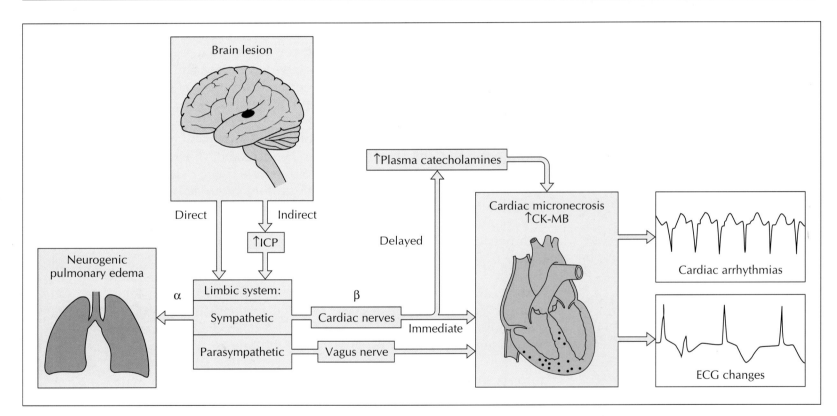

FIGURE 6-1. Electrocardiographic (ECG) changes and the emergence of cardiac arrhythmias have long been recognized as accompaniments of acute cerebral events [11]. In addition, stimulation of the central nervous system (CNS) has been shown to provoke malignant arrhythmias [18]. While the hypothalamus appears to play a central role in the cardiac manifestations associated with intracranial lesions, numerous other regions of the CNS also seem

to contribute, the most prominent of which are the limbic system and its connections, such as the cingulate gyrus, orbital frontal region, amygdala, thalamus, and midbrain [11,18]. The autonomic nervous system, particularly the sympathetic nervous system, also plays an integral role. CK-MB—MB fraction of creatine kinase; ICP—intracranial pressure. (*Adapted from* Norris [11]; with permission.)

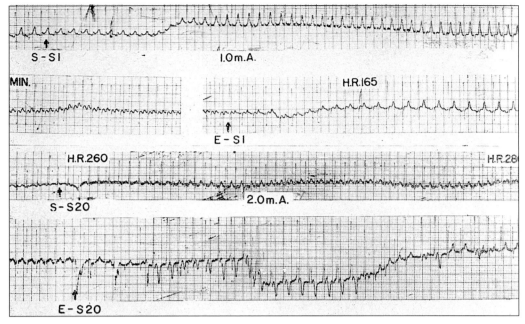

subsequently became inverted. After 20 successive stimulations, symmetrically inverted T waves with Q-T prolongation can be seen (after E-S20) [19]. This study, as well as others [20], demonstrates that both the hypothalamus and the sympathetic nervous system play a role in the development of the typical cardiac pathology associated with central neurologic lesions. In animal experiments, direct hypothalamic stimulation has induced varying degrees of ECG abnormalities [19]. When stimulation was applied after C2 transection, these abnormalities were not seen, although they were still present after vagotomy. On autopsy, more than one third of the animals who had undergone bilateral hypothalamic stimulation showed some of the typical cardiac findings seen on necropsy of patients dying of acute cerebral events—*ie*, small subendocardial hemorrhages and loss of myocardial cross-striations. (*Adapted from* Melville and coworkers [19]; with permission.)

FIGURE 6-2. Electrocardiogram (ECG) during repeated, bilateral, direct stimulation of the lateral hypothalamus of a cat. Each stimulation lasted 60 seconds and was repeated at 3-minute intervals. During the first stimulation (starting at S-S1 and ending at E-S1), the precordial lead shows marked ST-segment elevation and tall peaked T waves that

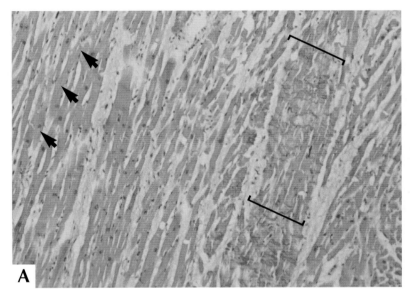

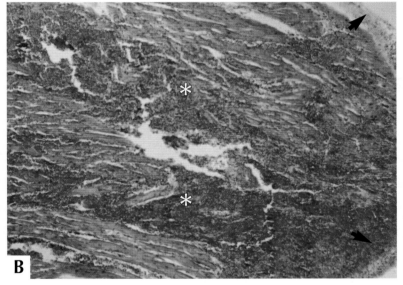

FIGURE 6-3. Acute cerebral events have been associated with cardiac pathologic changes in both animal and human studies [19–21]. Although early reports failed to show any evidence of significant cardiac pathology [22], later ones indicated a variety of abnormalities. Evidence of myocytolysis has been observed in as many as 62% of patients dying of intracerebral lesions, and the pathologic changes occurred as early as 6 hours after the neurologic insult [23]. **A,** Photomicrograph of ventricular myocardium with an area of contraction band necrosis (*in brackets*), also referred to as coagulative myocytolysis. Abnormal myocytes can be seen on the right, while normal ones are on the left (*arrows*). **B,** Pathologic specimen showing an area of left ventricular subendocardium with interstitial hemorrhage but without myocyte necrosis. In addition to myocytolysis and subendocardial hemorrhage (*asterisks*), interstitial edema, round cell infiltrates, and a diffuse micronecrotic mottling known as "myofibrillar degeneration" have been described in patients with subarachnoid hemorrhage [1,24,25]. The clinical significance of these abnormalities remains unclear. Some of these pathologic changes can also occur in the presence of catecholamine excess, hypoxia, hemorrhagic shock, direct electrical injury, and hypokalemia [12]. (*Arrows* indicate endocardium.) (Hematoxylin and eosin stain, ×40.) (*Adapted from* Kolin and coworkers [23]; with permission.)

HEART DISEASE IN THE PRESENCE OF NEUROLOGIC DISEASE
6.3

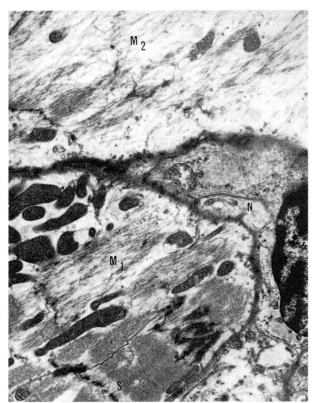

FIGURE 6-4. Electron micrograph showing portions of two injured myocardial cells from an animal study (×15,974) [21]. Stimulation of the mesencephalic reticular formation of cats can result in significant cardiac pathologic change, including cytoplasmic swelling with indistinct cross-striations and myocyte necrosis. Normal striations (S) can be seen here in the bottom portion of one myocardial cell; in the midportion, a focal area is distinguished by loss of striations and by granular myofibrils (M_1) adjacent to a small nerve (N) that contains agranular vesicles. In the upper cell, the entire cytoplasm shows loss of striations. Granular-appearing myofibrils (M_2) are also evident [21]. Of interest, the intracardiac nerves containing norepinephrine granules occasionally appeared near the regions of myocardium that exhibited the most striking pathologic changes, suggesting that myocardial necrosis may in part be secondary to the effect of local epinephrine release. These observations support the hypothesis that cardiac injury is secondary to autonomic neurologic activation. (*Adapted from* Greenhoot and Reichenbach [21]; with permission.)

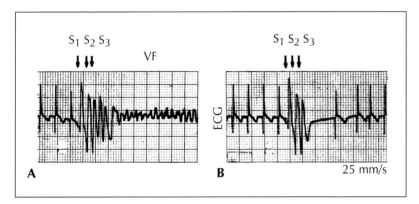

FIGURE 6-5. Electrocardiographic (ECG) effects of ventricular stimulation with (**A**) and without (**B**) concomitant stellate ganglion stimulation in a dog. The search for the origin of arrhythmias in the setting of an acute cerebral event has led investigators to the autonomic nervous system. Animal studies in which the right ventricle is pulsed with concomitant stellate ganglion stimulation have provoked ventricular fibrillation (VF) in 60% of animals tested when compared with a nonstimulated control group that did not develop VF. Moreover, stimulation of the left stellate ganglion has generated nonspecific ST-segment and T-wave abnormalities as well as Q-T prolongation in 100% of animals studied, whereas right stellate ganglion stimulation resulted in these changes in less than half the cases [26]. In the experiment shown here, three stimuli were delivered in close succession to the animal's right ventricle. By varying the timing and intensity of the third stimulus, changes in cardiac electrical stability can be examined. The tracing in *panel B* demonstrates three extrastimuli followed by resumption of the underlying rhythm. The tracing in *panel A* shows the onset of VF when the same stimuli are accompanied by stellate ganglion stimulation [27]. Therefore, the autonomic nervous system—and more specifically the sympathetic nervous system—plays an important role in the genesis of arrhythmias and ECG abnormalities in the presence of acute cerebral accidents. (*Adapted from* Verrier and coworkers [27]; with permission.)

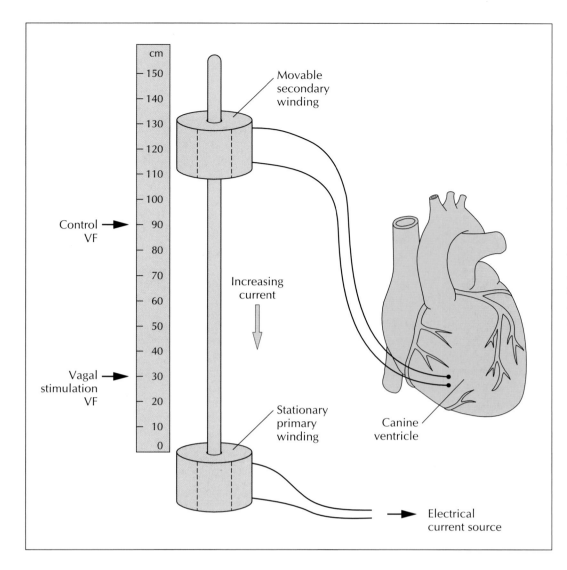

FIGURE 6-6. Studies to elucidate the role of the parasympathetic nervous system in the origin of arrhythmias date back to 1859, when Einbrodt attempted to provoke ventricular fibrillation (VF) in dogs by directly stimulating the ventricle with and without vagal stimulation [28]. As shown here, fibrillation occurred when the stimulation coils were 90 cm apart. As the coils were approximated, the threshold for VF could be estimated. During vagal stimulation, the spacing between the coils could be narrowed to 30 cm before fibrillation occurred [29]. Thus, the vagus protected against VF. Since these findings have not been confirmed *in vivo*, the exact role of the isolated parasympathetic nervous system in the presence of acute cerebral accidents remains unclear [30]. (*Adapted from* Lown and Verrier [29]; with permission.)

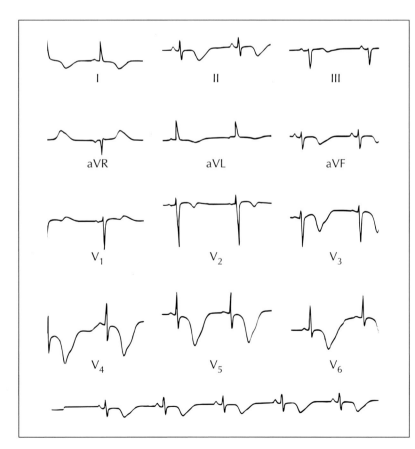

FIGURE 6-7. Electrocardiogram (ECG) from a 45-year-old woman with a subarachnoid hemorrhage. ECG abnormalities are reported in as many as 60% to 90% of patients with acute cerebral events or head trauma [1–3]. The classic finding is deeply, symmetrically inverted (neurogenic) T waves (shown here in leads V_3 to V_6) that are associated with prolongation of the Q-T interval. Other frequently reported changes include "U" waves, ST-segment depression and elevation, and tall upright T waves [1–8]. Since most studies have not analyzed ECG recordings prior to the catastrophic neurologic event, some of the reported ECG abnormalities may have been pre-existing [1–8]. Although an association between frontal lobe injury and "neurogenic" T waves has been suggested [1], it has been difficult to correlate specific ECG abnormalities with a discrete neurologic lesion.

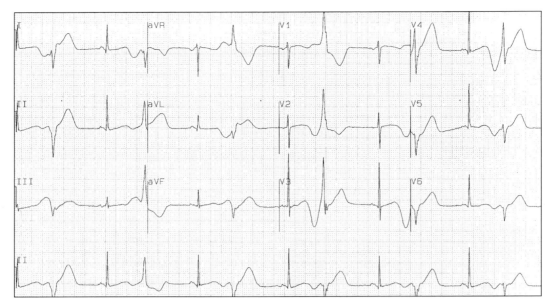

Figure 6-8. Electrocardiogram from a young woman who presented with a subarachnoid hemorrhage. Cardiac bradyarrhythmias and tachyarrhythmias are also seen with intracranial disease or injury. Occasional premature atrial and ventricular depolarizations have been well described, as have more complex dysrhythmias such as atrial fibrillation, wandering atrial pacemaker, multifocal atrial tachycardia, nonsustained and sustained ventricular tachycardia, and ventricular fibrillation. The rhythm here is sinus, with frequent multiform ventricular ectopic beats in a bigeminal pattern. The Q-T interval is 0.548 second, which is markedly prolonged. The "neurogenic" T waves are masked by the premature ventricular beats but are still prominent in leads V_3 and V_4. (Courtesy of Howard Warner, MD, Temple University, Philadelphia, PA.)

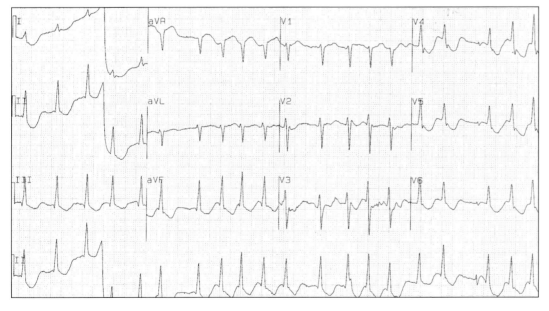

Figure 6-9. Atrial fibrillation (AF) in a patient recovering from a subarachnoid hemorrhage. The T waves are deeply inverted, although not symmetric. An association between AF and brainstem hemorrhage has been suggested [1], with a reported incidence of AF as high as 31% in association with acute cerebrovascular events [31]. However, since the onset of AF can be the inciting event for a cerebrovascular accident, it is often difficult to establish the chronologic order of events.

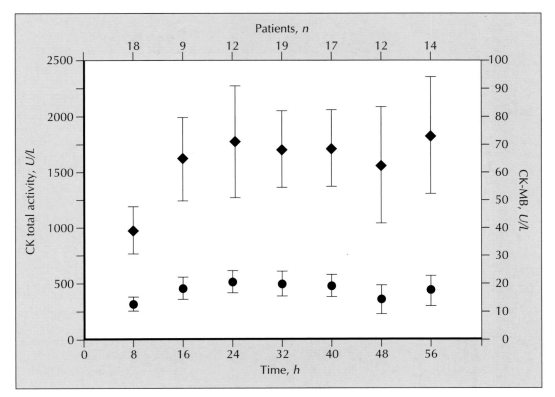

FIGURE 6-10. Mean levels (±SE) of total creatine kinase (CK) (*diamonds*) and the myocardial isoenzyme CK-MB (*circles*) in a group of patients with an acute cerebral event. The upper limits of normal for these values are 132 U/L and 6.6 U/L, respectively. CK peaked at 56 hours [32]. Further evidence of myocardial necrosis in association with acute cerebral events is this rise in serum CK and, more specifically, CK-MB levels. Elevations are seen in 93% of patients after severe head trauma [32,33]. In contrast to the rise in CK-MB seen in acute myocardial infarction, the levels after a neurologic event rise progressively, peaking on the third or fourth day, and may remain elevated (albeit only slightly) for several days [20,21]. The fact that this rise is late and persistent suggests a low-grade, subacute process compatible with myocytolysis at the cellular level. (*Adapted from* Hackenberry and coworkers [32]; with permission.)

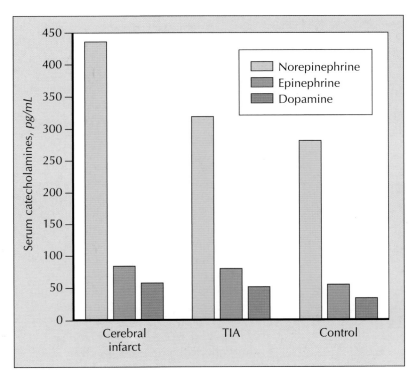

FIGURE 6-11. Rise in catecholamine levels in patients who had suffered a cerebral infarction (*n*=74) or a transient ischemic attack (TIA) (*n*=18) compared with a control group (*n*=33), after adjustments for age and blood pressure [34]. The mean adjusted norepinephrine concentration in the patients with stroke remained significantly higher, while epinephrine and dopamine did not increase as much. Elevations in serum catecholamines are associated with TIAs and cerebral infarcts [34] and are felt to be higher than those expected on the basis of age, presence of hypertension, stress, or severity of stroke [33]. The rise in catecholamines is most pronounced in the first few days after the stroke, with a gradual return to normal after 1 or 2 weeks [33,35,36]. With the recent improvement in catecholamine assay techniques, investigators can now analyze further the role of the sympathetic nervous system in the cardiac manifestations of acute cerebral events [11]. (*Adapted from* Myers and coworkers [34]; with permission.)

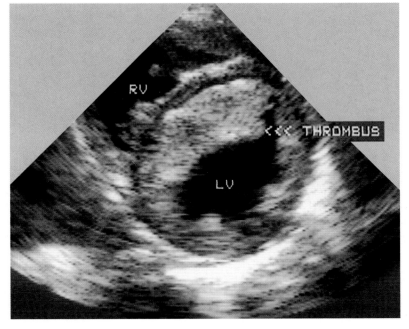

FIGURE 6-12. Echocardiogram from a patient with a subarachnoid hemorrhage. A mural thrombus (*arrowheads*) occupies a large portion of the ventricular cavity. Efforts to correlate the biochemical and histologic changes associated with acute central nervous system events have led to the review of echocardiographic findings in patients with subarachnoid hemorrhage. Left ventricular (LV) wall motion abnormalities have been noted in approximately one third of patients, none of whom had a previous history of cardiac disease. In addition, mural thrombi were described occasionally. The presence of wall motion abnormalities identifies a subset of patients with more severe neurologic disease and a higher mortality [13]. RV—right ventricle.

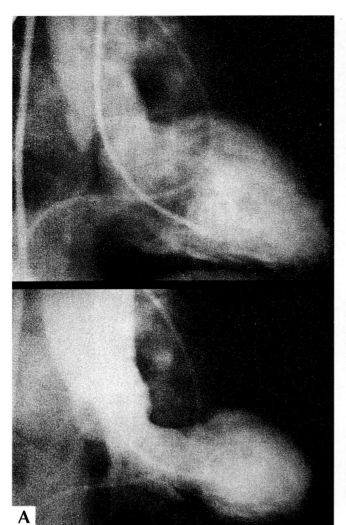

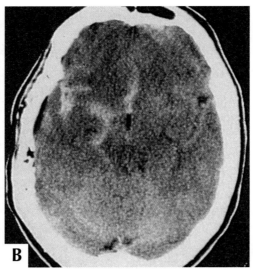

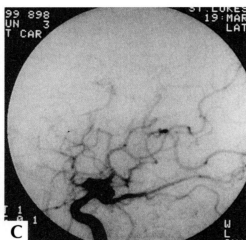

FIGURE 6-13. Left ventricular (LV) wall motion abnormalities associated with acute cerebrovascular events may not be permanent, as is evident in this case of a 64-year-old woman with no previous history of cardiac disease who presented with an acute change in mental status preceded by symptoms of nausea and vomiting [37]. Because of hypotension and elevated ST segments in leads I and aVL, with diffuse ST-segment and T-wave abnormalities in the precordial leads, right and left cardiac catheterization was carried out. Findings on hemodynamic and coronary angiography were normal; however, the left ventriculogram showed anterior, septal, and apical akinesis with an ejection fraction of 30% to 35% (**A**). Since her mental status remained abnormal, a head computed tomogram was obtained that revealed a subarachnoid hemorrhage (**B**). The source was identified on cerebral angiography as a right internal carotid aneurysm (**C**). After successful surgical repair, LV function returned to normal, as determined by echocardiography. (*Adapted from* Handlin and coworkers [37]; with permission.)

RESULTS OF THALLIUM SCANNING AS A FUNCTION OF ECG ABNORMALITY

ECG ABNORMALITY	POSITIVE (*n*=6)	NEGATIVE (*n*=13)
ST-T wave changes	2	2
Diffuse, deeply inverted T waves	2	4
Inverted T waves	2	6
Nonspecific*	1	4
Prolonged Q-T$_C$ interval†	0	1
Q waves	0	2
U waves		

*ST-segment depression or elevation of 25 to 50 μV in middle of ST segment across several leads.
†Corrected for heart rate.

FIGURE 6-14. Data from 19 patients suggesting that a positive thallium scan (present in six) correlates poorly with clinical history, electrocardiographic (ECG) pattern, and neurologic condition [14]. All 19 patients had recently suffered a subarachnoid hemorrhage. Although thallium defects and possibly ischemia are frequently observed after a subarachnoid bleed, no specific ECG abnormalities can be said to identify patients with a positive thallium scan. (*Adapted from* Szabo and coworkers [14]; with permission.)

CARDIAC PRESENTATION SUGGESTING POOR OUTCOME AFTER ACUTE NEUROLOGIC EVENT

Hypertension and bradycardia (Cushing's response) [38]

Sinus tachycardia [7]

Large, negative P wave in lead V_1 (P-mitrale) [32]

Nonspecific ST-segment and T-wave abnormalities [4]

"U" waves [39]

Prolongation of the Q-T interval [39]

Ventricular arrhythmias [4]

Elevation of creatine phosphokinase [2]

Echocardiographic wall motion abnormalities [13]

FIGURE 6-15. Although nonspecific, some of the cardiac and electrocardiographic (ECG) manifestations of acute cerebral events have been correlated with prognosis. Extensive ECG and echocardiographic changes probably indicate severe underlying neurologic disease and are markers of a poor outcome, although they may not be the initiating mechanism of death.

A. APPROACH TO THE PATIENT WITH ACUTE NEUROLOGIC SYMPTOMS

HISTORY	CARDIOVASCULAR PHYSICAL EXAMINATION
Symptoms of underlying cardiac disease predating neurologic event	Vital signs
Previous cardiac disease	Carotid pulses, upstroke and flow
Risk factors for CAD	CVP, pulmonary rales, or signs of CHF
Current cardiac medications	Heart sounds, gallops, or murmurs
Any substance abuse, including alcohol and cocaine	Embolic events (eg, petechiae)
	Peripheral pulses
	ECG (see panel B)

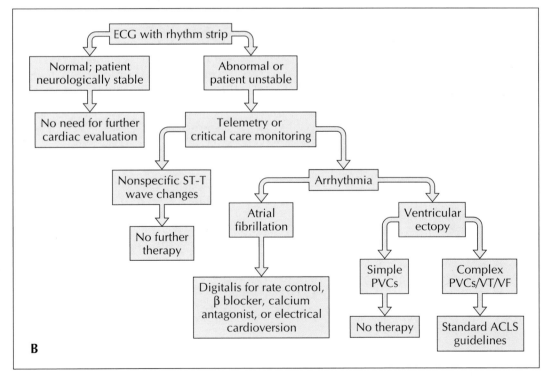

B

the degree to which the creatine phosphokinase MB fraction (CK-MB) is elevated may help to distinguish the origin of the initial event, particularly when the ECG is markedly abnormal and the patient is unable to give an adequate history. Second, given the transient nature of left ventricular dysfunction, an echocardiogram may yield limited information, as noted elsewhere in this chapter (see Fig. 6-13), but can supplement a history of antecedent heart failure. Furthermore, in patients with previously established ventricular dysfunction, the ejection fraction itself has prognostic value [41]. When both cardiac and neurologic diseases coexist, and when the etiology of the neurologic manifestation is unclear, an echocardiogram should be obtained to rule out an intracardiac source (eg, thrombus, valvular endocarditis). Finally, the best therapeutic approach to arrhythmias must include a thorough clinical evaluation.

If atrial fibrillation is compromising the patient's status, the ventricular rate can be controlled with digitalis, a β blocker (if no contraindications exist), or a calcium antagonist (eg, verapamil). Should these pharmacologic measures fail and acute decompensation ensue, electrical cardioversion can be employed. The therapy for complex ventricular arrhythmias (eg, ventricular tachycardia/fibrillation [VT/VF]) should follow advanced cardiac life support (ACLS) guidelines [42]. It should be recognized that these arrhythmias probably indicate significant underlying neurologic pathology and that in such cases the response to therapy may be limited. However, there is some evidence to suggest that early administration of β blockers can prevent myocardial damage in the presence of acute neurologic events [21,43]. CAD—coronary artery disease; CHF—congestive heart failure; CVP—central venous pressure; PVCs—premature ventricular contractions.

FIGURE 6-16. Approach to the cardiologic evaluation of a patient who presents with an acute cerebral event. Such an evaluation should serve only as a guide, since many of the cardiac diagnostic tools commonly employed may yield nonspecific findings that are not clinically significant. **A,** Patient history and cardiovascular physical examination. **B,** Electrocardiography (ECG).

Although the patient's clinical status, both neurologic and cardiac, is the best guide to management, several observations are worthy of mention. First, a myocardial infarction can mask as a stroke secondary to an acute reduction in cerebral blood flow [40]. Patterns and

NONMYOTONIC DYSTROPHIES

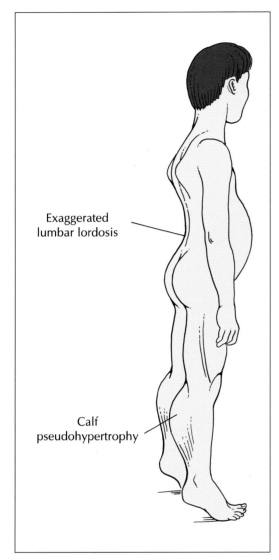

FIGURE 6-17. *Duchenne muscular dystrophy* is a progressive sex-linked disorder that affects myocardial muscle as well as skeletal muscle [44]. The population prevalence is 3/100,000. Clinical manifestations appear in the second year of life and consist of a clumsy, waddling gait, with early pseudohypertrophy of the calves and exaggerated lumbar lordosis. Weakness increases with age, requiring leg braces and ultimately resulting in the patient being wheelchair-bound [45]. Patients usually succumb to pulmonary complications and infection with dystrophy of respiratory muscles, although cardiac disease can also be the cause of sudden, unexpected death. (*Adapted from* Brooke [45]; with permission.)

Exaggerated
lumbar lordosis

Calf
pseudohypertrophy

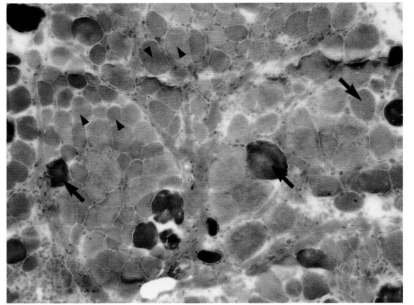

FIGURE 6-18. Skeletal muscle specimen showing an increase in connective tissue (stained blue) and variations in fiber size (*arrowheads*), with evidence of phagocytosis (*arrows*). Duchenne muscular dystrophy is caused by an abnormality of the dystrophin gene located at Xp21 [46]. (Gomori trichrome stain.) (*Adapted from* Hoffman and coworkers [46]; with permission.)

CARDIAC MANIFESTATIONS IN DUCHENNE MUSCULAR DYSTROPHY

Physical examination
  Systolic impulse at left sternal border
  Short midsystolic murmur at 2nd left ICS
  Loud P_2
Electrocardiogram
  Intra- and interatrial conduction defects
  Short P-R interval
  RAD and/or LPHB
  Tall right precordial R wave; increased R/S
    amplitude ratios
  Deep Q (I, aVL, and V_{5-6})
Arrhythmias
  Paroxysmal and inappropriate sinus
    tachycardia
  Atrial flutter
  PACs; intermittent/sustained atrial ectopic rhythms
  Simple and complex PVCs
Echocardiography (*see* Fig. 6-22)
  Cardiomyopathy (posterobasal segments)
  MVP
Thallium SPECT
  Perfusion defects (posteroapical wall)

FIGURE 6-19. Cardiac manifestations of Duchenne muscular dystrophy. An abnormally small antero-posterior chest diameter is responsible for the prominent systolic impulse at the left sternal edge. The systolic mitral murmur is caused by a definitive pathologic entity, *ie*, dystrophic papillary muscle and adjacent ventricular myocardium [47]. Persistent sinus tachycardia has long been described in Duchenne dystrophy [48]. Atrial conduction is abnormal, as evidenced by intra- and interatrial conduction abnormalities as well as atrial flutter. Atrioventricular (AV) conduction is accelerated, probably at the AV node. The QRS complex can be abnormal, with right ventricular delay and the rightward axis deviation (RAD) of a left posterior fascicular heart block (LPHB). Interest has focused on the abnormal precordial Q waves and an anterior shift in QRS forces. In patients with Duchenne muscular dystrophy, single-photon emission computed tomography (SPECT) using thallium-201 has shown solitary perfusion defects, which most commonly involve the posterior wall and less commonly, the apical wall. Since the plasma membrane is primarily affected in muscular dystrophy, altered sarcoplasmic permeability could lead to reduced thallium uptake and hence perfusion defects. Thus, LV fibrosis may be of significance in Duchenne dystrophy, and SPECT imaging may serve as a useful clinical screening tool [49]. ICS—intercostal space; MVP—mitral valve prolapse; P_2—pulmonic component of second heart sound; PACs—premature atrial contractions; PVCs—premature ventricular contractions.

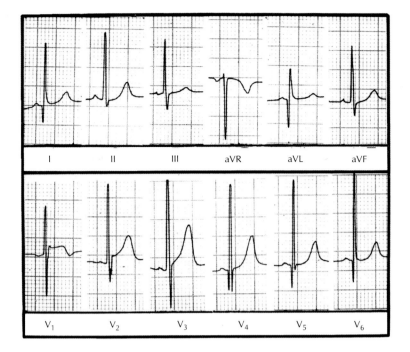

FIGURE 6-20. Typical electrocardiogram from a 10-year-old boy with Duchenne muscular dystrophy. The P-R interval is short (100 ms in lead II). Deep, narrow Q waves can be seen in leads I, aVL, and V$_{4-6}$, and the QRS precordial axis is shifted anteriorly. (*Adapted from* Perloff [48]; with permission.)

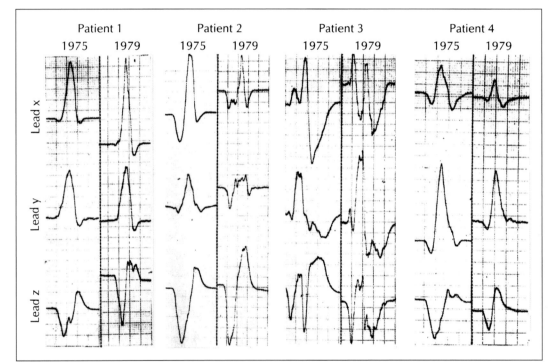

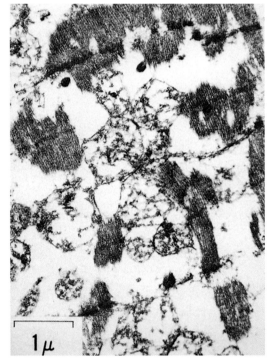

FIGURE 6-21. High-frequency notching on QRS complexes has been described in Duchenne muscular dystrophy, as is evident in these electrocardiograms from four different patients [50]. These tracings from x, y, and z leads are shown in pairs, taken 4 years apart, for each patient. Patients 2 and 3 both showed a marked increase in high-frequency notching, while patient 1 showed a less prominent increase. Patient 4 showed a decrease in notching despite an increase in disease severity. QRS notching increases with increasing severity of the disease until the terminal stages, when high-frequency notching tends to decrease. The source of the notching is not well known, but theories include Purkinje block and activation across rather than along myocardial fibers [51,52]. (*Adapted from* Ishikawa and coworkers [50]; with permission.)

FIGURE 6-22. Ultrastructure of a posterior papillary muscle in Duchenne muscular dystrophy showing multifocal and confluent areas of total loss of thick and thin myofilaments, resulting in a "moth-eaten" appearance (×10,000). Electron microscopic studies indicate that myofibrillar lysis with loss of thick and thin myofilaments represents the classic pathology in the cardiomyopathy of Duchenne dystrophy. Myocardial thinning and fibrosis are most prominent in the posterobasal wall of the left ventricle. The mitral valve prolapse reported in patients with Duchenne dystrophy appears to be caused by the same dystrophic changes seen in ventricular muscle and involves the papillary muscles. In postmortem studies, examination of valve leaflets, chordae tendineae, and annulus have failed to show any morphologic abnormalities [53]. (*Adapted from* Sanyal and coworkers [54]; with permission.)

CARDIAC MANIFESTATIONS IN BECKER MUSCULAR DYSTROPHY

ECG findings
  His bundle and infranodal conduction abnormalities with
  fascicular or complete heart block
  Pathologic Q waves in anterolateral leads
  Increased QRS voltage in right and middle precordial leads (V_{1-4})
  RVH or LVH
  Atrial arrhythmias
Anatomic findings
  Four-chamber cardiac dilatation
  Focal subendocardial fibrosis and fatty replacement of
  myocardium
  Absence of gross coronary lesions
  Systolic MVP

FIGURE 6-23. Cardiac manifestations of *Becker's muscular dystrophy.* In contrast to Duchenne dystrophy, the sex-linked muscular dystrophy described by Becker is characterized by a delayed age of onset and slower progression, so survival into middle age is not uncommon [45]. The incidence of cardiac abnormalities rises after adolescence and becomes more clinically significant during the third decade of life. As many as 50% of patients with Becker's dystrophy will develop some type of cardiac abnormality [15,55]. In addition, the rate of progression of cardiac disease does not always parallel the skeletal muscle involvement [16]. The cardiomyopathy can be fatal [44], and these patients are now considered suitable candidates for cardiac transplantation [16]. LVH—left ventricular hypertrophy; MVP—mitral valve prolapse; RVH—right ventricular hypertrophy.

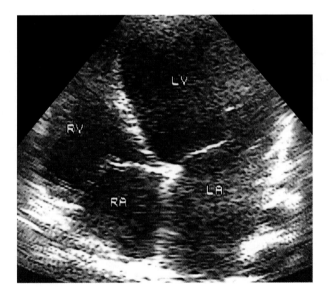

FIGURE 6-24. Echocardiogram from a 26-year-old man with Becker's muscular dystrophy showing four-chamber dilatation, with an ejection fraction of 10%. The patient presented at age 11 years with classic motor difficulties on climbing stairs and standing up from a sitting position. He did relatively well until age 24, when he presented with fatigue and dyspnea on exertion. Clinically, he was in heart failure with dilatation of all four chambers and was treated with digoxin, diuretics, and angiotensin-converting enzyme inhibitors. The symptoms of failure subsided, and he remained functional for 2 years until he noted increasing fatigue both with activity and at rest, early satiety, and orthopnea. He is currently listed as a candidate for cardiac transplantation. LA—left atrium; LV—left ventricle; RA—right atrium; RV—right ventricle.

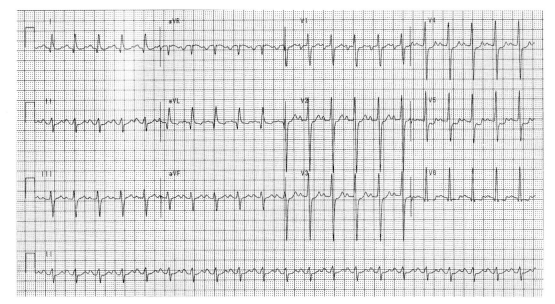

FIGURE 6-25. Electrocardiogram from the patient described in Fig. 6-25 showing sinus tachycardia. There is left axis deviation with voltage criteria for left ventricular hypertrophy and concomitant ST-segment and T-wave changes. Prominent Q waves can be seen in leads I and aVL. The left atrium is enlarged, as evidenced by a prominent negative component of the P wave in lead V₁.

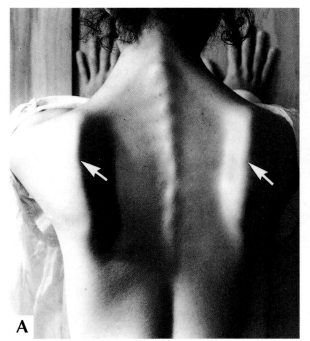
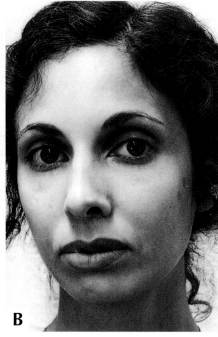

A **B**

FIGURE 6-26. *Facioscapulohumeral muscular dystrophy* (Landouzy-Déjèrine) is inherited as an autosomal-dominant disorder with an incidence of 3 to 10 per million. The clinical presentation can vary widely, ranging from mild facial muscle weakness to more progressive weakness of the shoulders and arms (**A**), resulting in winging of the scapulae (*arrows*). The typical myopathic facies shows dimpling at the corners of the mouth, resembling the enigmatic "Mona Lisa smile" (**B**) [56]. (*Adapted from* Stevenson and coworkers [56]; with permission.)

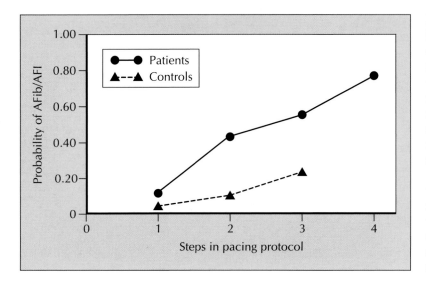

FIGURE 6-27. Atrial fibrillation/flutter is much more easily provoked by atrial stimulation in patients with facioscapulohumeral muscular dystrophy than in a control group [56]. The cumulative incidence of initiation of atrial fibrillation (AFib) or flutter (AFl) for each step in the pacing protocol is shown for patients and controls. Steps 1 to 3 involve high right atrial pacing (at cycle lengths of 600, 500, and 400 ms), while step 4 involves pacing at additional sites in the right atrium at the same cycle lengths. The most worrisome of the cardiac manifestations of facioscapulohumeral muscular dystrophy is atrial standstill or paralysis, as described in early reports of this disease [56,57]. Criteria for the diagnosis of atrial paralysis include loss of P waves, atrial immobility on fluoroscopy, and absence of an atrial response to direct electrical stimulation. More recently, however, there is reason to believe that the permanent atrial standstill previously reported may have been associated with the phenotypically similar Emery-Dreifuss syndrome [56]. (*Adapted from* Stevenson and coworkers [56]; with permission.)

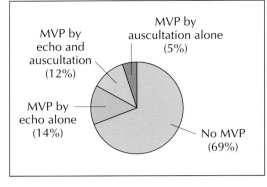

FIGURE 6-28. Cardiac manifestations of *Erb's limb-girdle dystrophy*. This type of dystrophy is characterized by progressive weakness of the hips and shoulders until the patient becomes wheelchair-bound. The disorder is inherited as an autosomal-recessive trait in segregated populations [45]. Mild manifestations of the syndrome often make definitive diagnosis difficult. Involvement of the heart is infrequent and not severe and is manifest primarily by arrhythmias. Rare sporadic cases of cardiomyopathy have been reported [15]. AV—atrioventricular. (*Adapted from* Perloff [15]; with permission.)

FIGURE 6-29. *Charcot-Marie-Tooth disease*, also known as peroneal muscular atrophy, is characterized by distal leg weakness and involvement of the muscles innervated by the peroneal nerve. Among 68 patients with a diagnosis of Charcot-Marie-Tooth disease, palpitations were the most frequent cardiac complaint (present in 22%); three of these patients had documented mitral valve prolapse (MVP) [58]. In 5% of the patients, the presence of MVP was based on auscultatory evidence alone. Prolapse was diagnosed by echocardiography in 26% and by both echocardiography and auscultation in 12%. Left anterior hemiblock was present in only 4% of the group, ST-segment changes in 7.5%, and supraventricular arrhythmias in 3%. Electrocardiographic (ECG) abnormalities, however, were infrequent in patients under the age of 50 and were not more frequent in patients older than 50 when compared with a normal population [58]. Currently, no firm association has been established between the presence of Charcot-Marie-Tooth disease and cardiomyopathy. There appears to be no correlation between disease severity and cardiac abnormalities (such as MVP) and ECG changes [59]. (*Adapted from* Isner and coworkers [58]; with permission.)

FIGURE 6-30. Cardiac manifestations of *Emery-Dreifuss syndrome*. This syndrome has been recognized as a distinct sex-linked neuromuscular disease associated with progressive involvement of the humeral and/or scapular muscles as well as weakness of the peroneal muscles. Cardiac involvement is common and places the patient at risk for sudden death, presumably owing to complete heart block [45]. The hallmark of such involvement has been described as atrial paralysis [60]. AV—atrioventricular.

MYOTONIC DYSTROPHY

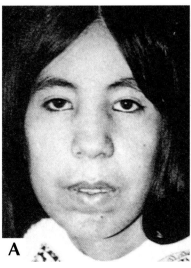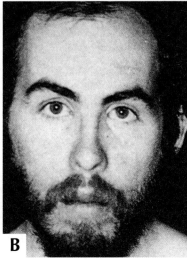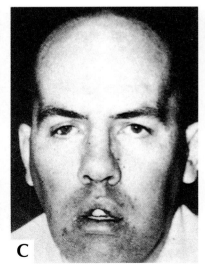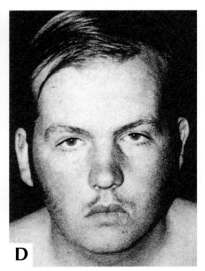

FIGURE 6-31. Myotonic dystrophy, originally described by Steinert in 1909 [61], is inherited as an autosomal-dominant disorder at a prevalence of 3 to 5 per 1000 and is thus a relatively common neuromuscular disorder. **A** through **D,** The syndrome consists of weakness of the flexor muscles of the neck, giving the face a "sagging" appearance. Muscle stimulation provokes the typical myotonic response. Frontal baldness and premature graying of the hair have also been described [45]. (*Adapted from* Brooke [45]; with permission.)

CARDIAC MANIFESTATIONS OF MYOTONIC DYSTROPHY

Involvement of specialized tissues
  Sinus node
  Conduction system (AV node, His-Purkinje system)
  Arrhythmias
Involvement of the myocardium
  Dystrophy (uncommon)
  Myotonia (unproven) (mitral valve prolapse)

FIGURE 6-32. Cardiac manifestations of myotonic dystrophy. Cardiac involvement in these patients is well known and is reflected primarily by abnormalities in conduction, the His-Purkinje system being the primary site of involvement [62]. Death from a cardiac cause is almost always sudden, in the form of complete atrioventricular (AV) block. However, ventricular arrhythmias as the cause of sudden death cannot be totally overlooked [63]. Cardiac muscle involvement is less common but has been described in the form of a dystrophy involving all four chambers. Myocardial dystrophy may serve as the site of both atrial and ventricular arrhythmias but rarely causes heart failure. (*Adapted from* Perloff and coworkers [62]; with permission.)

ABNORMAL ECG IN MYOTONIC DYSTROPHY BY AGE AND SEVERITY

| | DISEASE SEVERITY | | | |
PATIENT AGE, Y	MILD (n=6)	MODERATE (n=12)	SEVERE (n=23)	TOTAL (n=41)
29	2	3	3	8
30–39	2	2	6	10
40–49	2	5	2	9
50–59	0	2	12	14

FIGURE 6-33. Distribution of 41 patients with myotonic dystrophy and abnormal electrocardiograms (ECGs) by age and severity [64]. Early published reports concerning myotonic dystrophy noted the presence of a slow pulse. It was not until ECG became routine, however, that the associated cardiologic manifestations were recognized. The proportion of patients with ECG abnormalities increases with increasing disease severity. In one series, the ECG was found to be abnormal in 35% of patients with mild disease, 50% with moderate disease, and 96% with severe disease. (*Adapted from* Olofsson and coworkers [64]; with permission.)

FIGURE 6-34. Electrocardiogram (ECG) showing QS in leads V$_{1-3}$ and first-degree atrioventricular block (P-R interval, 0.21 s) in a patient with myotonic dystrophy. The most common ECG abnormalities in this condition include prolongation of the P-R interval and QRS complex and left fascicular block, which indicate involvement of the His-Purkinje system. Arrhythmias include atrial fibrillation, atrial flutter, and premature ventricular beats. They are often associated with more severe stages of the neuromuscular disease and may indicate myocardial dysfunction. Ambulatory Holter monitoring is in order when conduction abnormalities are observed on the resting ECG [65]. (*Adapted from* Perloff and coworkers [62]; with permission.)

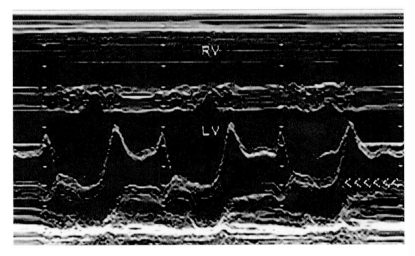

FIGURE 6-35. Echocardiogram in mitral valve prolapse (MVP) associated with myotonic dystrophy showing "bowing" motion of the posterior leaflet (*arrowheads*). Various myopathies have been associated with this disorder. Whether a true association exists between the presence of MVP and a myopathy or whether it is purely a chance occurrence is still in question. At least two families have been reported with concomitant myotonic dystrophy and MVP [17,66]. Because both entities have been associated with arrhythmias, their coexistence may identify a group at high risk for significant arrhythmias and/or syncope. LV—left ventricle; RV—right ventricle.

CARDIAC FINDINGS IN FA

	PATIENTS WITH FA (n=10)	CONTROL SUBJECTS (n=10)	P VALUE
Heart rate, *bpm*	102±17	76±12	<0.001
Blood pressure, *mm Hg*	114±9/73±9	122±8/73±5	<0.05/NS
IVS, *mm*	13±2	8±1	<0.001
LVPW, *mm*	13±3	8±1	<0.001
Aortic diameter, *mm*	23±4	24±3	NS
Left atrium, *mm*	27±5	27±2	NS
EDD, *mm*	35±6	47±6	<0.001
ESD, *mm*	22±6	32±5	<0.001
% change in D*	40±9	33±5	<0.05

*Percent change in LV minor axis diameter with systole.

FIGURE 6-36. Results of a study comparing 10 patients with Friedreich's ataxia (FA) with 10 healthy control subjects in terms of the functional, morphologic, and histologic characteristics of the heart [67]. FA is a spinocerebellar degenerative disease inherited as an autosomal-recessive trait [46]. Onset is usually in the first or second decade of life. It is more common in males and progresses relentlessly, with worsening of ataxia and muscle weakness of all extremities. Heart disease is present in 50% to 90% of patients by the time of their death [68]. Although cardiac involvement may be occult, a combination of electrocardiography and echocardiography will identify 95% of patients with such abnormalities [69]. Whether the cardiac abnormalities described in FA are related to the genetic abnormality or to the spinocerebellar degeneration is not entirely clear [70]. Compared with control subjects, patients with ataxia have an increased heart rate and decreased blood pressure. In addition, the left ventricular walls were hypertrophied in a symmetric fashion, resulting in a small left ventricular cavity. However, the ventricular walls moved normally, and systolic anterior motion of the mitral valve, previously described in other studies, was not evident. Of interest, asymmetric septal hypertrophy, formerly noted by others [71], was not present in this series of patients. EDD—end-diastolic diameter; ESD—end-systolic diameter; IVS—interventricular septum; LVPW—left ventricular posterior wall. (*Adapted from* Unverferth and coworkers [67]; with permission.)

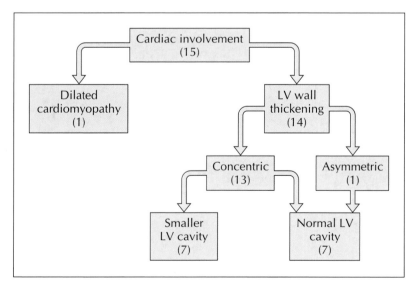

FIGURE 6-37. Summary of echocardiographic findings in 15 of 25 patients with Friedreich's ataxia (FA) who demonstrated some cardiac abnormality [70]. Since several groups of investigators had reported asymmetric septal hypertrophy in patients with FA [67,68], these patients were studied in order to better categorize this particular cardiac anomaly. Only one patient had evidence of dilated cardiomyopathy. Of the remaining 14, 13 had concentric left ventricular (LV) hypertrophy and only one had asymmetric dimensions. Thus, cardiac manifestations of FA do not seem commonly to involve asymmetric septal hypertrophy [69]. (*Adapted from* Gottdiener and coworkers [70]; with permission.)

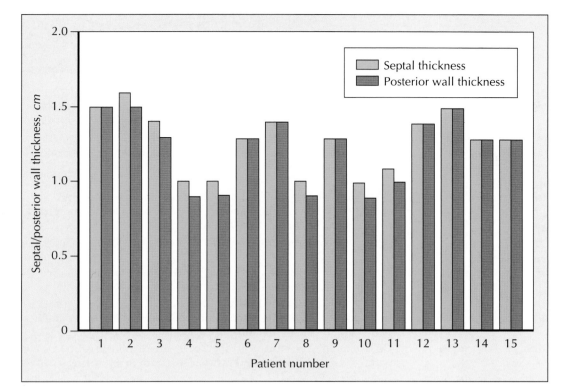

FIGURE 6-38. Further evidence of the type of cardiomyopathy (asymmetric versus symmetric) seen in patients with Friedreich's ataxia (FA) [72]. Fifteen patients with a known diagnosis of FA, all of whom had either electrocardiographic or echocardiographic abnormalities, were studied. Sixty-seven percent had hypertrophic cardiomyopathy, defined as septal and posterior wall thickness exceeding 1.3 cm, which was symmetric in all cases. Only one patient had paradoxic septal motion with a diffuse cardiomyopathic process. In all the patients, the septal wall/posterior wall ratio was approximately 1.0. One patient also had mitral valve prolapse. (*Adapted from* Pasternac and coworkers [72]; with permission.)

CATECHOLAMINE LEVELS AND WALL THICKNESS IN FA

STAGE OF FA	INCREASED FREE CATECHOLAMINES/ENHANCED ADRENERGIC FUNCTION, n/n					INCREASED WALL THICKNESS, n/n
	NE	E	NE+E	DOPAMINE	TOTAL	
0 (n=3)	1	1	—	—	2/3	2/3
I (n=4)	1	—	2	—	3/4	4/4
II (n=9)	2	1	—	1	4/9	6/9
III (n=4)	3	—	1	—	4/4	4/4
IV (n=3)	1	—	1	—	2/3	2/3
Total (n=23)	8	2	4	1	15/23 (65%)	18/23 (78%)

FIGURE 6-39. Inappropriate sinus tachycardia has been described in patients with Friedreich's ataxia (FA). Since both concentric left ventricular (LV) hypertrophy and sinus tachycardia may be due in part to elevated catecholamines, 23 patients with FA of varying severity were classified according to degree of severity (stages 0 to IV). These patients were then compared with a control group of 35 subjects. Fifteen of the 23 patients (65%) showed definitive increases in adrenergic function. In 12 of the 23 (52%), the increase in catecholamines primarily involved norepinephrine. In the 12 patients who had both enhanced adrenergic function and LV hypertrophy, disease severity ranged from 0 to 4. Increases in catecholamine levels were more prominent in patients with severe neurologic disease. Only one patient had both normal catecholamine levels and normal wall thickness. Four patients had enhanced adrenergic function without LV hypertrophy. E—epinephrine; NE—norepinephrine. (*Adapted from* Pasternac and coworkers [73]; with permission.)

We gratefully acknowledge the invaluable assistance of
Howard Warner, MD, Bruce Goldman, MD, Geraldo Torres, MD,
and Ray Gonzales, Echo Tech, who donated figures from their personal files.

REFERENCES

1. Yamour BJ, Sridharan MR, Rice JF, *et al.*: Electrocardiographic changes in cerebrovascular hemorrhage. *Am Heart J* 1980, 99:294–300.

2. Dimant J, Grob D: Electrocardiographic changes and myocardial damage in patients with acute cerebrovascular accidents. *Stroke* 1977, 8:448–455.

3. Lavy S, Yaar I, Melamed E, *et al.*: The effect of acute stroke on cardiac functions as observed in an intensive stroke care unit. *Stroke* 1974, 5:775–780.

4. VanderArk GD: Cardiovascular changes with acute subdural hematoma. *Surg Neurol* 1975, 3:305–308.

5. Stolar I, Hsu I, Katz R, *et al.*: P wave changes in intracerebral hemorrhage: clinical, echocardiographic, and CT scan correlation. *Am Heart J* 1984, 107:784–785.

6. Eisalo A, Perasalo J, Halonen PI: Electrocardiographic abnormalities and some laboratory findings in patients with subarachnoid hemorrhage. *Br Heart J* 1972, 34:217–226.

7. Melin J, Fogelholm R: Electrocardiographic findings in subarachnoid hemorrhage. *Acta Med Scand* 1983, 213:5–8.

8. Hunt D, McRae C, Zapf P: Electrocardiographic and serum enzyme changes in subarachnoid hemorrhage. *Am Heart J* 1969, 77:479–488.

9. Tropp GJ, Manning GW: Electrocardiographic changes simulating myocardial ischemia and infarction associated with spontaneous intracranial hemorrhage. *Circulation* 1960, 22:25–38.

10. Kennedy FB, Pozen TJ, Gabelman EH, *et al.*: Stroke intensive care— an appraisal. *Am Heart J* 1970, 80:188–196.

11. Norris JW: Effects of cerebrovascular lesions on the heart. *Neurol Clin* 1983, 1:87–101.

12. Reichenbach D, Benditt EP: Myofibrillar degeneration: a response of the myocardial cell to injury. *Arch Pathol* 1968, 85:189–199.

13. Pollick C, Cujec B, Parker S, *et al.*: Left ventricular wall motion abnormalities in subarachnoid hemorrhage: an echocardiographic study. *J Am Coll Cardiol* 1988, 12:600– 605.

14. Szabo MD, Crosby G, Hurford WE, *et al.*: Myocardial perfusion following acute subarachnoid hemorrhage in patients with an abnormal electrocardiogram. *Anesth Analg* 1993, 76:253–258.

15. Perloff JK: The heart in neuromuscular disease. *Curr Probl Cardiol* 1986, 11:513–557.

16. Quinlivan RM, Dubowitz V: Cardiac transplantation in Becker muscular dystrophy. *Neuromuscul Disord* 1992, 2:165–167.

17. Strasberg B, Kanakis C, Dhingra RC, *et al.*: Myotonia dystrophica and mitral valve prolapse. *Chest* 1980, 78:845–848.

18. Oppenheimer SM, Cechetto DF, Hachinski VC: Cerebrogenic cardiac arrhythmias. *Arch Neurol* 1990, 47:513–519.

19. Melville KI, Blum B, Shister HE, *et al.*: Cardiac ischemic changes and arrhythmias induced by hypothalamic stimulation. *Am J Cardiol* 1963, 12:781–791.

20. Hunt D, Gore I: Myocardial lesions following experimental intracranial hemorrhage: prevention with propranolol. *Am Heart J* 1972, 83:232–236.

21. Greenhoot JH, Reichenbach DD: Cardiac injury and subarachnoid hemorrhage: a clinical, pathological, and physiological correlation. *J Neurosurg* 1969, 30:521–531.

22. Wasserman F, Choquette G, Cassinelli R, *et al.*: Electrocardiographic observation in patients with cerebrovascular accidents. *Am J Med Sci* 1956, 231:502–510.

23. Kolin A, Norris JW, Hachinski VC: Myocardial lesions in acute stroke: a pathological study. *Can J Neurol Sci* 1980, 7:321–328.

24. Koskelo P, Punsar S, Sipila W: Subendocardial hemorrhage and ECG changes in intracerebral bleeding. *BMJ* 1964, 1:1479–1480.

25. Reichenbach DD, Benditt EP: Catecholamines and cardiomyopathy: the pathogenesis and potential importance of myofibrillar degeneration. *Hum Pathol* 1970, 1:125–148.

26. Yanowitz F, Preston JB, Abildskov JA: Possible role of unilateral changes in sympathetic tone in the production of neurogenic electrocardiographic abnormalities [abstract]. *Circulation* 1965, 31/32(suppl II):223.

27. Verrier RL, Thompson PL, Lown B: Ventricular vulnerability during sympathetic stimulation: role of heart rate and blood pressure. *Cardiovasc Res* 1974, 8:602–610.

28. Einbrodt: Akademie der Wissenschaften (Wien). Sitzungsbedichte 1859, 38:345-359.

29. Lown B, Verrier RL: Neural activity and ventricular fibrillation. *N Engl J Med* 1976, 294:1165–1170.

30. Kolman BS, Verrier RL, Lown B: The effect of vagus nerve stimulation upon vulnerability of the canine ventricle: role of sympathetic-parasympathetic interactions. *Circulation* 1975, 52:578–585.

31. Goldstein DS: The electrocardiogram in stroke: relationship to pathophysiological type and comparison with prior tracings. *Stroke* 1979, 10:253–259.

32. Hackenberry LE, Miner ME, Rea GL, *et al.*: Biochemical evidence of myocardial injury after severe head trauma. *Crit Care Med* 1982, 10:641–644.

33. Norris JW, Hachinski VC, Myers MG, *et al.*: Serum cardiac enzymes in stroke. *Stroke* 1979, 10:548–553.

34. Myers MG, Norris JW, Hachinski VC, *et al.*: Plasma norepinephrine in stroke. *Stroke* 1981, 12:200–204.

35. Kanda T, Gotoh F, Yamamato M, *et al.*: Serum dopamine beta-hydroxylase activity in acute stroke. *Stroke* 1979, 10:168–173.

36. Meyer JS, Stoica E, Pascu I, *et al.*: Catecholamine concentrations in CSF and plasma of patients with cerebral infarction and hemorrhage. *Brain* 1973, 96:277–288.

37. Handlin LR, Kindred LH, Beauchamp GD, *et al.*: Reversible left ventricular dysfunction after subarachnoid hemorrhage. *Am Heart J* 1993, 126:235–240.

38. Schneider RC: Craniocerebral trauma. In *Correlative Neurosurgery*, 2nd ed. Edited by Kahn EA, Crosby EC, Schneider RC, *et al.*. Springfield, IL: Charles C Thomas; 1969:533–596.

39. Cruickshank JM, Neil-Dwyer G, Brice J: Electrocardiographic changes and their prognostic significance in subarachnoid hemorrhage. *J Neurol Neurosurg Psychiatry* 1974, 37:755–759.

40. Bean WB: Masquerade of myocardial infarction. *Lancet* 1977, 1:1044–1045.

41. Sanz G, Castaner A, Betriu A, *et al.*: Determinants of prognosis in survivors of myocardial infarction. *N Engl J Med* 1982, 306:1065–1069.

42. Emergency Cardiac Care Committee and Subcommittees, American Heart Association: Guidelines for cardiopulmonary resuscitation and emergency cardiac care. *JAMA* 1992, 268:2171–2302.

43. Neil-Dwyer G, Walter P, Cruickshank JM, *et al.*: Effect of propranolol and phentolamine on myocardial necrosis after subarachnoid hemorrhage. *BMJ* 1978, 2:990–992.

44. Perloff JK, de Leon AC Jr, O'Doherty D: The cardiomyopathy of progressive muscular dystrophy. *Circulation* 1966, 33:625–648.

45. Brooke MH: *A Clinician's View of Neuromuscular Diseases*, 2nd ed. Baltimore: Williams and Wilkins; 1986.

46. Hoffman EP, Brown RH Jr, Kunkel LM: Dystrophin: the protein product of the Duchenne muscular dystrophy locus. *Cell* 1987, 51:919–928.

47. Sanyal SK, Johnson WW, Dische MR, *et al*.: Dystrophic degeneration of papillary muscle and ventricular myocardium. *Circulation* 1980, 62:430–438.

48. Perloff JK: Cardiac rhythm and conduction in Duchenne's muscular dystrophy: prospective study of 20 patients. *J Am Coll Cardiol* 1984, 3:1263–1267.

49. Yamamoto S, Sotobata I, Indo T, *et al*.: Evaluation of myocardial involvement in muscular dystrophy with thallium-201 emission computed tomography. *Kaku Igako* 1986, 23:773–782.

50. Ishikawa K, Shirato C, Yotsukura M, *et al*.: Sequential changes in high frequency notches QRS complexes in progressive muscular dystrophy of the Duchenne type—a 3-year follow-up study. *J Electrocardiol* 1982, 15:23–30.

51. Oppenheimer BS, Rothchild MS: Electrocardiographic changes associated with myocardial involvement. *JAMA* 1917, 69:429–431.

52. VanderArk CR, Reynolds EW: Genesis of high frequency notching of QRS complexes in vivo cardiac model. *Circulation* 1975, 51:257–262.

53. Nigro G, Cosmi LI, Politano L, *et al*.: The incidence and evolution of cardiomyopathy in Duchenne muscular dystrophy. *Int J Cardiol* 1990, 26:271–277.

54. Sanyal SK, Johnson WW, Thapar MK, *et al*.: An ultrastructural basis for electrocardiographic alterations associated with Duchenne's progressive muscular dystrophy. *Circulation* 1978, 57:1122–1129.

55. Vrints C, Mercelis R, Vanagt E, *et al*.: Cardiac manifestations of Becker-type muscular dystrophy. *Acta Cardiol* 1983, 38:479–486.

56. Stevenson WG, Perloff JK, Weiss JN, *et al*.: Facioscapulohumeral muscular dystrophy: evidence for selective, genetic electrophysiologic cardiac involvement. *J Am Coll Cardiol* 1990, 15:292–299.

57. Baldwin BJ, Talley RC, Johnson C, *et al*.: Permanent paralysis of the atrium in a patient with facioscapulohumeral muscular dystrophy. *Am J Cardiol* 1973, 31:649–653.

58. Isner JM, Hawley RJ, Weintraub AM, *et al*.: Cardiac findings in Charcot-Marie-Tooth disease. *Arch Intern Med* 1979, 139:1161–1165.

59. Dyck PJ, Swanson CJ, Nishimura RA, *et al*.: Cardiomyopathy in patients with hereditary motor and sensory neuropathy. *Mayo Clin Proc* 1987, 62:672–675.

60. Dickey RP, Ziter FA, Smith RA: Emery-Dreifuss muscular dystrophy. *J Pediatr* 1984, 104:555–559.

61. Steinert H: Uber das klinische und anatomische Bild des Muskelschwundes der Myotoniker. *Dtsch Z Nervenh* 1909, 37:38.

62. Perloff JK, Stevenson WG, Roberts NK, *et al*.: Cardiac involvement in myotonic muscular dystrophy (Steinert's disease): a prospective study of 25 patients. *Am J Cardiol* 1984, 54:1074–1081.

63. Grigg LE, Chan W, Mond HG, *et al*.: Ventricular tachycardia and sudden death in myotonic dystrophy: clinical, electrophysiologic and pathologic features. *J Am Coll Cardiol* 1985, 6:254–256.

64. Olofsson B-O, Forsberg H, Andersson S, *et al*.: Electrocardiographic findings in myotonic dystrophy. *Br Heart J* 1988, 59:47–52.

65. Forsberg H, Olofsson B-O, Andersson S, *et al*.: Twenty-four-hour electrocardiographic study in myotonic dystrophy. *Cardiology* 1988, 75:241–249.

66. Winters SJ, Schreiner B, Griggs RC, *et al*.: Familial mitral valve prolapse and myotonic dystrophy. *Ann Intern Med* 1976, 85:19–22.

67. Unverferth DV, Schmidt WR, Baker PB, *et al*.: Morphologic and functional characteristics of the heart in Friedreich's ataxia. *Am J Med* 1987, 82:5–9.

68. Sutton MGS, Olukotun AY, Tajik AJ, *et al*.: Left ventricular function in Friedreich's ataxia. An echocardiographic study. *Br Heart J* 1980, 44:309–316.

69. Child JS, Perloff JK, Bach PM: Cardiac involvement in Friedreich's ataxia. *J Am Coll Cardiol* 1986, 7:1370–1377.

70. Gottdiener JS, Hawley RJ, Maron BJ, *et al*.: Characteristics of the cardiac hypertrophy in Friedreich's ataxia. *Am Heart J* 1982, 103:525–531.

71. Smith ER, Sangalang VE, Heffernan LP, *et al*.: Hypertrophic cardiomyopathy: the heart disease of Friedreich's ataxia. *Am Heart J* 1977, 94:428–434.

72. Pasternac A, Krol R, Petitclerc C, *et al*.: Hypertrophic cardiomyopathy in Friedreich's ataxia: symmetric or asymmetric? *J Canad Sci Neurol* 1980, 7:379–382.

73. Pasternac A, Wagniart P, Olivenstein R, *et al*.: Increased plasma catecholamines in patients with Friedreich's ataxia. *J Canad Sci Neurol* 1982, 9:195–203.

ALCOHOL AND HEART DISEASE

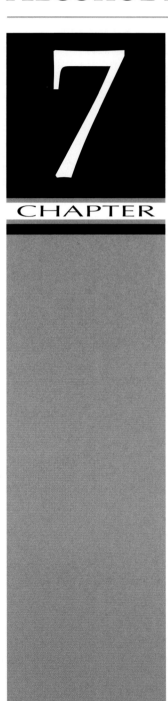

7

CHAPTER

Jonathan R. Lindner

Chronic, excessive alcohol intake has numerous cardiovascular manifestations that are largely nonspecific. These may result from the direct toxic effects of alcohol as well as from harmful additives, associated nutritional deficiencies, and electrolyte imbalances. The incidence of alcoholic cardiovascular disease has been difficult to estimate owing to patient denial, failure of clinicians to elicit a complete social history, and the lack of specific characteristic features, essentially making the diagnosis of these disorders one of exclusion.

The *dilated, congestive cardiomyopathy* associated with alcohol abuse is thought to be due to the direct toxic effects of alcohol and its metabolites, such as acetaldehyde. Although detrimental neurohumoral responses are also thought to contribute to the pathogenesis, their exact mechanism of action remains unclear. Few pathologic and clinical features distinguish alcoholic cardiomyopathy from idiopathic, postpartum, or other cardiomyopathies, although certain laboratory and physical findings may suggest a history of significant alcohol abuse. In the past, epidemics of a more fulminant form of cardiomyopathy have been attributed to the addition of cobalt salts to beer.

Arrhythmias are common in patients with or without overt cardiomyopathy. These include atrial arrhythmias, ventricular arrhythmias, and, rarely, conduction disorders. Atrial arrhythmias, especially atrial fibrillation, may be seen after a binge of heavy drinking, even in persons without a history of chronic alcohol consumption. This phenomenon is widely referred to as the "holiday heart syndrome." Alcohol intake is also associated with hypertension, which is thought to result from several direct vascular effects and sympathetic nervous system activation. The most often recognized nutritional disorder associated with alcoholism is beriberi, manifested as peripheral vasodilation and high-output heart failure. Other dietary factors, such as selenium deficiency, may play a role in the development of congestive cardiomyopathy.

Complete abstinence may reverse the signs and symptoms of congestive heart failure in patients with alcoholic cardiomyopathy. Abstinence also dramatically ameliorates the associated arrhythmias and hypertension, while thiamine replacement essentially reverses beriberi heart disease. Although recent studies have shown that moderate alcohol intake can have a beneficial effect on lipid profiles and risk for myocardial infarction, any recommendations regarding this preventive strategy must be tempered by knowledge of the multitude of possible detrimental effects associated with heavy alcohol use.

ALCOHOL AND THE HEART

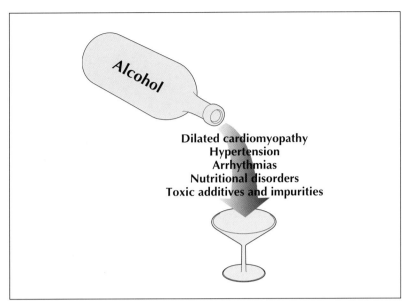

FIGURE 7-1. Cardiovascular manifestations of chronic alcohol abuse. Ethanol has multiple detrimental effects on the cardiovascular system. Alcohol consumption is one of the most frequent identifiable causes of dilated cardiomyopathy, accounting for up to 20% to 30% of cases in certain US populations [1]. Toxic impurities or additives, such as cobalt (to stabilize the foam in beer), have been known to precipitate a more severe, fulminant form of heart failure. Hypertension is both an acute and a chronic effect of heavy alcohol use, and dramatic elevations in blood pressure may occur on withdrawal [2]. Arrhythmias may be seen with or without cardiomyopathy and are most often supraventricular, although they may be of ventricular origin, especially during withdrawal. Nutritional disorders associated with the alcoholic syndrome, such as the thiamine deficiency syndrome beriberi, are also important in the genesis of heart failure.

DILATED CARDIOMYOPATHY

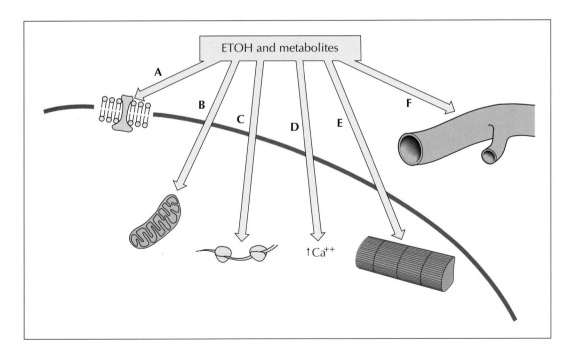

FIGURE 7-2. Pathophysiology of dilated cardiomyopathy. Although the direct effects of alcohol (ETOH) and its metabolite acetaldehyde are not completely understood, several possible mechanisms have been described. **A,** Membranes are damaged and phospholipid composition is altered, while sodium/potassium ATPase and other important cell surface transporters are inhibited. **B,** Mitochondrial function is impaired; important examples of this are decreased fatty acid oxidation and the uncoupling of oxidative phosphorylation [4]. **C,** Myocardial protein synthesis is depressed [3]. **D,** The flux of calcium increases and is thought to result from inhibition of the calcium-ATPase pump [3]. **E,** There is interference with calcium-modulated excitation-contraction coupling [5]. **F,** Various detrimental neurohumoral events are also known to ensue [2].

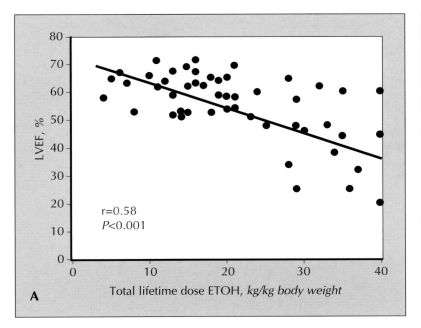

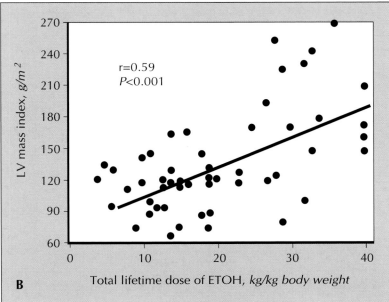

A

B

FIGURE 7-3. Correlation between cumulative alcohol (ETOH) intake and cardiomyopathy [6]. **A,** Myocardial dysfunction in alcoholics, as measured by echocardiography and technetium radionuclide angiocardiography, is largely dependent on the cumulative dose of ethanol. For all patients with depressed left ventricular ejection fraction (LVEF), etiologies of heart failure other than alcohol were excluded. **B,** LV mass also correlates with total lifetime consumption of alcohol. Cardiac decompensation typically occurs in people 30 to 55 years of age who have ingested at least 80 g of alcohol on a near-daily basis for 10 years or longer [7].

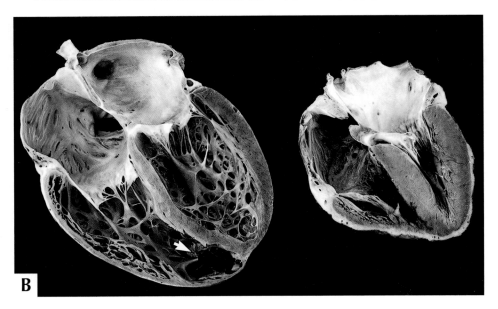

A

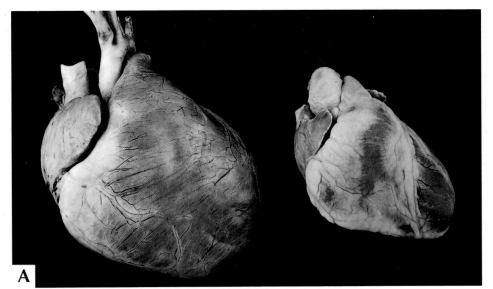

B

FIGURE 7-4. The macroscopic pathologic appearance of a normal heart (*right*) and a cardiomyopathic heart due to alcohol abuse. **A,** Anterior view showing an enlarged, globular heart of alcoholic cardiomyopathy compared with a normal specimen (*right*). **B,** All chambers are dilated, and although wall thickness is normal, ventricular mass is increased. A mural thrombus can be seen in the right ventricular apex (*arrow*). (*Adapted from* Edwards [8]; with permission.)

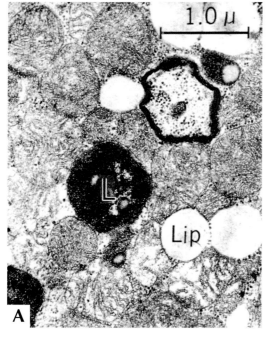

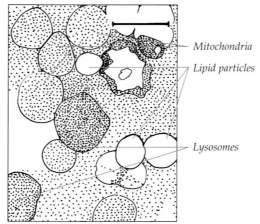

Mitochondria

Lipid particles

Lysosomes

FIGURE 7-5. Several histologic features differentiate alcoholic from idiopathic dilated cardiomyopathy. Some of the more prominent features of alcoholic cardiomyopathy are lipid infiltration (**A**), intracellular myocyte edema (**B**), interstitial fibrosis (**C**), myocyte necrosis (**D**), (*continued*)

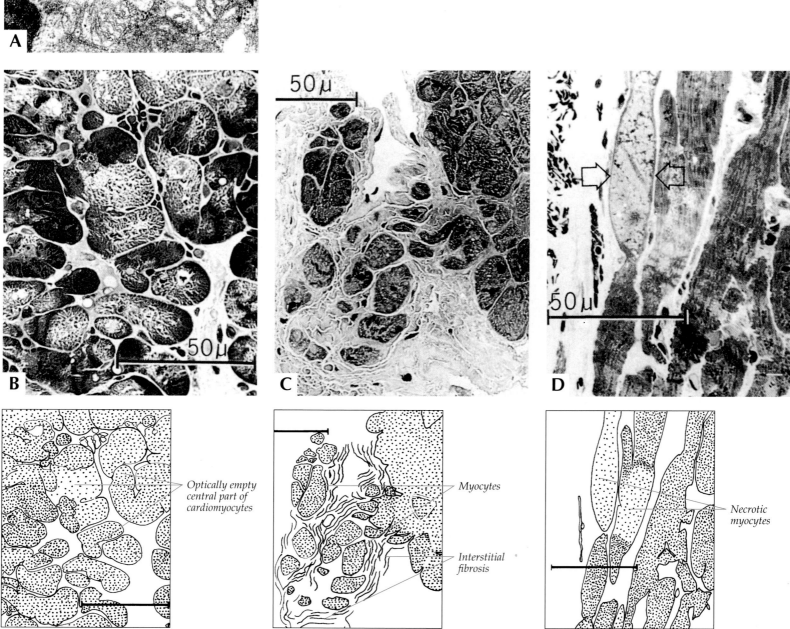

Optically empty central part of cardiomyocytes

Myocytes

Interstitial fibrosis

Necrotic myocytes

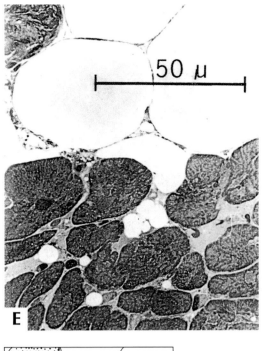

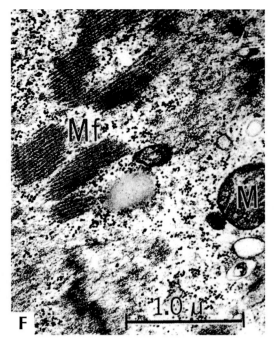

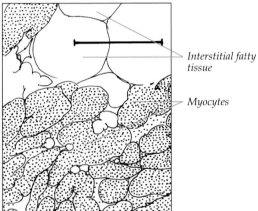

Interstitial fatty
tissue

Myocytes

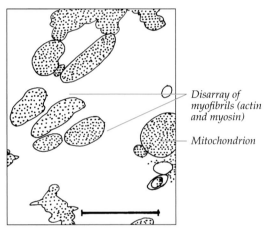

Disarray of
myofibrils (actin
and myosin)

Mitochondrion

FIGURE 7-5. (*continued*) fatty tissue in the interstitium (**E**), and myofibrillar disarray and lysis (**F**). Lipomatous degeneration is a prominent feature in alcoholic cardiomyopathy, especially late in the disease. Lysosomal accumulation and mitochondrial proliferation, both of which are shown in *panel A*, may also be seen frequently [9]. The degree of fibrosis is variable and is thought to be a less prominent feature than in idiopathic cardiomyopathy [10]. The myofibrils (actin and myosin) in *panel F* lack their usual hexagonal arrangement; this finding is more common in patients with cobalt-beer cardiomyopathy [9]. (*Adapted from* Tsiplenkova and coworkers [11]; with permission.)

CLINICAL AND LABORATORY FINDINGS IN ALCOHOLIC AND NONALCOHOLIC CARDIOMYOPATHY			
	ALCOHOLIC	NONALCOHOLIC	*P* VALUE
Clinical findings, *% of patients*			
Dyspnea	100	100	NS
Left heart failure	100	100	NS
Skeletal muscle myopathy	83	Unknown	Unknown
Right heart failure	61	56	NS
Palpitations	38	38	NS
Chest pain	31	38	NS
Laboratory findings			
LVEF, %	27	32	NS
GGT, *10–75 IU/mL*	263	80	0.004
ALT, *5–40 IU/mL*	153	46	0.137
MCV, *80–98 fL*	97	89	0.001

FIGURE 7-6. Diagnosis of alcoholic cardiomyopathy. Alcoholic and idiopathic forms of cardiomyopathy differ little in their clinical characteristics [12]. However, a coexistent skeletal myopathy is a common feature in alcoholic cardiomyopathy and occurs in a dose-dependent fashion [6]. Several laboratory abnormalities that reflect chronic or acute alcohol use are seen more commonly in ethanol-induced disease. The strongest correlations are with mean corpuscular volume (MCV), which increases with chronic alcohol use, and gamma glutamyltranspeptidase (GGT), which correlates with the total amount of ethanol recently ingested [12]. Clinical features other than cardiovascular ones may suggest an alcoholic etiology, such as evidence of cirrhosis, pancreatitis, gastritis, and various disorders of the central and peripheral nervous system. ALT—alanine aminotransferase; LVEF—left ventricular ejection fraction.

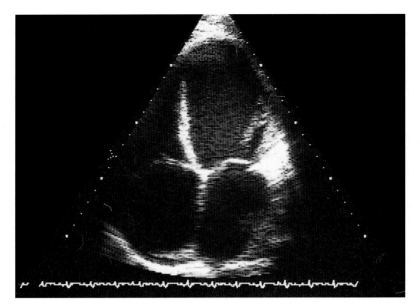
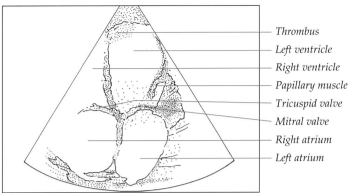

FIGURE 7-7. Apical four-chamber view on two-dimensional echocardiography showing enlargement of all cardiac chambers. Left ventricular (LV) end-diastolic dimension is 89 mm, with an end-systolic dimension of 78 mm. The LV apical shadow may reflect either artifact or thrombus, which is sometimes seen in association with poor ventricular function. Early in the course, before severe dilatation, the LV posterior wall and interventricular septum are often thickened [13]. LV mass by echocardiography usually precedes the decline in systolic function [14]. Echocardiography can be a useful adjunct in assessing the degree to which ventricular function is impaired and can also be employed to exclude other causes of heart failure, such as valvular or coronary artery disease.

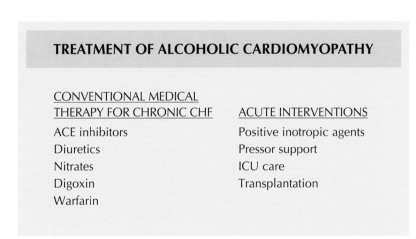

FIGURE 7-8. Medical therapy for alcoholic cardiomyopathy includes the medications conventionally used in congestive heart failure (CHF), such as angiotensin-converting enzyme (ACE) inhibitors, diuretics, and nitrates. Digoxin may also be used, although patients with this disorder seem to be particularly susceptible to digoxin toxicity [13]. Thromboembolic events are reduced with warfarin, but patient reliability and danger of traumatic falls should be considered when this drug is prescribed. Acute interventions during end-stage cardiomyopathy include therapies provided in the intensive care unit (ICU), such as positive inotropic agents (*eg*, dobutamine), pressors (*eg*, dopamine), and other forms of supportive care. The decision for transplantation must be made on a case-by-case basis by an experienced transplant team.

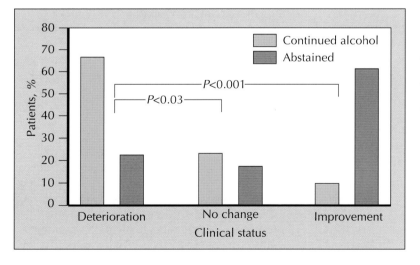

FIGURE 7-9. Total abstinence is the most important therapeutic goal in alcoholic cardiomyopathy. In this study, patients were divided into those who continued imbibing alcohol and those who abstained. Average follow-up was 41 months, and the percentage of patients who deteriorated, improved, or showed no change in functional classification was determined for each cohort. Abstinence is associated with improvement, whereas deterioration occurs in most who continue to drink. Of note, all those whose condition deteriorated died during the follow-up period [15].

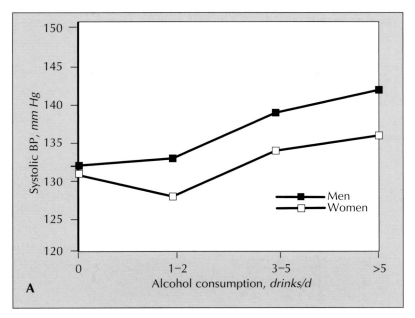

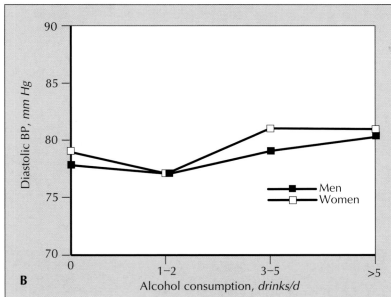

FIGURE 7-10. Association between daily alcohol intake and systolic (**A**) and diastolic (**B**) blood pressure. When the drinking habits of approximately 84,000 persons were examined, moderate-to-heavy ethanol intake was found to be associated with higher systolic and diastolic blood pressures. This effect was independent of gender, age, race, smoking status, obesity, and caffeine use [16]. Some data suggest that blood pressure may be lowered slightly with light alcohol use.

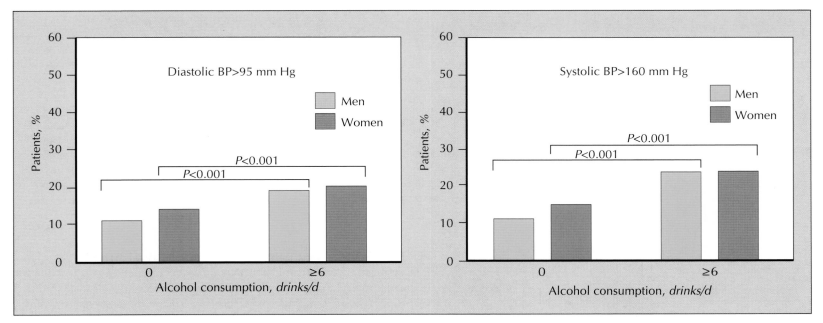

FIGURE 7-11. Association between alcoholism and hypertension. The number of patients with diastolic and systolic hypertension is significantly increased with long-term, heavy ethanol ingestion [16]. As shown here, at the time of their routine health check-up among 23,811 patients, the incidence is almost doubled in each group. (Nondrinkers: men = 7238, women = 14,453; ≥ 6 drinks/d: men = 1683, women = 437.) Again, this finding was independent of gender, age, race, smoking status, obesity, and caffeine use. It has also been shown that hypertension in the active alcoholic is less responsive to antihypertensive medications [1], but cessation of heavy alcohol use may normalize blood pressure in many cases [2].

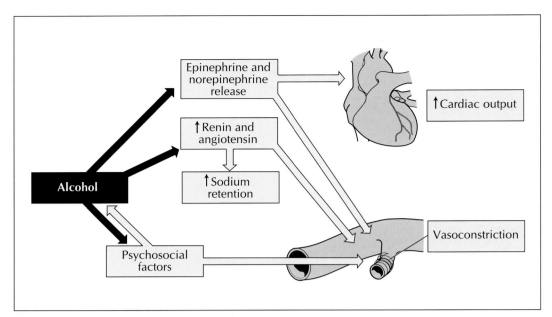

FIGURE 7-12. Proposed mechanisms of blood pressure elevation in chronic alcohol abuse. Heavy ethanol intake has been implicated in the release of epinephrine and norepinephrine from the adrenal medulla and peripheral nervous system, which increases cardiac output and vasomotor tone. Smooth muscle sensitivity to these neurotransmitters is augmented by alcohol intake [1]. Higher plasma levels of renin and angiotensin have been observed, which may lead to increased vasomotor tone and sodium retention [1]. Ethanol also has a direct vasopressor effect thought to be a result of elevated intracellular calcium concentration and possibly decreased local magnesium concentration [2,17]. In addition, psychosocial factors affecting the alcoholic must not be discounted.

ARRHYTHMIAS

RHYTHM DISTURBANCES WITH ETHANOL ABUSE

| | DRINK(S)/d, % | | | |
ARRHYTHMIA(S)	≥ 6	≤1	P VALUE	RELATIVE RISK
AF	1.1	0.5	0.02	2.3
Atrial flutter	0.6	0.2	0.05	3.0
SVT	0.4	0.1	0.03	5.0
AF, atrial flutter, SVT	1.6	0.7	< 0.01	2.3

FIGURE 7-13. Supraventricular arrhythmias are by far the most commonly encountered rhythm disturbances in ethanol abuse. In this study, alcoholics (n = 1322) had a significantly higher incidence of atrial fibrillation (AF), atrial flutter, and supraventricular tachycardia (SVT) on routine screening than did age-, gender-, and race-matched controls (n = 2644) [18]. This effect is independent of smoking status, valvular disease, coronary artery disease, hypertension, presence of cardiomyopathy, and pulmonary disease. It is estimated that alcohol causes or contributes to AF in up to 35% of new cases [19] and is responsible for a large proportion of recurrences [20,21]. Ettinger *et al.* defined "holiday heart syndrome" after observing 32 separate dysrhythmic episodes in patients with chronic ethanol use that occurred shortly after intensified ingestion [22], and this syndrome may even be seen in people without a background of chronic alcohol abuse [19,20]. Although the concept of the holiday heart has recently been challenged, electrophysiologic studies have demonstrated a substantially decreased threshold for atrial arrhythmias after acute, heavy intake [23].

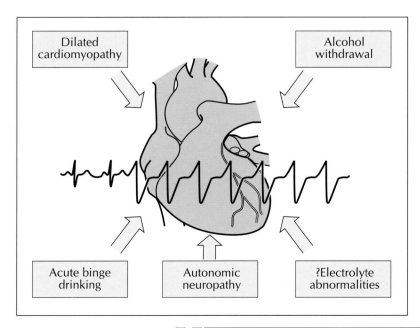

FIGURE 7-14. Although not as common as atrial arrhythmias, ventricular arrhythmias and an excess frequency of sudden deaths are known to occur in persons who abuse alcohol [1,23,24]. This is especially true in patients with histologic evidence of myocardial damage and overt cardiomyopathy [1,25]. Decreased heart rate variability, which may represent vagal neuropathy, is common in alcoholics and may contribute to the susceptibility to sudden death [26]. Ventricular premature beats, ventricular tachycardia, and ventricular fibrillation may occur during the withdrawal period. These may be due in part to catecholamine excess and can be aggravated by electrolyte imbalances. An acute increase in alcohol ingestion has also been implicated as a cause of these arrhythmias in patients with and without apparent heart disease [23]. Rarely, various conduction disorders such as alcohol-related Mobitz blocks, complete heart block, and bundle branch block have been observed.

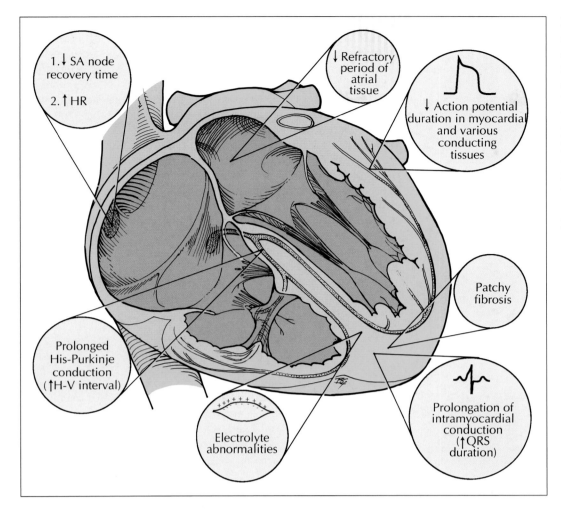

FIGURE 7-15. Proposed mechanisms for arrhythmogenesis [2,23]. Various alterations in normal cardiac conduction occur in alcoholics. One direct effect of alcohol is a decrease in action potential duration in the myocardium and various conducting tissues, shortening the effective refractory periods. This effect seems to be more pronounced in atrial tissue. Intramyocardial conduction is also prolonged and in some studies has been noted to increase QRS duration and His-Purkinje conduction. Patchy fibrosis may result in re-entry phenomena. Ethanol-induced catecholamine effects include increased automaticity, decreased sinus node recovery time, and a subsequent increase in heart rate (HR). Electrolyte disturbances, including hypomagnesemia and hypokalemia, may lower the arrhythmogenic threshold. Ethanol's inhibitory effects on sodium-potassium transport may explain some of the electrophysiologic events noted above. SA—sinoatrial.

NUTRITIONAL DISORDERS AND TOXIC ADDITIVES

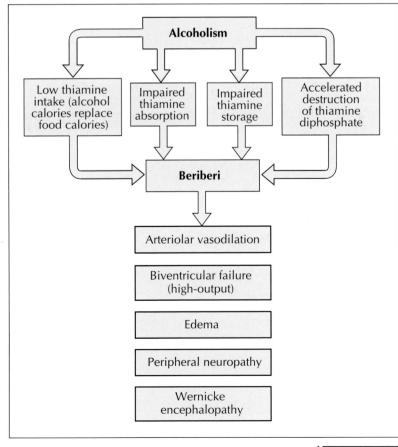

FIGURE 7-16. The major nutritional cardiovascular consequence of alcohol abuse is thiamine deficiency, or *beriberi*. Often, alcohol intake replaces the ingestion of food, resulting in a low thiamine intake. Active and passive gastrointestinal absorption of thiamine is impaired by high ethanol intake, as is thiamine storage in the skeletal muscles, heart, liver, kidneys, and brain. Thiamine degradation by thiaminases is accelerated at the same time as thiamine requirements increase owing to the high carbohydrate content of beer and wine. The typical clinical manifestations occur in only a minority of individuals, and genetic susceptibility may play a role.

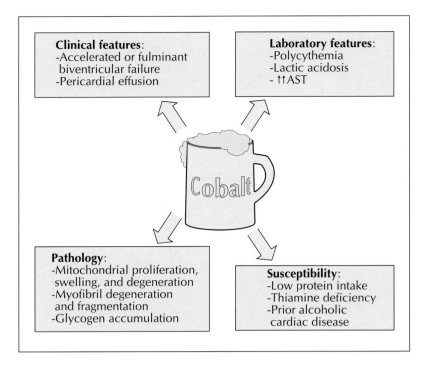

Clinical features:
-Accelerated or fulminant biventricular failure
-Pericardial effusion

Laboratory features:
-Polycythemia
-Lactic acidosis
- ↑↑AST

Pathology:
-Mitochondrial proliferation, swelling, and degeneration
-Myofibril degeneration and fragmentation
-Glycogen accumulation

Susceptibility:
-Low protein intake
-Thiamine deficiency
-Prior alcoholic cardiac disease

FIGURE 7-17. The only recent major cardiac toxicity involving a harmful additive in an alcoholic beverage was the outbreak of *cobalt-beer cardiomyopathy* in the mid-1960s. Outbreaks occurred in several regions (Quebec, Belgium, Nebraska, and Minnesota) and were attributed to the cardiotoxic effect of adding cobalt to beer to stabilize the foam. Cobalt cardiomyopathy progresses rapidly and is commonly accompanied by a pericardial effusion. One of the unique laboratory features of this syndrome is polycythemia, although high alkaline serum transaminase (AST) levels and lactic acidosis are also quite common. Although no distinguishing features of cobalt cardiomyopathy are evident on gross or light microscopy, most cardiac pathologic specimens reveal certain findings on electron microscopy (*see* Fig. 7-18). Pre-existing alcoholic cardiovascular disease or poor nutritional status seems to predispose to the disorder. With the removal of the cobalt additive the condition disappeared.

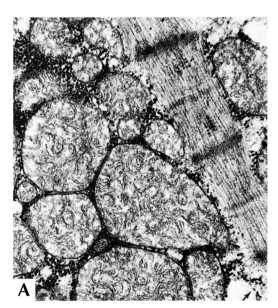
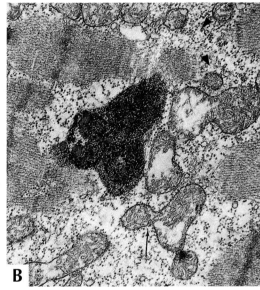

FIGURE 7-18. Pathologic changes in cobalt-beer cardiomyopathy [27]. **A,** Abundant, enlarged, and polymorphic mitochondria demonstrating early degeneration of the cristae. Glycogen granules are abundant, with a paucity of myofibers (×8730). **B,** Granular, amorphous material fills the mitochondria, some of which may contain cobalt (×19,200). Fragmented myofibrils (*arrowheads*) are identifiable. *Arrow* indicates budding mitochondria. (*Adapted from* Alexander and coworkers [27]; with permission.)

REFERENCES

1. Regan TJ: Alcohol and the cardiovascular system. *JAMA* 1990, 264:377–381.

2. Davidson DM: Cardiovascular effects of alcohol. *West J Med* 1989, 151:430–439.

3. Regan TJ, Morvai V: Experimental models for studying the effects of ethanol on the myocardium. *Acta Med Scand* 1987, 717(suppl):107–113.

4. Laposta EA, Lange LG: Presence of nonoxidative ethanol metabolism in human organs commonly damaged in ethanol abuse. *Science* 1986, 231:497–499.

5. Guarnieri T, Lakatta EG: Mechanism of myocardial contractile depression by clinical concentrations of ethanol. *J Clin Invest* 1989, 85:1462–1467.

6. Urbano-Marquez A, Estruch R, Navarro-Lopez F, *et al.*: The effects of alcoholism on skeletal and cardiac muscle. *N Engl J Med* 1989, 320:409–415.

7. Burch GE, Gilles TD: Alcoholic cardiomyopathy: concept of the disease and its treatment. *Am J Med* 1971, 50:141–145.

8. Edwards WD: Cardiomyopathies. *Hum Pathol* 1987, 18:625–635.

9. Ferrans VJ: Pathologic anatomy of the dilated cardiomyopathies. *Am J Cardiol* 1989, 64:9C–11C.

10. Teragaki M, Kazuhide T, Takeda T: Clinical and histologic features of alcohol drinkers with congestive heart failure. *Am Heart J* 1993, 125:808–817.

11. Tsiplenkova VG, Vikhert AM, Cherpachenko NM: Ultrastructural and histochemical observations in human and experimental alcoholic cardiomyopathy. *J Am Coll Cardiol* 1986, 8(suppl A):22A–32A.

12. Wang RY, Alterman AI, McLellan AT: Alcohol abuse in patients with dilated cardiomyopathy. *Arch Intern Med* 1990, 150:1079–1082.

13. McCall D: Alcohol and the cardiovascular system. *Curr Probl Cardiol* 1987, 12:355–414.

14. Matthews EC, Gardin JM, Henry WL, *et al.*: Echocardiographic abnormalities in chronic alcoholics with and without overt congestive heart failure. *Am J Cardiol* 1981, 47:570–578.

15. Demakis JG, Proskey A, Rahimtoola SH: The natural course of alcoholic cardiomyopathy. *Ann Intern Med* 1974, 80:293–297.

16. Klatsky AL, Friedman GD, Siegelaub AB, *et al.*: Alcohol consumption and blood pressure. *N Engl J Med* 1977, 296:1194–1200.

17. Vasdev S, Inder PG, Sampson CA, *et al.*: Ethanol induced hypertension in rats: reversibility and role of intracellular calcium. *Artery* 1993, 20:19–43.

18. Cohen EJ, Klatsky AL, Armstrong MA: Alcohol use and supraventricular arrhythmia. *Am J Cardiol* 1988, 62:971–973.

19. Lowenstein SR, Gabow PA, Cramer J, *et al.*: The role of alcohol in new-onset atrial fibrillation. *Arch Intern Med* 1983, 143:1882–1885.

20. Koskinen P, Kupari M, Leiononen H: Role of alcohol in recurrences of atrial fibrillation in persons less than 65 years of age. *Am J Cardiol* 1990, 66:954–958.

21. Kupari M, Koskinen P: Time of onset of supraventricular tachyarrhythmias in relation to alcohol consumption. *Am J Cardiol* 1991, 67:718–722.

22. Ettinger PO, Wu CF, DeLaCruz C, *et al.*: Arrhythmias and the "holiday heart": alcohol-associated cardiac rhythm disorders. *Am Heart J* 1978, 95:555–562.

23. Greenspon AJ, Schaal SF: Electrophysiologic studies of alcohol effects in alcoholics. *Ann Intern Med* 1983, 98:135–139.

24. Lithell H, Aberg H, Selinus I, *et al.*: Alcoholic intemperance and sudden death. *BMJ* 1987, 294:1456–1458.

25. Vikhert AM, Tsiplenkova VG, Cherpachenko NM: Alcoholic cardiomyopathy and sudden cardiac death. *J Am Coll Cardiol* 1986, 8(suppl A):3A–11A.

26. Malpas SC, Whiteside EA, Maling TJB: Heart rate variability and cardiac autonomic function in men with chronic alcohol dependence. *Br Heart J* 1991, 65:84–88.

27. Alexander CS: Cobalt-beer cardiomyopathy. *Am J Med* 1972, 53:395–417.

CARDIAC EFFECTS OF ELECTROLYTE DISORDERS, DRUGS, AND TOXINS

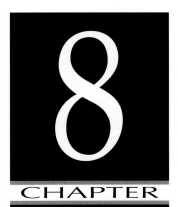

8

CHAPTER

Richard A. Lange and L. David Hillis

Electrolyte disorders, drugs, and toxins can adversely affect cardiac conduction, coronary perfusion, and function of the myocardium and cardiac valves. In general, electrolyte disorders primarily affect the heart's conduction properties. Changes in serum sodium and magnesium concentrations do not usually cause changes on the electrocardiogram (ECG); however, changes in serum potassium and calcium concentrations may cause profound ECG changes and life-threatening arrhythmias. Psychotropic medications (phenothiazines or lithium) also affect the ECG, even when drug concentrations are in the therapeutic range. At high concentrations, these drugs have also been associated with conduction abnormalities, ventricular arrhythmias, and sudden death.

As cocaine use has steadily increased in the United States, the incidence of cocaine-induced cardiovascular complications, including myocardial ischemia and infarction, left ventricular hypertrophy, arrhythmias, cardiomyopathy, and endocarditis, has risen. Cocaine may cause myocardial ischemia by increasing myocardial oxygen demands (*ie*, heart rate and systemic arterial pressure) and/or decreasing myocardial oxygen supply because of coronary vasoconstriction, platelet aggregation, thrombus formation, or accelerated atherosclerosis. Hypertrophy of the left ventricle has been demonstrated in some chronic cocaine users, and myocarditis and cardiomyopathy have been described in others. All of these cardiac conditions may predispose cocaine users to serious arrhythmias. In addition, cocaine has electrophysiologic properties similar to those of quinidine and may, therefore, cause significant arrhythmias in patients with underlying cardiac disease.

A variety of cardiovascular complications occur in uremic patients and are a major source of morbidity and mortality. Congestive heart failure is common and may be due to diastolic dysfunction, a high-output state, or dilated cardiomyopathy. Diastolic dysfunction may result from myocardial fibrosis and hypertrophy, which are commonly observed in patients with end-stage renal disease. A high-output state may be observed in the uremic patient with anemia or an arteriovenous fistula. Multiple etiologies may contribute to systolic dysfunction, including hypervolemia, hypertension, metabolic disturbances, toxins, nutritional factors, and coronary artery disease. Many patients with end-stage renal disease develop pericarditis and pericardial effusion; the hemodynamic consequences of the latter depend on the size of the effusion and its rate of accumulation. Myocardial calcification is seen in patients with chronic renal disease and may involve the valves or cardiac conduction system, causing valvular stenosis or regurgitation and atrioventric-ular block. As a result of the electrolyte abnormalities and dilated cardiomyopathy associated with uremia, atrial and ventricular arrhythmias are common. Finally, myocardial ischemia is common in uremic patients, even those with angiographically normal coronary arteries.

ELECTROLYTES AND DRUGS

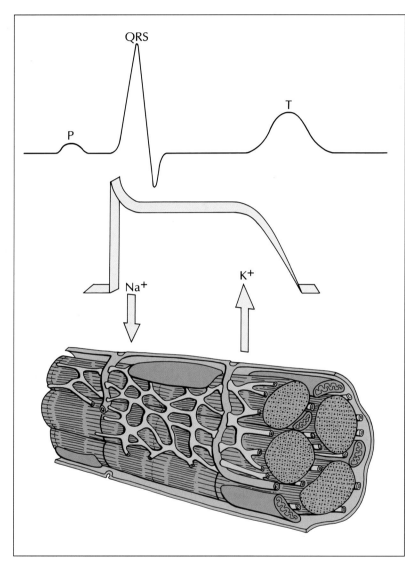

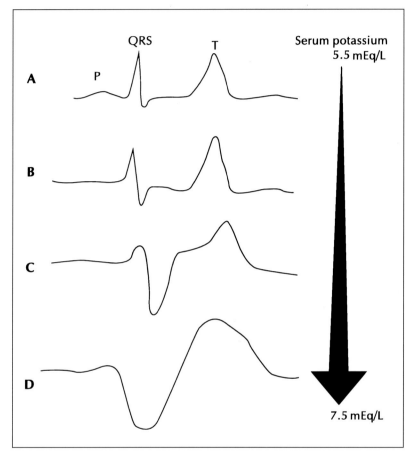

FIGURE 8-2. The ECG changes associated with hyperkalemia. These changes are affected by the rate of development and duration of hyperkalemia and do not correlate precisely with the serum potassium concentration. The earliest change observed with hyperkalemia is the appearance of tall, peaked T waves (**A**). As the serum potassium concentration increases, the P wave decreases in amplitude and may disappear (**B**), the QRS widens with intraventricular conduction delay, and the ST segment becomes elevated (**C**). Progressive widening of the QRS complex results in a "sinusoidal waveform" (**D**) that may degenerate into atrioventricular block and ventricular fibrillation.

FIGURE 8-1. Ion movement during myocardial excitation. The conduction of electrical impulses and myocardial excitation is dependent on the movement of sodium ions (Na^+) and potassium ions (K^+) across the cell membrane. The potassium concentration is high and the sodium concentration is low in the intracellular space, whereas the opposite is true in the extracellular space. Depolarization—reflected in the QRS complex—occurs when there is a rapid influx of sodium into the cell, and repolarization—reflected in the T wave—occurs when there is an efflux of potassium from the cell. Although the surface electrocardiogram (ECG) is not appreciably affected by physiologic changes in serum sodium concentration, hypokalemia and hyperkalemia may cause marked ECG changes in humans [1].

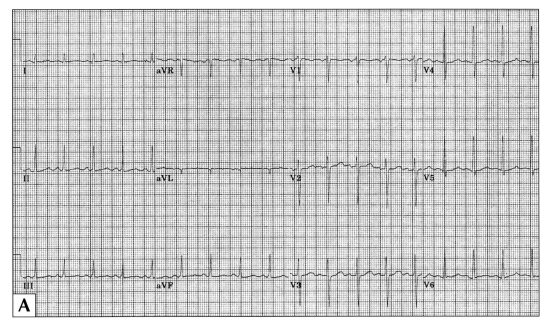

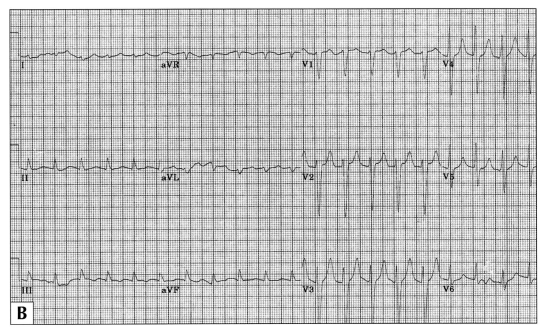

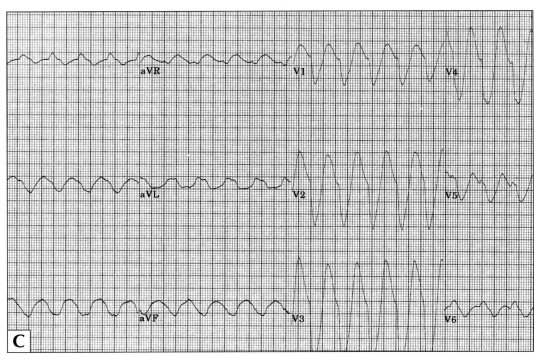

FIGURE 8-3. Twelve-lead ECG tracings obtained over 48 hours in a patient with renal failure and hyperkalemia who refused hemodialysis. **A,** Initially, the ECG and serum potassium were normal. **B,** With hyperkalemia, the T waves become tall and peaked, the QRS complex widens, and the P wave disappears. **C,** At a serum potassium concentration of 9.2 mEq/L, the ECG shows a "sine wave" pattern.

FIGURE 8-4. Life-threatening hyperkalemia can occur with uremia; the administration of potassium-sparing diuretics (*ie*, spirono-lactone, amiloride) or potassium supplements, especially in the setting of a low cardiac output or mild-to-moderate renal impairment; diabetic ketoacidosis; and severe burns or trauma.

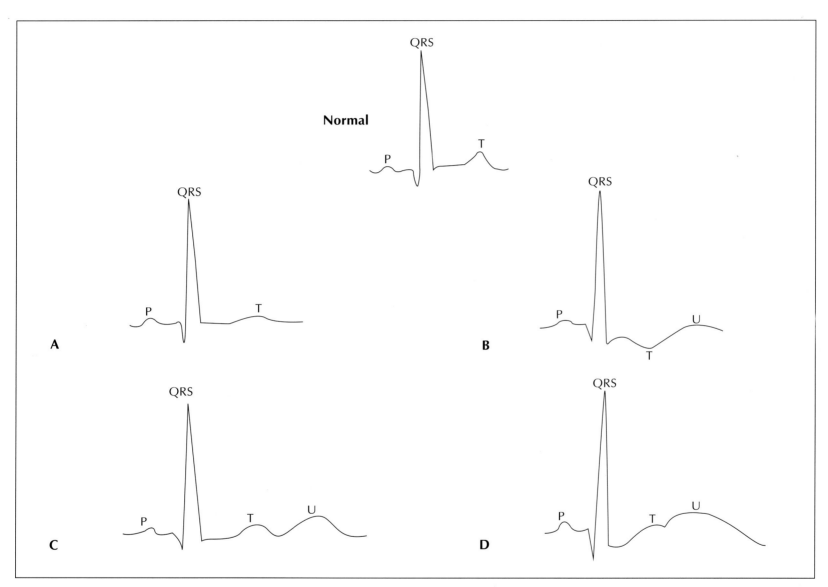

FIGURE 8-5. As with hyperkalemia, the ECG changes associated with hypokalemia also depend on the rate of development and duration of potassium depletion and do not correlate precisely with the serum potassium concentration. The most common patterns include T-wave flattening (**A**); concave depression of the ST segment, sometimes with T-wave inversion (**B**); and the appearance of prominent U waves (**C**). When the prominent U wave is superimposed on the descending portion of the T wave, it may be mistaken for a prolonged Q-T interval (**D**).

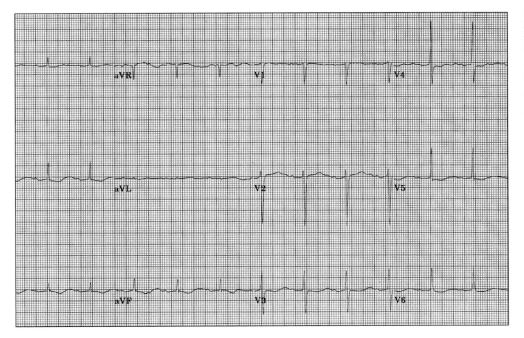

FIGURE 8-6. Twelve-lead ECG in a patient with hypokalemia showing concave depression of the ST segment inferiorly and laterally, diffuse flattening of the T wave, and prominent U waves. If the U wave is confused with a T wave, the tracing would be mistakenly identified as having a prolonged Q-T interval.

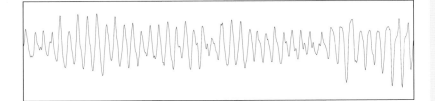

FIGURE 8-7. A number of arrhythmias have been associated with hypokalemia [2], including paroxysmal atrial tachycardia with block, first- and second-degree heart block, atrioventricular dissociation, ventricular tachycardia and fibrillation, and torsades de pointes (shown here). Originally described as a "twisting of the points," this rhythm is intermediate between ventricular tachycardia and fibrillation. Antiarrhythmic drugs, psychotropic drugs, and electrolyte abnormalities (ie, hypokalemia and hypocalcemia) may also precipitate this life-threatening arrhythmia [2,3].

CAUSES OF LETHAL HYPOKALEMIA

Diuretic use
Gastrointestinal potassium loss
Renal tubular acidosis
Cushing's syndrome
Insulin treatment

FIGURE 8-8. Life-threatening hypokalemia is most commonly due to diuretic therapy with inadequate potassium supplementation. Severe hypokalemia may also be seen in patients with vomiting, diarrhea, renal tubular acidosis, or Cushing's syndrome and in diabetics who receive insulin treatment for ketoacidosis.

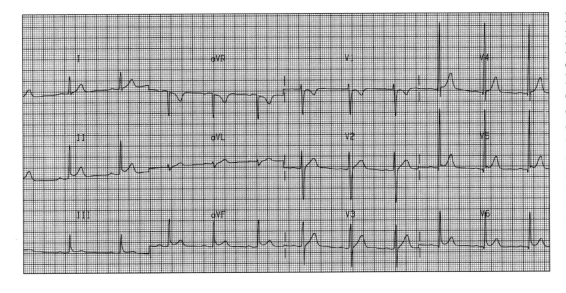

FIGURE 8-9. Electrocardiographic changes in hypercalcemia. This 20-year-old patient had hyperparathyroidism and a serum calcium concentration of 11.7 mg/dL. In hypercalcemia, the ST segment is shortened or absent, and the Q-T interval is correspondingly shortened. The QRS complex, P wave, and T wave are not usually changed. Although hypercalcemia does not usually cause significant arrhythmias, rapid intravenous administration of calcium may induce lethal ventricular arrhythmias, especially in patients taking digoxin or with hypokalemia.

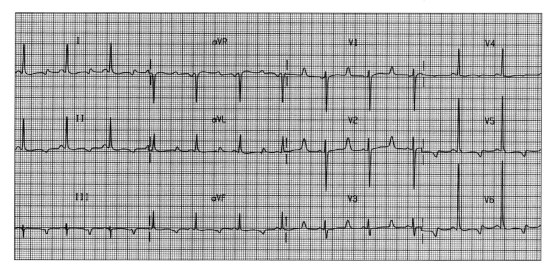

FIGURE 8-10. Electrocardiographic changes with hypocalcemia. When the serum ionized calcium concentration becomes low, the ST segment lengthens, leading to prolongation of the Q-T interval. The T-wave morphology may change (peaking, flattening, and inversion have all been described), but the QRS complex, P waves, and P-R interval are unchanged.

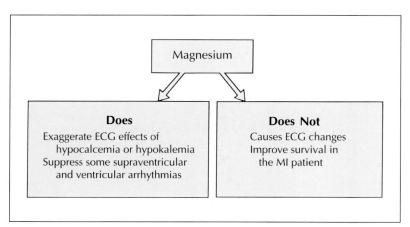

FIGURE 8-11. Effects of magnesium on the ECG. Changes in serum magnesium concentration alone do not usually affect the ECG [4]. Magnesium deficiency often occurs in the setting of potassium or calcium depletion and may exaggerate their electrophysiologic effects. However, isolated depletion of magnesium does not cause ECG changes. Although intravenous magnesium has been used empirically to suppress a variety of supraventricular and ventricular arrhythmias, recent studies have shown that intravenous magnesium does not reduce in-hospital arrhythmias or short-term mortality in the patient with acute myocardial infarction (MI).

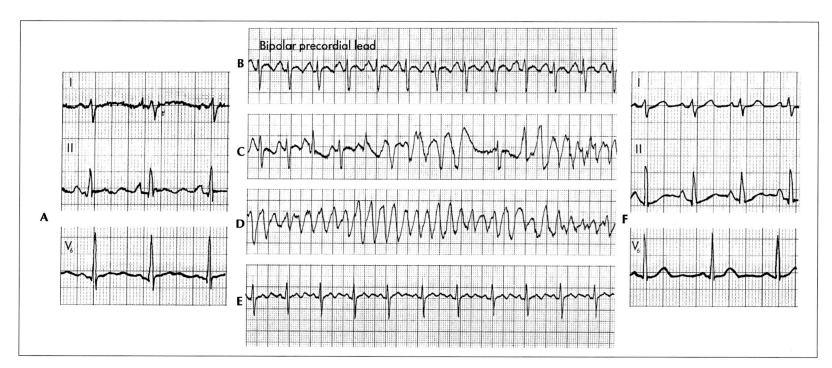

FIGURE 8-12. Electrocardiographic changes associated with the use of a phenothiazine, which is widely used to treat psychosis. In this 25-year-old woman, the initial ECG (**A**), obtained 3 hours after ingestion of 1000 mg of thioridazine, demonstrates prolongation of the Q-T interval (0.52 second) and a prominent U wave. Over the first 8 hours the patient had sinus tachycardia (**B**). Shortly thereafter, she developed nonsustained ventricular tachycardia (**C**) and then sustained polymorphic ventricular tachycardia (torsades de pointes) (**D**). Following two direct-current countershocks, the rhythm stabilized (**E**). Three days later, the ECG and intervals were normal (**F**). The electrophysiologic effects of the phenothiazines—thioridazine (Mellaril,

Sandoz, East Hanover, NJ), chlorpromazine (Thorazine, Smithkline Beacham, Philadelphia, PA), and trifluoperazine (Stelazine, Smithkline Beacham)—are dose-related and similar to those of the class IA antiarrhythmic agents. In low doses, these drugs cause flattening of the T wave, Q-T interval prolongation, and a prominent U wave. ECG changes may be observed in up to 50% of hospitalized patients receiving therapeutic doses of phenothiazines and are most marked with thioridazine, less marked with chlorpromazine, and least obvious with trifluoperazine [5,6]. In high doses, all may cause ventricular fibrillation and tachycardia [7,8]. (*Adapted from* Sandøe and Sigurd [2]; with permission.)

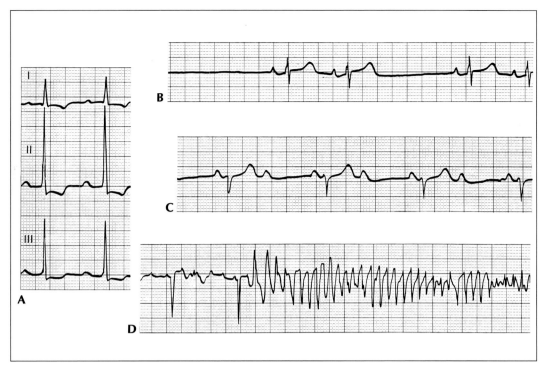

FIGURE 8-13. Effects of lithium on the ECG. T-wave abnormalities are present in 20% to 30% of patients taking lithium (A); these are benign and resolve when the drug is discontinued [9]. Sinus node dysfunction (B) and atrioventricular block (C) have been reported in those taking therapeutic doses [10]. Ventricular tachycardia and sudden death (D) have occurred with toxic doses as well as in an occasional patient with therapeutic lithium levels [11,12]. The fact that lithium displaces intracellular potassium ions most likely accounts for its electrophysiologic effects. (*Adapted from* Sandøe and Sigurd [2]; with permission.)

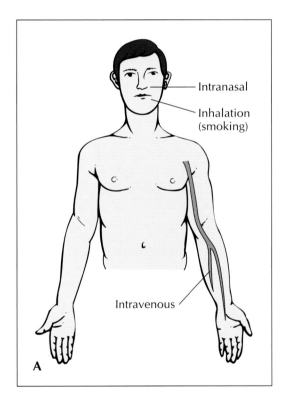

B. PHARMACOKINETICS OF COCAINE			
ROUTE	ONSET OF ACTION	PEAK EFFECT	DURATION
Intranasal	1–5 min	10–20 min	60–90 min
Inhalation (smoking)	3–5 s	1–3 min	5–15 min
Intravenous	10–60 s	3–5 min	20–60 min

FIGURE 8-14. Extent of cocaine abuse in the United States. A, Routes of administration. B, Pharmacokinetics. Over the past 15 years, the use of cocaine has increased dramatically. This drug can be administered by a variety of routes (*ie*, intranasal [topical], intravenous, or inhaled [smoked]), is readily available and affordable, and is thought to be a "safe" drug. At least 30 million Americans have used cocaine at least once, 5 million use it regularly, 1 million are addicted to it, and 5000 use it for the first time daily. Cocaine is the most commonly used illicit drug among patients entering emergency departments and is estimated to account for 5% to 10% of all emergency room visits. It is well absorbed from all mucous membranes. The route of administration determines its onset of action, time of peak effect, and duration of action.

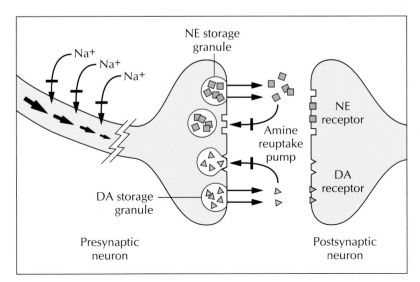

FIGURE 8-15. Cocaine's mechanism of action. When applied locally, cocaine acts as an anesthetic. It blocks the initiation and propagation of electrical signals within nerves by interfering with sodium (Na^+) permeability during depolarization. When administered systemically, cocaine blocks the reuptake of norepinephrine (NE) and dopamine (DA) at the presynaptic nerve terminal. The excess of these neurotransmitters at postsynaptic sites accounts for cocaine's sympathomimetic effects.

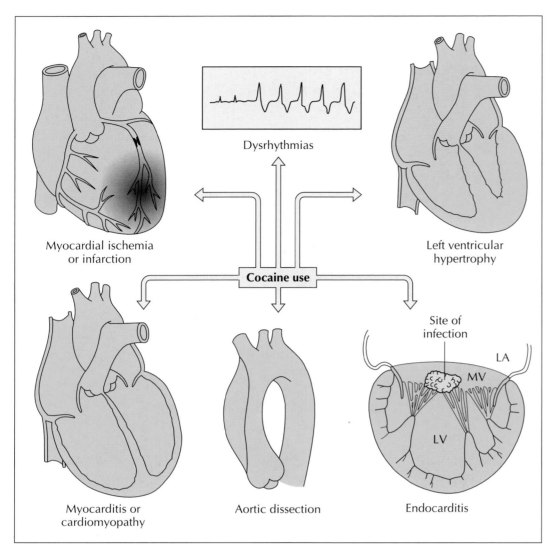

Myocardial ischemia or infarction

Dysrhythmias

Left ventricular hypertrophy

Cocaine use

Myocarditis or cardiomyopathy

Aortic dissection

Site of infection

LA

MV

LV

Endocarditis

FIGURE 8-16. Cardiovascular complications associated with cocaine use. Myocardial ischemia and infarction following cocaine use may result from increased myocardial oxygen demands and/or a decrease in myocardial blood flow [13]. Supraventricular and ventricular dysrhythmias may occur as a result of cocaine's sympathomimetic effects, its Na^+-blocking effects, or cocaine-induced myocardial ischemia or infarction. Left ventricular hypertrophy, acute myocarditis, and congestive cardiomyopathy have been reported in chronic cocaine users [14]. Severe hypertension resulting from the sympathomimetic effects of cocaine has led to aortic dissection. In comparison with other illicit drugs, intravenous cocaine use has been reported to be an independent risk factor for the development of endocarditis. LA—left atrium; LV—left ventricle; MV—mitral valve.

CLINICAL CHARACTERISTICS OF PATIENTS WITH COCAINE-INDUCED MI

Young age (mean age, 34 years)

Male gender

Minimal or no risk factors for coronary artery disease

Occurs with habitual, recreational, or first-time use

Onset of symptoms within minutes to hours of cocaine use

Associated with all routes of administration and with large or small doses of cocaine

FIGURE 8-17. Clinical characteristics of patients with cocaine-induced myocardial infarction (MI). Patients are typically young, and 90% are male. Most (65% to 70%) smoke cigarettes but have no other risk factor for atherosclerotic coronary artery disease [15]. Myocardial ischemia usually occurs within minutes of drug ingestion but has been reported up to 15 hours after ingestion. The occurrence of MI is unrelated to the dose, route of administration, or frequency of use of cocaine.

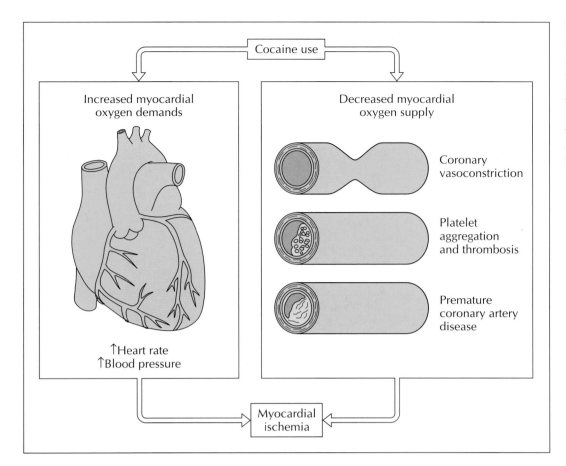

FIGURE 8-18. Cocaine may cause myocardial ischemia via several mechanisms. As a result of its sympathomimetic effects, cocaine increases myocardial oxygen demands by elevating heart rate and blood pressure. Concomitantly, cocaine may reduce myocardial oxygen supply by causing coronary vasoconstriction [16], platelet aggregation, and/or premature atherosclerotic coronary artery disease.

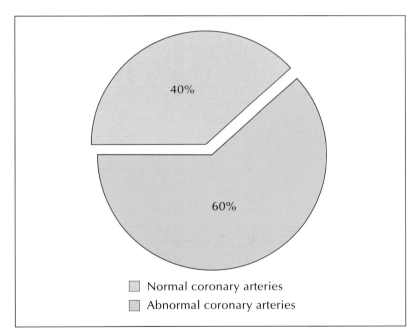

FIGURE 8-19. Coronary anatomy in subjects with cocaine-induced myocardial infarction (MI). In approximately half the patients with reported cocaine-associated MI, coronary anatomy has been visualized on angiography or postmortem examination. Many (40%) had no evidence of coronary artery disease; thus, MI was most likely caused by cocaine-induced coronary vasoconstriction and/or thrombus formation [15].

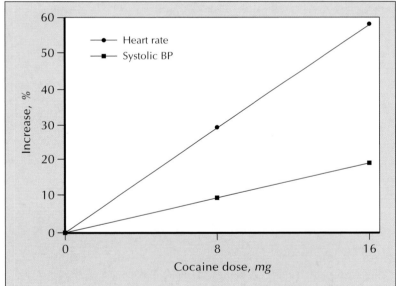

FIGURE 8-20. Myocardial oxygen demands after cocaine use. Both heart rate and systemic arterial blood pressure (BP) increase in a dose-dependent fashion when cocaine is administered intravenously. In patients with atherosclerotic coronary artery disease and a fixed myocardial oxygen supply, this increase in myocardial oxygen demand may precipitate myocardial ischemia.

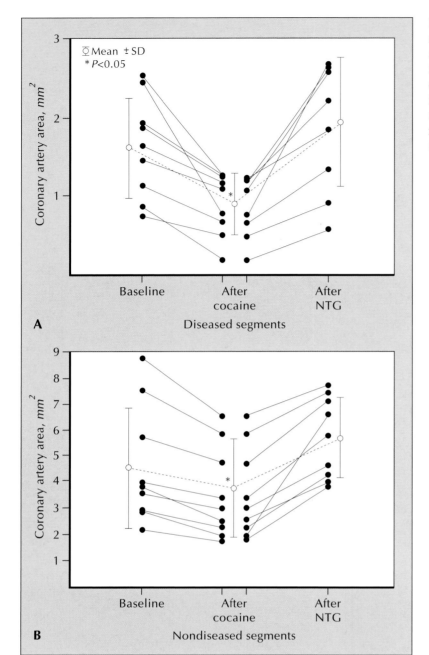

FIGURE 8-21. Cocaine-induced coronary vasoconstriction. Cross-sectional areas of diseased (**A**) and nondiseased (**B**) coronary arteries in 18 patients who received intranasal cocaine (2 mg/kg) followed by sublingual nitroglycerin (NTG) (0.4 mg). Cocaine caused constriction in both nondiseased and diseased vessels, but its effects were particularly marked in the arterial segments with atherosclerotic disease [17]. NTG reversed cocaine-induced coronary vasoconstriction in both diseased and nondiseased segments. (*Adapted from* Flores and coworkers [18]; with permission.)

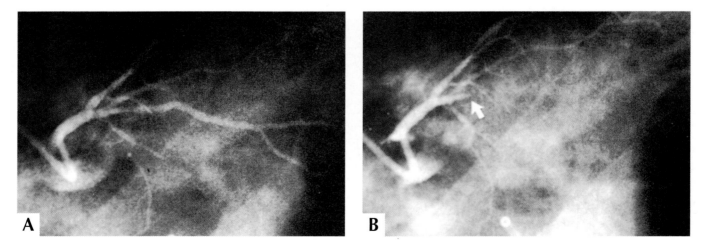

FIGURE 8-22. Effect of β-adrenergic blockade on cocaine-induced coronary vasoconstriction. Such vasoconstriction is mediated—at least in part—by adrenergic stimulation, in that it is reversed by α-adrenergic blockade (with phentolamine) but potentiated by treatment with the β-blocker propranolol [16,19]. Arteriography of the left coronary artery in a patient who received a β-blocker after cocaine use. The left anterior descending artery was mildly constricted after cocaine (**A**) and completely occluded (*arrow*) after propranolol (**B**). (*Adapted from* Lange and coworkers [19]; with permission.)

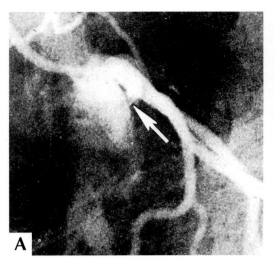 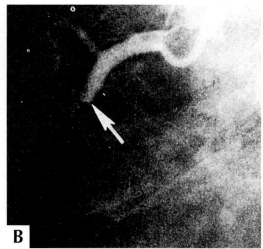

FIGURE 8-23. Cocaine-induced coronary artery occlusion. Coronary arteriography in a 38-year-old man with no previous cardiac history who had a myocardial infarction 15 minutes after intravenous cocaine use [20]. Simultaneously, the patient had acute thrombosis (*arrows*) of the left anterior descending coronary artery (**A**) and right coronary artery (**B**). (*Adapted from* Stenberg and coworkers [20]; with permission.)

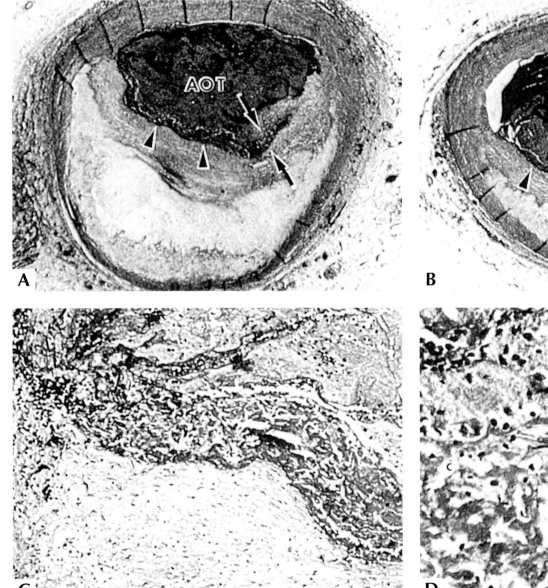

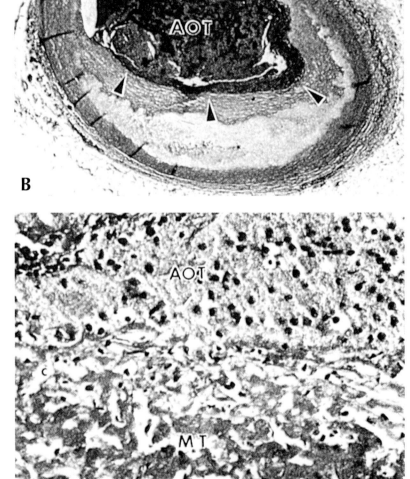

FIGURE 8-24. Coronary artery histology in a cocaine user [20]. In the left (**A**) and right (**B**) coronary arteries, there is a disrupted atherosclerotic plaque (*arrows*), an organizing mural thrombus (*arrowheads*), and an acute occlusive thrombus (AOT). Higher magnification (**C**) reveals loose connective tissue in the atherosclerotic plaque (*bottom*), a thin layer of organizing thrombus (*middle*), and an occlusive thrombus (*top*). A large number of platelets can be seen in the acute occlusive thrombus (**D**). *In vitro* studies have shown that cocaine causes increased platelet aggregation [21]. Premature atherosclerosis, thrombus formation, and platelet deposition are commonly observed in patients who have died from cocaine-induced myocardial infarction. MT—mural thrombus. (*Adapted from* Stenberg and coworkers [20]; with permission.)

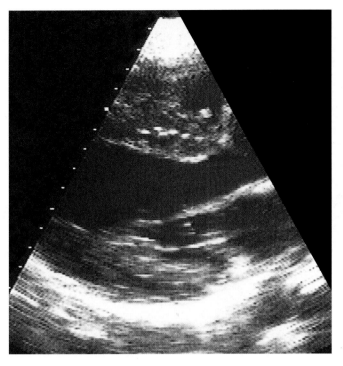

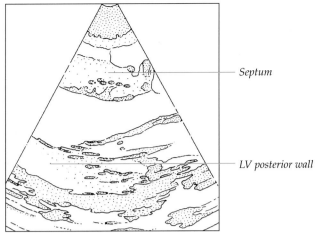

Septum

LV posterior wall

FIGURE 8-25. Left ventricular (LV) hypertrophy in a cocaine user. A two-dimensional echocardiogram demonstrates hypertrophy of the LV septum and posterior wall in a chronic cocaine user. Chronic use of cocaine is associated with increased LV mass and wall thickness [22], which may provide a substrate for the development of myocardial ischemia and/or arrhythmias in cocaine abusers.

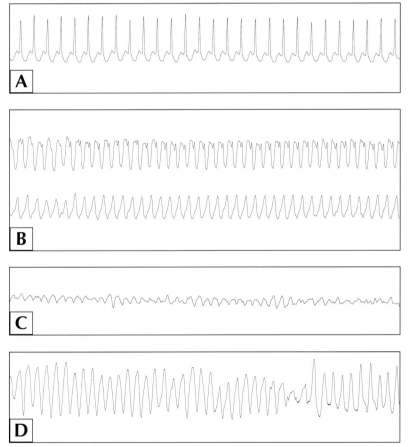

A

B

C

D

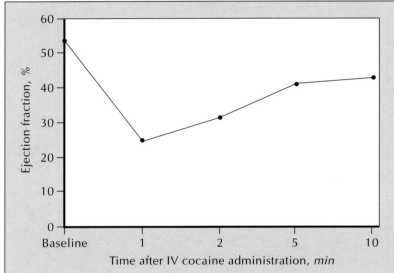

FIGURE 8-27. Cardiomyopathy with cocaine use. Dilated cardiomyopathy has been described in chronic cocaine users, and transient, severe myocardial dysfunction has been described after acute cocaine ingestion [23]. Studies in conscious animals have shown that intravenous (IV) cocaine (4 mg/kg) rapidly depresses left ventricular function—*ie*, the ejection fraction fell from 53% to 25% 1 minute after the drug was administered [24]. Presumably, cocaine similarly affects myocardial function in humans. (*Adapted from* Fraker and coworkers [24]; with permission.)

FIGURE 8-26. Cardiac arrhythmias associated with cocaine use. Large doses of cocaine prolong the P-R interval, QRS, and Q-T interval, acting like a class I antiarrhythmic agent. Supraventricular tachycardia (**A**), ventricular tachycardia (**B**), ventricular fibrillation (**C**), and asystole have been reported after cocaine use in the absence of myocardial ischemia. Heart block, bundle branch block, and torsades de pointes (**D**) have been reported in the setting of cocaine-induced myocardial ischemia [13].

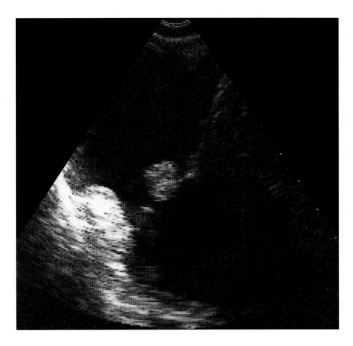

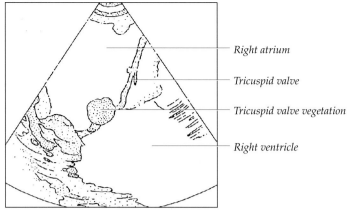

Right atrium

Tricuspid valve

Tricuspid valve vegetation

Right ventricle

FIGURE 8-28. Transesophageal echocardiogram in a patient with tricuspid valve endocarditis. Endocarditis is a relatively frequent infection in intravenous drug abusers [25], with involvement of the tricuspid valve especially common. *Staphylococcus* is most often the offending organism, followed by *Streptococcus* and gram-negative organisms.

TOXINS (UREMIA)

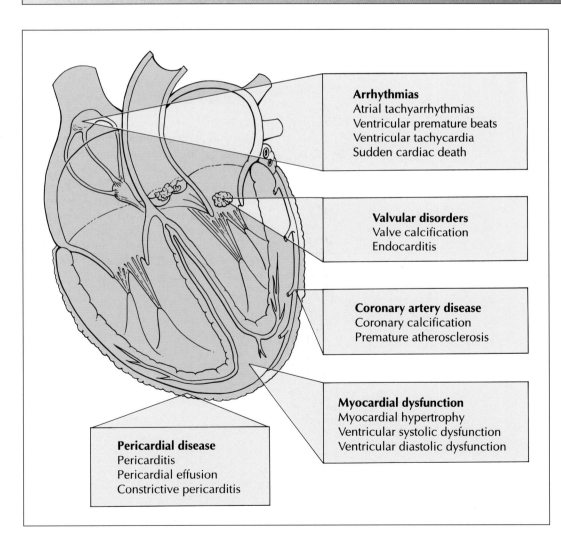

Arrhythmias
Atrial tachyarrhythmias
Ventricular premature beats
Ventricular tachycardia
Sudden cardiac death

Valvular disorders
Valve calcification
Endocarditis

Coronary artery disease
Coronary calcification
Premature atherosclerosis

Myocardial dysfunction
Myocardial hypertrophy
Ventricular systolic dysfunction
Ventricular diastolic dysfunction

Pericardial disease
Pericarditis
Pericardial effusion
Constrictive pericarditis

FIGURE 8-29. Cardiovascular disease accounts for more than 50% of the morbidity and mortality in patients with end-stage renal disease. Patients with chronic renal failure (uremia) may develop a variety of cardiovascular diseases including arrhythmias, valvular disorders, coronary artery disease, myocardial dysfunction, and pericardial disease [26–39].

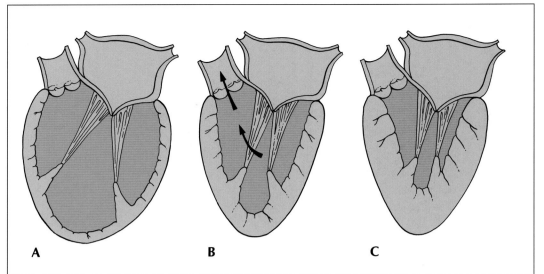

FIGURE 8-30. Congestive heart failure in the patient with uremia may result from the following: **A,** Systolic dysfunction (*ie,* dilated or congestive cardiomyopathy); **B,** A high-output state (*eg,* from anemia, arteriovenous fistula); or **C,** Diastolic dysfunction (left ventricular [LV] hypertrophy [27,29]). **D,** These disease states can be differentiated based on cardiac output, systemic vascular resistance, LV ejection fraction, wall thickness, and volumes.

D. DISEASE DIFFERENTIATION

	DILATED CARDIOMYOPATHY	HIGH-OUTPUT STATE	DIASTOLIC DYSFUNCTION
Cardiac output	Decreased	Increased	Normal
Systemic vascular resistance	Increased	Decreased	Normal or increased
LV ejection fraction	Decreased	Normal or decreased	Normal
LV wall thickness	Decreased	Normal	Increased
LV volumes	Increased	Increased	Normal

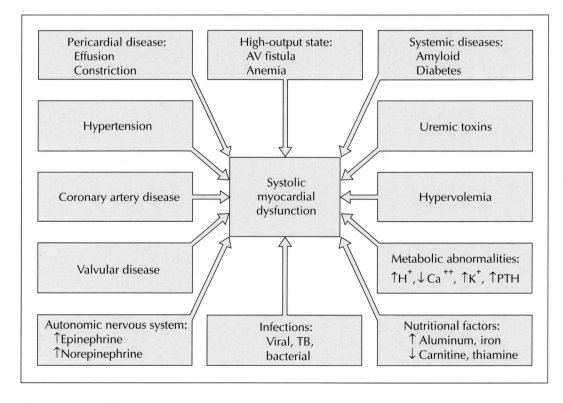

FIGURE 8-31. Left ventricular systolic dysfunction is common in uremic patients, and a number of factors may contribute to its development [29–33]. Noninvasive imaging techniques (*eg,* radionuclide ventriculography, echocardiography) or contrast left ventriculography demonstrates dilatation of the cardiac chambers and reduced ejection fraction in these patients. AV—arteriovenous; PTH—parathyroid hormone; TB—tuberculosis.

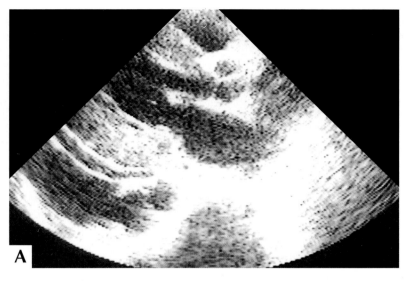

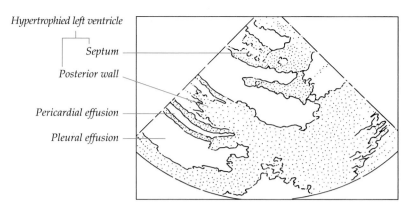

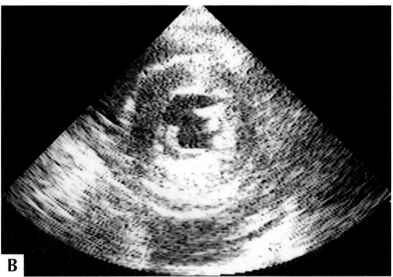

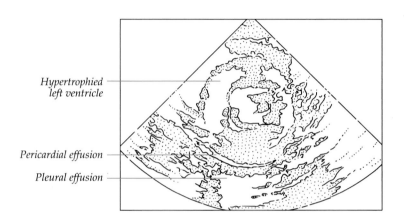

FIGURE 8-32. Two-dimensional echocardiograms (parasternal long-axis [A] and short-axis [B] views) in a uremic patient. Hypertrophy of the left ventricle is due to chronic volume overload and systemic arterial hypertension. Even though systolic function is normal, congestive heart failure may develop in these patients because the ventricle is stiff and noncompliant (*ie*, diastolic function is impaired) [28]. Pericardial and pleural effusions are evident. Chest pain in the absence of epicardial coronary artery disease is common because the number of capillaries is not adequate to supply the hypertrophied myocardium. Furthermore, the capacity of the arterioles to dilate and augment coronary flow is reduced, resulting in a decrease in coronary flow reserve [34,35].

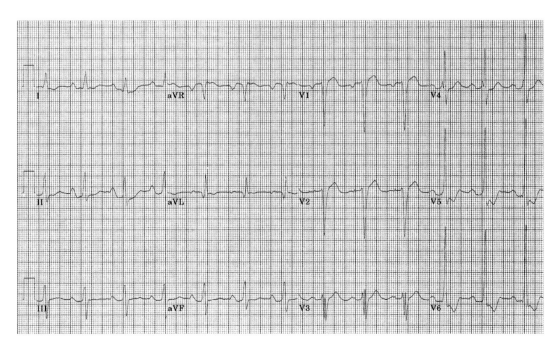

FIGURE 8-33. Twelve-lead ECG of a patient with uremia showing left atrial and left ventricular hypertrophy. The P wave is wide and notched in the inferior leads. The QRS voltage is increased, and repolarization abnormalities can be seen throughout. Patients with left ventricular hypertrophy are predisposed to atrial and ventricular arrhythmias.

CLINICAL FEATURES OF UREMIC PERICARDITIS

SYMPTOMS	PHYSICAL FINDINGS
Chest pain	Fever
Nonspecific complaints	Friction rub
Fever	Pericardial effusion, resulting in
Nonproductive cough	Tachycardia
Dyspnea, tachypnea	Hypotension
Malaise	Pulsus paradoxus
Headache, myalgias	Jugular venous distension
	Left infrascapular egophony (Ewart's sign)
	Dampened maximal impulse
	Distant heart sounds
	Neurologic disorders (stupor, confusion, coma)

FIGURE 8-34. Clinical features of uremic pericarditis. Chest pain is most common and is present in approximately 65% of uremic patients with pericarditis. It may be quite severe and is typically worse when the patient is recumbent but improves when the patient is upright and leaning forward. Fever and nonspecific symptoms may also be present. On examination, a scratchy, high-frequency heart sound having one, two, or three components can be heard. Uremic pericarditis is almost always accompanied by pericardial effusion; related physical findings depend upon the size of the effusion and its rate of development as well as the compliance of the pericardial sac.

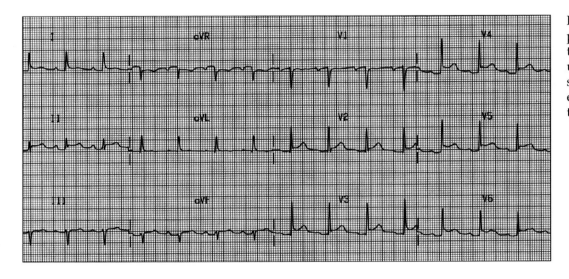

FIGURE 8-35. Electrocardiogram in uremic pericarditis. Pericarditis develops in 10% to 20% of patients in acute renal failure or undergoing chronic hemodialysis for end-stage renal disease. Diffuse ST-segment elevation and PR-segment depression are typical findings in such patients.

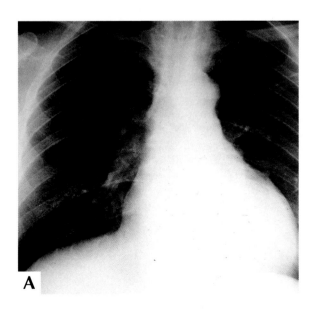

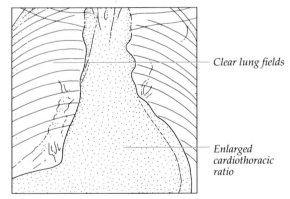

Clear lung fields

Enlarged cardiothoracic ratio

FIGURE 8-36. Chest radiograph in a uremic patient with pericardial effusion. **A,** With a moderate to large effusion, the cardiothoracic ratio is typically increased in the absence of pulmonary congestion, and the cardiac silhouette has a globular ("water-bottle") or triangular configuration. (*continued*)

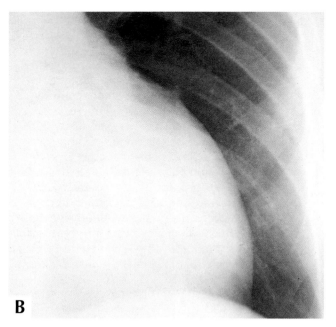

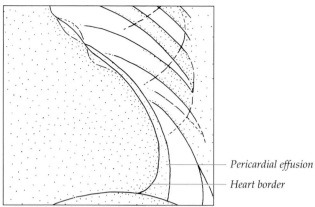

B

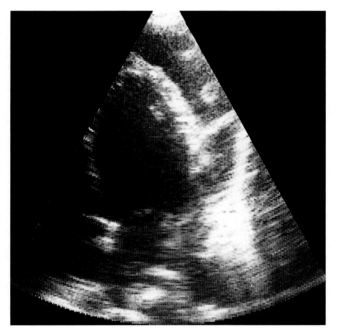

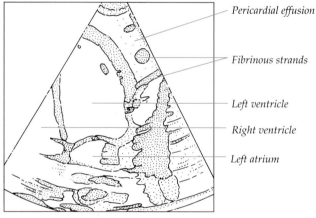

FIGURE 8-36. (*continued*) **B,** On closer inspection, the pericardial effusion can occasionally be seen extending past the heart border.

FIGURE 8-37. Two-dimensional echocardiogram (long-axis view) in a uremic patient with a large pericardial effusion. The presence and size of such effusions are best evaluated using this imaging modality. Uremic pericardial effusions are usually hemorrhagic, and fibrinous strands can often be seen. The hemodynamic significance of the effusion depends upon its volume and rate of accumulation and the compliance of the pericardial sac. Cardiac tamponade develops in 10% to 35% of uremic patients with pericardial effusion and can be identified on two-dimensional echocardiography by collapse of the right-sided heart chambers during diastole.

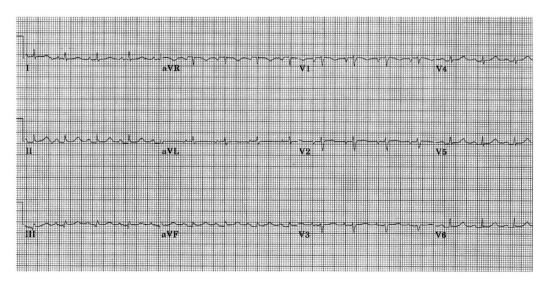

FIGURE 8-38. Electrocardiogram in a uremic patient with pericardial effusion. When the effusion is large, low-voltage QRS complexes may replace the tall (high-voltage) QRS complexes typical of the left ventricular hypertrophy that is usually present. In this patient, low-voltage QRS complexes and diffuse ST-segment elevation due to pericarditis are evident. In some patients, electrical alternans (*ie,* beat-to-beat variation in the heart axis) may also be seen.

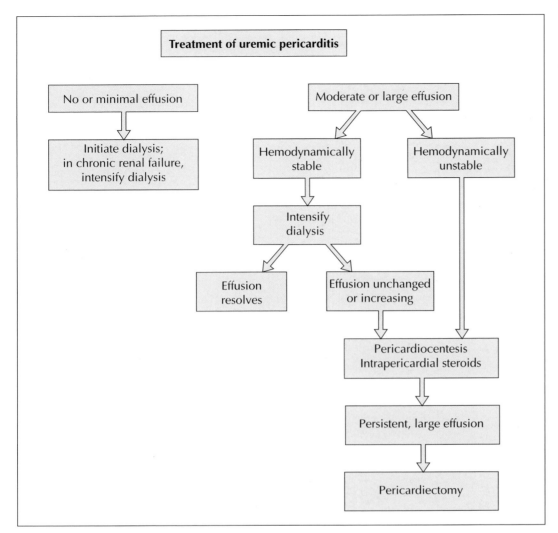

Treatment of uremic pericarditis

No or minimal effusion → Initiate dialysis; in chronic renal failure, intensify dialysis

Moderate or large effusion → Hemodynamically stable / Hemodynamically unstable

Hemodynamically stable → Intensify dialysis → Effusion resolves / Effusion unchanged or increasing

Effusion unchanged or increasing → Pericardiocentesis Intrapericardial steroids

Hemodynamically unstable → Pericardiocentesis Intrapericardial steroids

Pericardiocentesis Intrapericardial steroids → Persistent, large effusion → Pericardiectomy

FIGURE 8-39. Approach to treatment of uremic pericarditis. In the patient with acute renal failure, the presence of pericarditis (with or without pericardial effusion) is an indication to initiate dialysis. In the patient with chronic renal failure on maintenance dialysis, a large pericardial effusion is an indication to intensify dialysis by increasing its frequency and/or duration. Two-dimensional echocardiography should be used to follow the progress of therapy. If the patient is hemodynamically unstable or has a persistent, large pericardial effusion despite intensive dialysis, pericardiocentesis and intrapericardial instillation of steroids should be performed. If a large effusion persists, pericardiectomy is indicated [36].

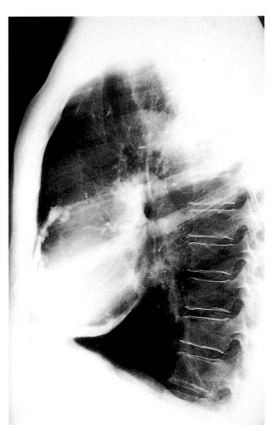

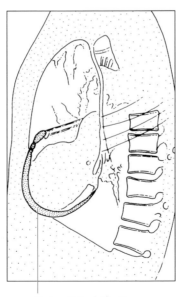

Pericardial calcification

FIGURE 8-40. Chest radiograph in constrictive pericarditis. Chronic constrictive pericarditis develops in less than 5% of patients with uremic pericarditis. In these patients, pericardial calcification may be observed on a routine chest radiograph. The lateral view is particularly useful for detecting calcification along the diaphragmatic and

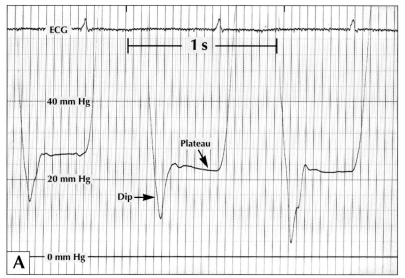

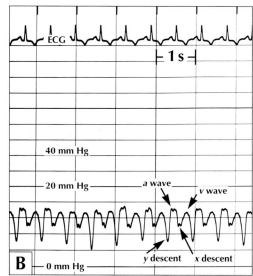

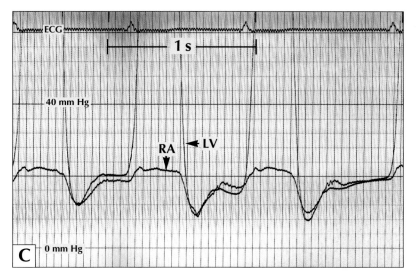

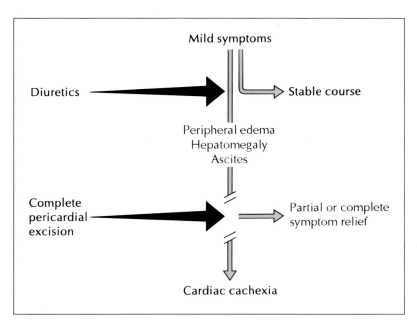

FIGURE 8-41. Hemodynamic effects of constrictive pericarditis. **A,** Left ventricular (LV) pressure tracing showing the characteristic "dip-and-plateau" configuration during diastole. The dip represents unimpeded emptying of atrial blood into the ventricle, and the plateau is due to a rapid rise in pressure as the constricting pericardium impairs LV filling. **B,** Right atrial (RA) pressure tracing showing a prominent *y* descent, which indicates that RA emptying is rapid and unimpeded during early diastole. **C,** Simultaneous LV and RA pressure recordings showing elevated and equalized pressures during diastole.

FIGURE 8-42. Management of constrictive pericarditis. Chronic constrictive pericarditis is a progressive and unrelenting disease. A minority of patients with mild symptoms and modestly elevated venous pressure may survive for many years on diuretic therapy. However, in most cases, increasing venous congestion leads to peripheral edema, hepatomegaly, ascites, and cardiac cachexia. Complete resection of the pericardium is required in these patients. Although this procedure carries a 15% mortality rate, over 90% of survivors show symptomatic improvement, and symptoms are relieved completely in 50%.

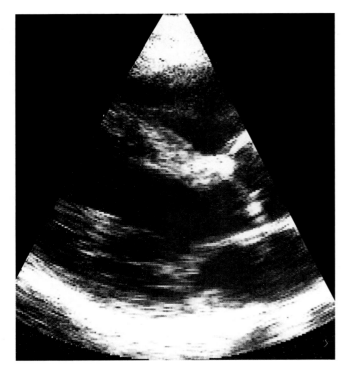
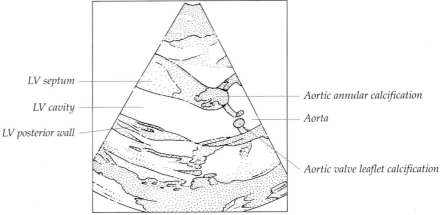

LV septum

LV cavity

LV posterior wall

Aortic annular calcification

Aorta

Aortic valve leaflet calcification

FIGURE 8-43. Valve calcification on two-dimensional echocardiography in a patient with uremia. Secondary hyperparathyroidism associated with chronic renal failure results in ectopic calcification that may involve the cardiac valves, conduction system, and epicardial coronary vessels [33]. Calcification most commonly involves the aortic valve (as in this patient) and mitral valve, affecting the annulus, cusps, and/or leaflets. Valve calcification may lead to infective endocarditis, aortic stenosis, or mitral regurgitation. LV—left ventricular.

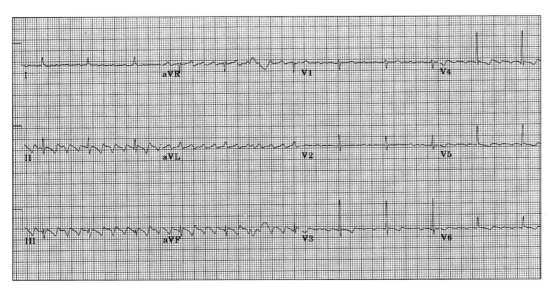

FIGURE 8-44. Atrial flutter in a patient with uremia. Supraventricular and ventricular arrhythmias are common in patients with end-stage renal disease and may be due to electrolyte or acid-base disturbances; pericardial disease; impaired ventricular systolic function; ventricular hypertrophy and diastolic dysfunction; calcification of the sinoatrial node, atrioventricular node, and conduction system; myocardial ischemia; accumulation of drugs normally excreted by the kidney; and hemodialysis.

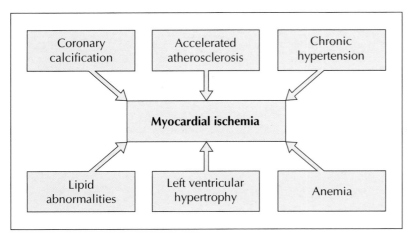

FIGURE 8-45. In the patient with uremia, coronary calcification, accelerated atherosclerosis, chronic hypertension, lipid abnormalities (elevated triglycerides and reduced high-density lipoprotein cholesterol), left ventricular hypertrophy, and anemia may contribute to the development of myocardial ischemia [37,38]. Those with coronary artery stenoses may undergo coronary artery surgery, albeit at an increased risk [39]. Coronary angioplasty is associated with a high incidence of restenosis in patients on chronic dialysis [40] and, therefore, is not usually performed.

REFERENCES

1. Chou T-C: Electrolyte imbalance. In *Electrocardiography in Clinical Practice*, ed 2. Edited by Chou T-C. Orlando: Grune & Stratton; 1986:563–585.

2. Sandøe E, Sigurd B: *Arrhythmia—A Guide to Clinical Electrocardiology.* Bingen: Publishing Partners Verlags GmbH; 1991:167.

3. Stratmann HG, Kennedy HL: Torsades de pointes associated with drugs and toxins: recognition and management. *Am Heart J* 1987, 113:1470–1482.

4. Surawicz B: Is hypermagnesemia or magnesium deficiency arrhythmogenic? *J Am Coll Cardiol* 1989, 14:1093–1096.

5. Fowler NO, McCall D, Chou T, *et al.*: Electrocardiographic changes and cardiac arrhythmias in patients receiving psychotropic drugs. *Am J Cardiol* 1976, 37:223–230.

6. Huston JR, Bell GE: The effect of thioridazine hydrochloride and chlorpromazine on the electrocardiogram. *JAMA* 1966, 198:16–20.

7. Kemper AJ, Dunlap R, Pietro DA: Thioridazine-induced torsades de pointes: successful therapy with isoproterenol. *JAMA* 1983, 249:2931–2934.

8. Hollister LE, Kosek JC: Sudden death during treatment with phenothiazine derivatives. *JAMA* 1965, 192:1035–1038.

9. Demers RG, Heniger GR: Electrocardiographic T-wave changes during lithium carbonate treatment. *JAMA* 1977, 218:381–386.

10. Montalescot G, Levy Y, Hatt PY: Serious sinus node dysfunction caused by therapeutic doses of lithium. *Int J Cardiol* 1984, 5:94–96.

11. Tilkian AG, Schroeder JS, Kao JJ, *et al.*: The cardiovascular effects of lithium in man: a review of the literature. *Am J Med* 1976, 61:665–670.

12. Brady HR, Horgan JH: Lithium and the heart: unanswered questions. *Chest* 1988, 93:166–169.

13. Lange RA, Willard JE: The cardiovascular effects of cocaine. *Heart Dis Stroke* 1993, 2:136–141.

14. Isner JM, Estes NAM III, Thompson PD, *et al.*: Acute cardiac events temporally related to cocaine use. *N Engl J Med* 1986, 315:1438–1443.

15. Minor RL Jr, Scott BD, Brown DD, *et al.*: Cocaine-induced myocardial infarction in patients with normal coronary arteries. *Ann Intern Med* 1991, 115:797–806.

16. Lange RA, Cigarroa RG, Yancy CW, *et al.*: Cocaine-induced coronary artery vasoconstriction. *N Engl J Med* 1989, 321:1557–1562.

17. Flores ED, Lange RA, Cigarroa RG, *et al.*: Effect of cocaine on coronary arterial dimensions in atherosclerotic coronary artery disease: enhanced vasoconstriction at sites of significant stenoses. *J Am Coll Cardiol* 1990, 16:74–79.

18. Brogan WC, Lange RA, Kim AS, *et al.*: Alleviation of cocaine-induced coronary vasoconstriction by nitroglycerin. *J Am Coll Cardiol* 1991, 18:581–586.

19. Lange RA, Cigarroa RG, Flores ED, *et al.*: Potentiation of cocaine-induced coronary vasoconstriction by beta-adrenergic blockade. *Ann Intern Med* 1990, 112:897–903.

20. Stenberg RG, Winniford WD, Hillis LD, *et al.*: Simultaneous acute thrombosis of two major coronary arteries following intravenous cocaine use. *Arch Pathol Lab Med* 1989, 113:521–524.

21. Kugelmass AD, Oda A, Monahan K, *et al.*: Activation of human platelets by cocaine. *Circulation* 1993, 88:876–883.

22. Brickner ME, Willard JE, Eichorn EJ, *et al.*: Left ventricular hypertrophy associated with drug abuse. *Circulation* 1991, 84:1130–1135.

23. Chokshi SK, Moore R, Pandian NG, *et al.*: Reversible cardiomyopathy associated with cocaine intoxication. *Ann Intern Med* 1989, 111:1039–1040.

24. Fraker TD, Temesy-Armos PN, Brewster PS, *et al.*: Mechanism of cocaine-induced myocardial depression in dogs. *Circulation* 1990; 81:1012–1016.

25. Chambers HF, Morris DL, Tauber MG, *et al.*: Cocaine use and the risk for endocarditis in intravenous drug users. *Ann Intern Med* 1987, 106:833–836.

26. Silberberg JS, Barre PE, Prichard SS, *et al.*: Impact of left ventricular hypertrophy on survival in end-stage renal disease. *Kidney Int* 1989, 36:286–290.

27. London GM, Fabiani F, Marchais SJ, *et al.*: Uremic cardiomyopathy: an inadequate left ventricular hypertrophy. *Kidney Int* 1987, 31:973–980.

28. Kramer W, Wizeman V, Lammlein G, *et al.*: Cardiac dysfunction in patients on maintenance hemodialysis. II. Systolic and diastolic properties of the left ventricle assessed by invasive methods. *Contrib Nephrol* 1986, 52:110–124.

29. Silberberg JS, Rahal DP, Patton DR, *et al.*: Role of anemia in the pathogenesis of left ventricular hypertrophy in end-stage renal disease. *Am J Cardiol* 1989, 64:222–224.

30. London GM, de Vernejoul MC, Fabiani F, *et al.*: Secondary hyperparathyroidism and cardiac hypertrophy in hemodialysis patients. *Kidney Int* 1987, 32:900–907.

31. Mall G, Huther W, Schneider J, *et al.*: Diffuse intermyocardiocytic fibrosis in uraemic patients. *Nephrol Dial Transplant* 1990, 5:39–44.

32. Burt RK, Gupta-Burt S, Suki WN, *et al.*: Reversal of left ventricular dysfunction after renal transplantation. *Ann Intern Med* 1989, 111:635–640.

33. Rostand SG, Sanders C, Kirk KA, *et al.*: Myocardial calcification and cardiac dysfunction in chronic renal failure. *Am J Med* 1988, 85:651–657.

34. Roig E, Betriu A, Castaner A, *et al.*: Disabling angina pectoris with normal coronary arteries in patients undergoing maintenance hemodialysis. *Am J Med* 1981, 71:431–434.

35. Brush JE Jr, Cannon RO III, Shenke WH, *et al.*: Angina due to coronary microvascular disease in hypertensive patients without left ventricular hypertrophy. *N Engl J Med* 1988, 319:1302–1307.

36. Rutsky EA, Rostand SG: Treatment of uremic pericarditis and pericardial effusion. *Am J Kidney Dis* 1987, 10:2–8.

37. Lindner A, Charra B, Sherrard DJ, *et al.*: Accelerated atherosclerosis in prolonged maintenance hemodialysis. *N Engl J Med* 1974, 290:697–701.

38. Attman P-O, Alaupovic P, Gustafson A: Serum apolipoprotein profile of patients with chronic renal failure. *Kidney Int* 1987, 32:368–375.

39. Deutsch E, Bernstein RC, Addonizio P, *et al.*: Coronary artery bypass surgery in patients on chronic hemodialysis. *Ann Intern Med* 1989, 110:369–372.

40. Kahn JK, Rutherford BD, McConahay DR, *et al.*: Short- and long-term outcome of percutaneous transluminal coronary angioplasty in chronic dialysis patients. *Am Heart J* 1990, 119:484–489.

THE ATHLETE'S HEART AND CARDIOVASCULAR DISEASE IN COMPETITIVE ATHLETES

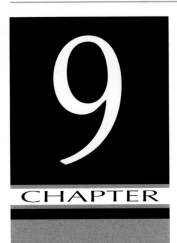

9

CHAPTER

Barry J. Maron

Long-term athletic training often leads to increases in left ventricular (LV) end-diastolic cavity dimension, wall thickness, and calculated mass, constituting what is commonly known as the "athlete's heart." This form of LV hypertrophy is regarded as "physiologic" because it appears to be related dynamically to the magnitude of athletic activity—ie, it increases with training and decreases with deconditioning. Alterations in the cardiac dimensions of trained athletes are variable in expression and also appear to be determined by the intensity and duration of the conditioning program as well as the type of sport in which they are engaged. Indeed, in primarily isometric (power) sports, increases in LV wall thickness are usually disproportionate to those in cavity size, although rarely is the wall thickness increased in absolute terms. On the other hand, in many isotonic (endurance) sports, the increases in cavity dimension associated with training are either disproportionate to or similar in magnitude to the increase in wall thickness.

When more substantial increases in absolute wall thickness are observed in selected elite athletes, it may pose the diagnostic dilemma of distinguishing between the clinically benign hypertrophy of "athlete's heart" and pathologic hypertrophy (*ie*, hypertrophic cardiomyopathy [HCM]). Several approaches have been suggested to aid in this differential diagnosis. Among the findings that support the diagnosis of HCM are an LV wall thickness of 15 mm or more and an LV cavity dimension less than 45 mm, documentation of HCM in a relative of the athlete, and a transmitral Doppler waveform consistent with impaired LV filling or relaxation. Findings that favor "athlete's heart" are regression of LV hypertrophy following a short period of deconditioning and an LV diastolic cavity dimension exceeding 55 mm.

Recently, the compelling problem of cardiovascular disease and sudden cardiac death in youthful trained athletes has become a subject of growing interest. In young competitive athletes, a variety of largely congenital cardiovascular disorders have been implicated as the principal causes of death on the athletic field, the most common being HCM, congenital anomalies of the coronary arteries, Marfan syndrome, myocarditis, and (in one series) right ventricular dysplasia. In most of these disorders, sudden death occurs in the setting of electrical instability and ventricular arrhythmias. In older athletes (over 35 years of age), sudden death is usually due to coronary artery disease.

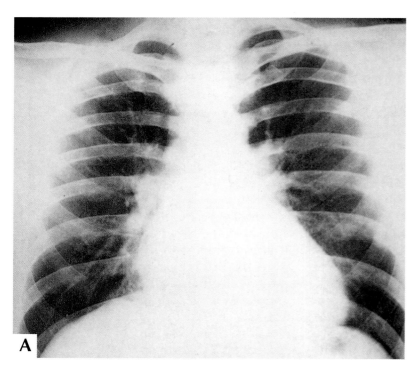

FIGURE 9-1. A, Chest radiograph from an athlete in 1959 (over a decade before the era of echocardiography) showing cardiac enlargement, believed to be due to increased volume. These radiographic changes were attributed to the effects of conditioning ("athlete's heart") rather than to structural cardiac disease. **B,** Associated electrocardiographic abnormalities, suggestive of left ventricular hypertrophy.

The entity of athlete's heart was first recognized in 1899 by Henschen, who measured cardiac size by carefully performed percussion in cross-country skiers. Therefore, almost 100 years ago, physiologic enlargement of the heart due to sports activity was described and thought to be capable of enhanced workload. (*Adapted from* Rost and Hollmann [1]; with permission.)

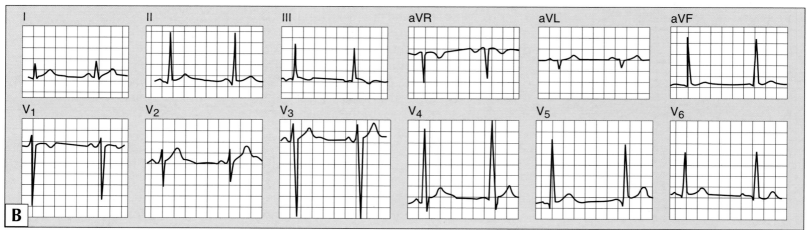

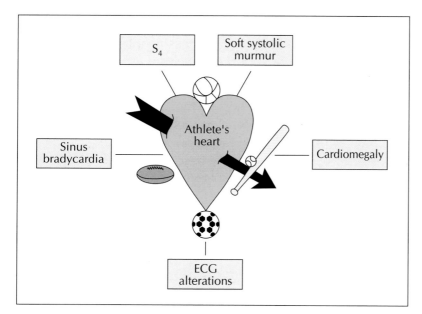

FIGURE 9-2. The "athlete's heart syndrome," as classically described, comprises the constellation of sinus bradycardia, cardiomegaly on chest radiography, and a variety of electrocardiographic (ECG) alterations, often accompanied by a soft systolic ejection murmur and fourth heart sound (S₄).

ADAPTATIONS TO EXERCISE TRAINING

PARAMETER	TYPE OF TRAINING	
	DYNAMIC	STATIC
O_2 consumption ($\dot{V}O_2$max)	↑↑↑↑	↑
Stroke volume	↑↑↑	No change
Cardiac output	↑↑↑	↑
Heart rate (maximal)	↑↑↑	↑
Blood pressure		
Systolic	↑↑	↑↑↑
Diastolic	↓	↑↑↑
Mean	↑	↑↑↑
End-diastolic LV volume	↑	No change
End-systolic LV volume	↓	No change
Systemic vascular resistance	↓↓↓	No change
O_2 extraction (A-$\dot{V}O_2$ diff$_{max}$)	↑↑	No change
Cardiac contractility	↑	↑

FIGURE 9-3. Physiologic cardiovascular adaptations to exercise training in athletes. Responses are shown to both dynamic conditioning (isotonic, endurance, or aerobic), such as distance running or swimming, and static training (isometric, power, or strength), such as weightlifting or wrestling. The cardiovascular adaptations to dynamic training in normal subjects have been well documented for over 25 years and classically include (during exercise) increases in maximal oxygen consumption, stroke volume, cardiac output, arteriovenous oxygen difference, and heart rate. The precise cardiovascular responses to static (isometric) training differ somewhat from those in endurance athletes, with less marked changes in maximal oxygen consumption, stroke volume, cardiac output, and left ventricular (LV) volume but more marked increases in blood pressure.

It should be emphasized, however, that athletes rarely engage in purely dynamic or purely static modes of training; for example, dynamic (endurance) athletes may lift weights as part of their training, while weightlifters sometimes include running as part of their regimen. All these cardiovascular alterations are produced by a complex set of central and peripheral mechanisms operating at the structural, metabolic, and regulatory levels. Furthermore, it should be emphasized that physical training has the potential to alter not only cardiac dimensions but also autonomic state, preload, and afterload. Therefore, it is often difficult to separate the effects of cardiac and extracardiac training on ventricular performance.

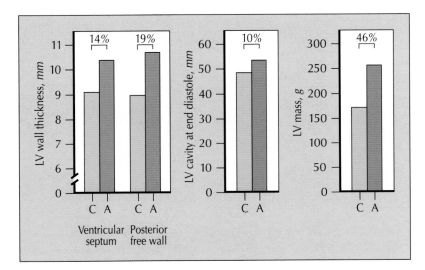

FIGURE 9-4. Global analysis of cardiac dimensional changes in trained athletes based on 25 cross-sectional studies comprising over 700 subjects [2]. Left ventricular (LV) dimensions derived from

M-mode echocardiographic studies in chronically conditioned athletes (A) (mostly men) and nonathlete controls (C) are compared in absolute terms in order to be more clinically relevant. However, it should be noted that published reports of cardiac dimensions in athletes are not infrequently normalized for body surface area, body weight, or lean body mass. Differences between the athlete and the nonathlete populations are significant but relatively small in absolute terms. Values for LV wall thickness and LV cavity dimension at end diastole in athletes exceed those of controls by about 10% to 20%, while differences in calculated LV mass are more substantial (*ie*, approaching 50%), and magnified because both wall thickness and cavity size are taken into account. Of note, an end-diastolic LV dimension 10% greater than that in sedentary control subjects corresponds to a ventricular volume difference of about 33%. A broad range of sporting disciplines and levels of training and achievement, as well as ages and backgrounds of the subjects, have been "lumped" together here for the purpose of generating a picture of the overall echocardiographic results. The percent difference between athletes and controls for each dimension is shown above the respective bars.

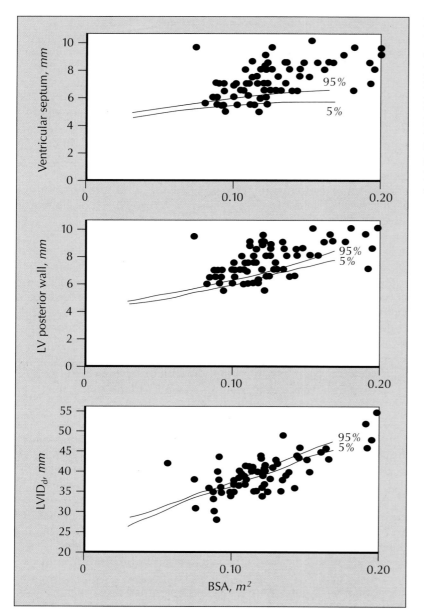

FIGURE 9-5. Alterations in cardiac dimensions associated with training may be induced early in childhood, even when the athletes are still maturing physically and their body habitus is not yet fully developed. Cardiac dimensions are shown for 77 competitive swimmers, 5 to 17 years of age, as assessed by echocardiography. Whereas measurements of ventricular septal and posterior left ventricular (LV) free wall thickness exceeded 95% confidence limits in most athletes, LV end-diastolic internal dimensions (LVID$_d$) were more frequently within normal limits. In only 30% of these athletes was the LV cavity size greater than normal. BSA—body surface area. (*Adapted from* Allen and coworkers [3]; with permission from the American Heart Association, Inc.)

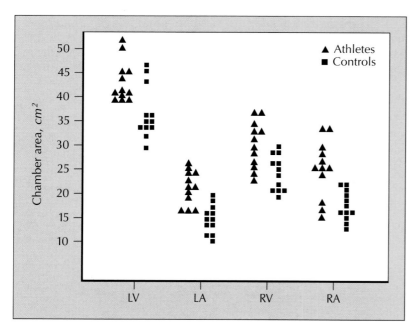

FIGURE 9-6. Chamber areas in endurance athletes and control subjects as measured in the four-chamber view for the left ventricle (LV), left atrium (LA), right ventricle (RV), and right atrium (RA). Although alterations in LV dimension have been emphasized as a frequent consequence of training, all four cardiac chambers are often enlarged. Enlargement of both ventricles and atria is relatively symmetric. (*Adapted from* Hauser and coworkers [4]; with permission).

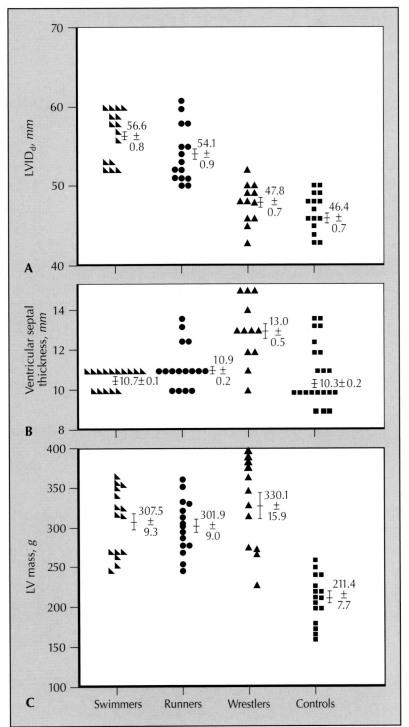

FIGURE 9-7. Initial echocardiographic study in college athletes showing the diversity of effects on cardiac dimensions induced by different sports and training regimens. Isometric (power) trained wrestlers had disproportionately increased wall thickness with respect to cavity dimension when compared with two groups of isotonic (dynamic) trained athletes (swimmers and runners). It may be convenient to regard dynamic training as inducing a left ventricular (LV) *volume* load and, in contrast, static training as inducing a *pressure* load. **A,** LV internal dimensions at end diastole (LVID$_d$). Data for swimmers and runners are statistically different from those of wrestlers and control subjects (P<0.001). **B,** Diastolic ventricular septal thicknesses. Data for wrestlers are statistically different from those of swimmers, runners, and control subjects (P<0.001). **C,** LV mass in swimmers, runners, and wrestlers is statistically different from that of control subjects (P<0.001). (*Adapted from* Morganroth and coworkers [5]; with permission from the American College of Physicians.)

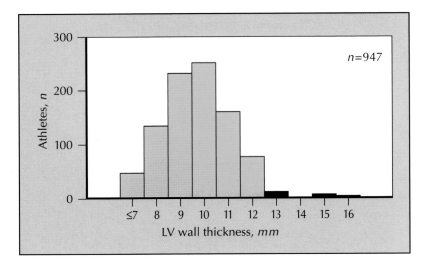

FIGURE 9-8. Distribution of maximal left ventricular (LV) wall thicknesses in 947 elite Italian athletes. *Orange* bars indicate wall thicknesses within the normal range; *black* bars indicate those athletes with increased thickness (≥13 mm). Therefore, of this large population of highly trained elite athletes, about 3% (limited to cyclists, rowers, and canoeists) have wall thicknesses within a range compatible with the diagnosis of hypertrophic cardiomyopathy. For athletes in these sports, the increase in LV wall thickness is disproportionate to that in cavity dimension (or internal cavity radius), possibly because of the greater isometric work required of the upper body. (*Adapted from* Pelliccia and coworkers [6]; with permission from the *New England Journal of Medicine*.)

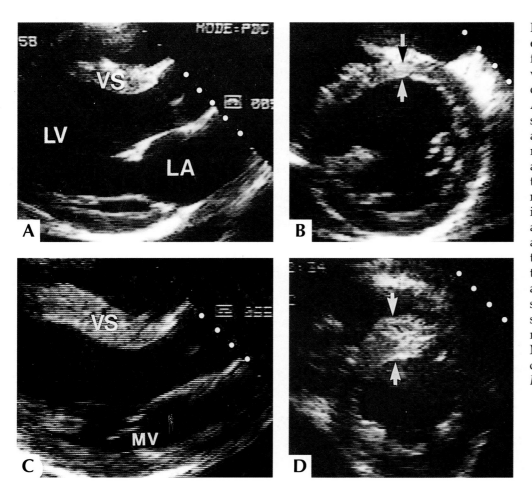

FIGURE 9-9. Stop-frame two-dimensional echocardiograms obtained during diastole from a 21-year-old cyclist with normal left ventricular (LV) wall thickness and a 25-year-old canoeist with thickening of the LV wall. **A,** Parasternal long-axis view in the cyclist showing normal anterior ventricular septal (VS) and posterior wall thicknesses (11 and 10 mm, respectively) and an enlarged LV cavity (61 mm) at end diastole. **B,** Short-axis view at the level of the papillary muscle in the same athlete showing normal thickness of all segments of the LV wall, including the anterior septum (*arrows*). **C,** Long-axis view in the canoeist showing a thickened anterior VS (16 mm) that exceeds the thickness of the posterior free wall; moderate enlargement of the LV cavity is also present. **D,** Short-axis view at the papillary muscle level in the same athlete showing localized thickening of the anterior septum (*arrows*), whereas the free wall and posterior septum are virtually normal. LA—left atrium; MV—mitral valve. (*Adapted from* Pelliccia and coworkers [6]; with permission from the *New England Journal of Medicine*.)

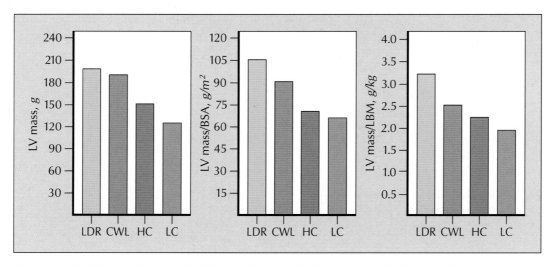

FIGURE 9-10. Comparison of *absolute* and *relative* left ventricular (LV) mass in athletes training in a dynamic sport (long-distance runners [LDR]) and a static one (competitive weightlifters [CWL]) and in appropriate heavyweight (HC) and lightweight (LC) control groups. Both dynamic and static training increase absolute LV mass to a similar degree. However, with static training the increase in LV mass is proportional to the increase in skeletal muscle mass, whereas with dynamic training the increase in LV mass is disproportionate to that in skeletal muscle mass. Therefore, only in highly trained competitive endurance athletes is LV mass significantly increased so that normalization with respect to body weight, body surface area (BSA), or lean body mass (LBM) does not alter this relationship. Also, LV mass was significantly larger in both runners and weightlifters in this study than in the respective control groups; normalization for LBM revealed that the weightlifters' mass was not significantly different from that of the heavyweight controls. (*Adapted from* Longhurst and coworkers [7]; with permission from the American Heart Association, Inc.)

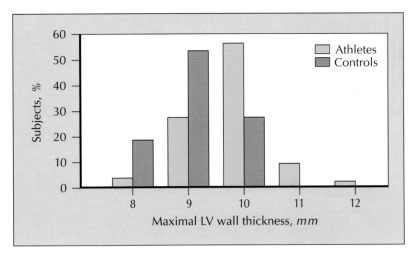

FIGURE 9-11. Power training per se does not constitute a particularly strong stimulus to increase *absolute* left ventricular (LV) wall

thickness. Distribution of absolute LV wall thicknesses in 100 athletes who trained systematically in a variety of sports involving pure power training over long periods of time (weight- and power-lifting, wrestling, bobsledding, and weight-throwing events) was compared with that in sedentary controls. The greatest wall thickness encountered was 12 mm, and only 12% of the athletes had thicknesses of 11 or 12 mm; however, wall thickening in such power athletes was disproportionate to cavity size (*ie*, internal cavity radius). Consequently, absolute increases in ventricular septal or posterior free wall thickness (≥13 mm) in elite athletes who train in power disciplines are unlikely to be due to conditioning and, by inference, are probably manifestations of primary LV hypertrophy (*ie*, hypertrophic cardiomyopathy). The cardiac dimensions presented here are in absolute terms for clinical relevance, although in the literature wall thicknesses reported in power athletes have frequently been normalized for body surface area, body weight, or lean body mass. (*Adapted from* Pelliccia and coworkers [8]; with permission.)

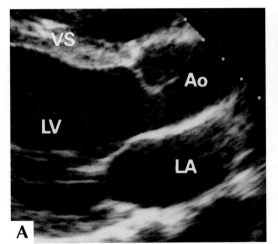
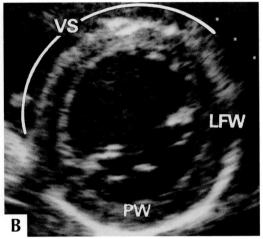

FIGURE 9-12. Alterations in echocardiographic dimensions associated with isometric (power) training. Two-dimensional (**A** and **B**) and M-mode (**C**) echocardiograms from a 20-year-old Olympic bobsledder with an increased body surface area of 2.02 m^2. Ventricular septal (VS) and posterior free wall (PW) thicknesses are normal (only 9 mm each), and left ventricular end-diastolic dimension (LVD) is mildly increased (57 mm). Calibration dots are 1 cm apart. Ao—aorta; LA—left atrium; LFW—lateral free wall. (*Adapted from* Pelliccia and coworkers [8]; with permission.)

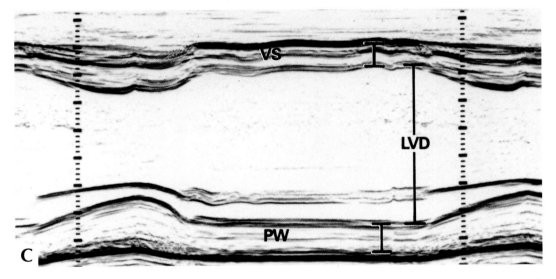

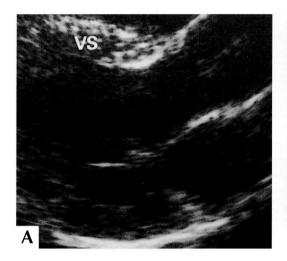

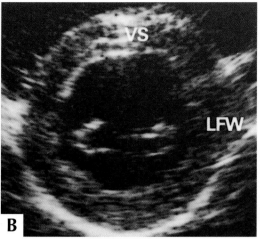

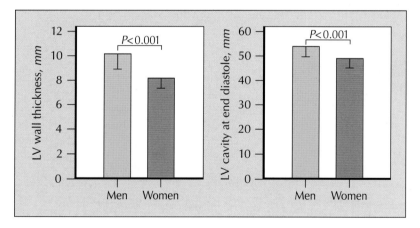

FIGURE 9-13. Alterations in echocardiographic dimensions associated with isometric (power) training. Two-dimensional (**A** and **B**) and M-mode (**C**) echocardiograms from a 24-year-old weightlifter with a body surface area of 2.32 m^2. Ventricular septal (VS) thickness is 12 mm, constituting the greatest wall thickness measurement identified a in study group of 100 purely power-trained athletes. Left ventricular end-diastolic dimension is mildly increased (*ie*, 56 mm). Calibration dots are 1 cm apart. LFW—lateral free wall. (*Adapted from* Pelliccia and coworkers [8]; with permission.)

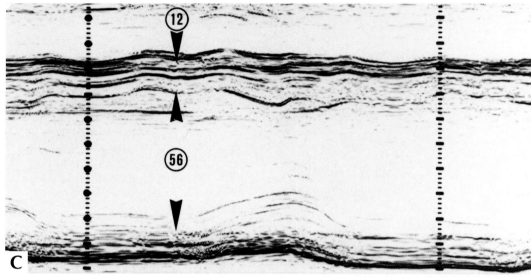

FIGURE 9-14. Data for 738 male and 607 female elite athletes participating in a variety of Olympic sports who show significantly different cardiac dimensions as a consequence of training. Left ventricular (LV) wall thickness and cavity dimension at end diastole were greater in the men than in the women, undoubtedly owing largely to differences in body size.

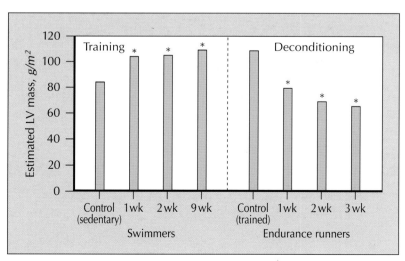

FIGURE 9-15. Serial echocardiographic data for estimated left ventricular (LV) mass (corrected for body surface area) showing an increase in mass with training and a decrease with deconditioning, owing largely to changes in LV cavity size. Subjects were eight competitive swimmers who trained for 9 weeks after a sedentary period and six endurance runners who trained for at least 3 months but later ceased their conditioning program. *Asterisks* indicate mean values obtained during training or deconditioning that were significantly different from those of respective control subjects (*P*<0.005). These results reflect the dynamic nature of the athlete's heart and substantiate the conclusion that the increase in LV mass is "physiologic" and thus a consequence of the training regimen. (*Adapted from* Ehsani and coworkers [9]; with permission.)

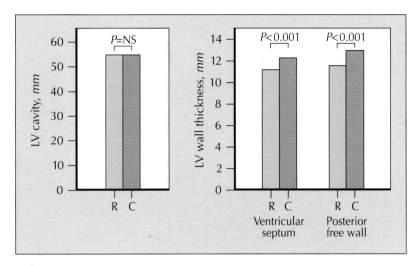

FIGURE 9-16. Dynamic changes in cardiac dimension associated with *spontaneously* occurring periods of conditioning and deconditioning, as assessed by echocardiography, in highly trained Belgian cyclists [10]. During the resting (R) and competitive (C) phases of their season, left ventricular (LV) cavity size did not change. However, LV mass changed significantly, primarily because the thickness of both the ventricular septum and the posterior wall increased during periods of training but decreased during periods of deconditioning.

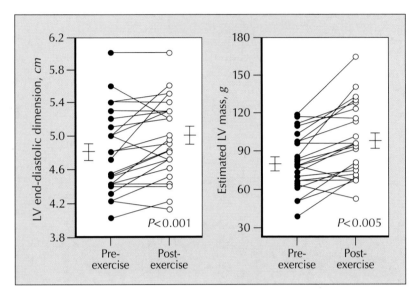

FIGURE 9-17. The acute dynamic changes in cardiac dimensions associated with conditioning can also be demonstrated in nontrained athletic subjects. Increases in transverse left ventricular (LV) end-diastolic dimension and calculated LV mass are shown here after a short-term (11-week) walk-jog-run exercise program. Compared with athletes exposed to long-term training, such short-term longitudinal studies (lasting less than 20 weeks) generally produce less impressive changes in LV volume. Mean values and standard deviations are shown for both the preexercise and postexercise evaluations. (*Adapted from* DeMaria and coworkers [11]; with permission from the American Heart Association, Inc.)

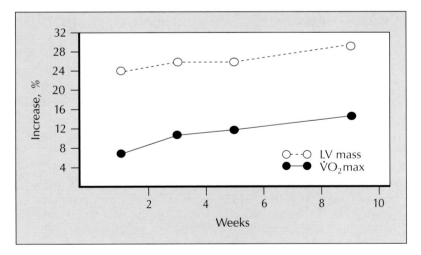

FIGURE 9-18. Sequential percent increase in maximal oxygen uptake ($\dot{V}O_2$max) associated with an increase in left ventricular (LV) mass during 9 weeks of intense physical training in competitive swimmers. (*Adapted from* Ehsani and coworkers [9]; with permission.)

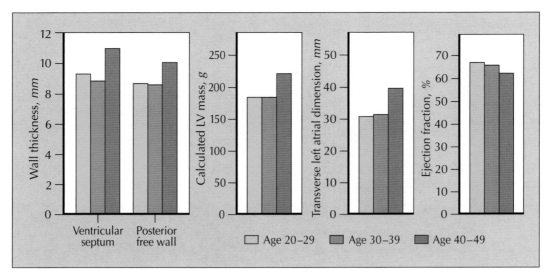

FIGURE 9-19. Alterations in cardiac dimensions based on M-mode echocardiographic data after particularly prolonged (*ie*, virtually lifelong) athletic conditioning in 60 competitive bicyclists [12]. Mean ventricular septal and posterior free wall thicknesses, calculated left ventricular (LV) mass, left atrial dimension, and ejection fraction are compared for bicyclists in three different age groups (20 to 29, 30 to 39, and 40 to 49 years of age). In the oldest age group the magnitude of LV hypertrophy was greater and the percent fractional shortening lower than in younger bicyclists, suggesting that the impact of (and adaptations to) training with respect to cardiac dimensions may continue or even progress over substantial portions of a lifetime.

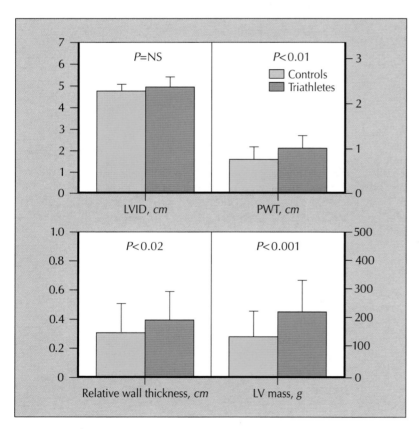

FIGURE 9-20. Effects on cardiac dimensions and mass associated with extreme (ultraendurance) forms of athletic training (*ie*, the triathlon). These triathletes trained for 20 to 40 hours per week, and the differences compared with control subjects are relatively mild (although statistically significant). These results suggest that the intensity of training is not always an absolute determinant of the magnitude of cardiac dimensional changes that result. LVID—left ventricular internal diameter; PWT—posterior wall thickness. (*Adapted from* Douglas and coworkers [13]; with permission.)

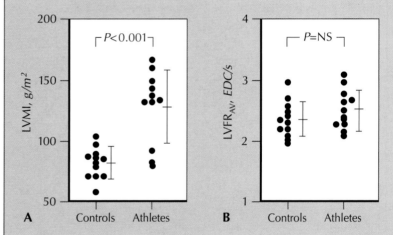

FIGURE 9-21. Left ventricular (LV) function in trained athletes. Although athletes have greater LV mass than sedentary controls, these two groups do not differ with respect to LV filling. **A,** Individual and mean values and standard deviations for LV mass index (LVMI) in the control subjects and the athletes (male distance runners). **B,** Individual and mean values and standard deviations for LV filling rates (LVFR$_{AV}$) for the two groups, as assessed with technetium-99m radionuclide angiography and expressed as end-diastolic counts per second (EDC/s) during the rapid filling phase of diastole. Digitized M-mode echocardiography and pulsed Doppler echocardiography have produced similar findings relative to LV filling in athletes under basal conditions. However, during exercise, LV filling indices may be enhanced. There is no evidence that training has any significant effect on contractile performance in athletes; if anything, training-induced bradycardia at rest may be associated with a negative inotropic effect, presumably reflecting decreased sympathetic drive. (*Adapted from* Granger and coworkers [14]; with permission from the American College of Cardiology.)

RESULTS OF HOLTER MONITORING IN 20 ENDURANCE ATHLETES AND 50 UNTRAINED CONTROL SUBJECTS

	LONG-DISTANCE RUNNERS, n(%)	UNTRAINED SUBJECTS, n(%)	P VALUE
Sinus nodal function			
Sinus tachycardia	17(85)	50(100)	<0.05
Sinus bradycardia	20(100)	50(100)	NS
Marked sinus bradycardia	17(85)	12(24)	<0.01
Moderate sinus arrhythmia	20(100)	43(86)	NS
Marked sinus arrhythmia	7(35)	25(50)	NS
Atrial arrhythmias			
APBs	20(100)	28(56)	<0.01
>100 APBs in 24 h	1(5)	1(2)	NS
Blocked APBs	2(10)	2(4)	NS
Atrial couplets	5(25)	0(0)	<0.01
Ectopic atrial tachycardia	2(10)	1(2)	NS
Ventricular arrhythmias			
VPBs	14(70)	25(50)	NS
>50 VPBs in 24 h	2(10)	1(2)	NS
Multifocal VPBs	4(20)	6(12)	NS
R-on-T phenomenon (VPBs)	0(0)	3(6)	NS
Ventricular couplets	0(0)	1(2)	NS
Ventricular tachycardia	0(0)	1(2)	NS
Atrioventricular block			
First-degree	9(45)	4(8)	<0.01
Second-degree, type I	8(40)	3(6)	<0.01

FIGURE 9-22. Arrhythmias in 20 endurance athletes (long-distance runners) and 50 untrained control subjects as evidenced by 24-hour ambulatory (Holter) electrocardiographic monitoring. These data substantiate that trained athletes do not differ from controls with respect to the prevalence of ventricular premature beats (VPBs), R-on-T phenomenon, ventricular couplets, or nonsustained ventricular tachycardia. In contrast, atrial premature beats (APBs) and first- and second-degree atrioventricular block are more common in athletes. (*Adapted from* Talan and coworkers [15]; with permission from the American College of Chest Physicians.)

DISTINCTION BETWEEN ATHLETE'S HEART AND PRIMARY LV HYPERTROPHY

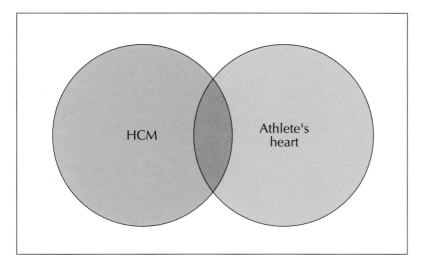

FIGURE 9-23. Athlete's heart (a "physiologic" state) and hypertrophic cardiomyopathy (HCM) (a primary cardiac disease that is the most common cause of sudden death in competitive athletes) are, in selected instances, difficult to distinguish based on morphologic appearance alone. This diagnostic dilemma arises when LV wall thickness is in the range of 13, 14, or possibly 15 mm, placing the athlete in the overlapping "gray zone" between the two conditions.

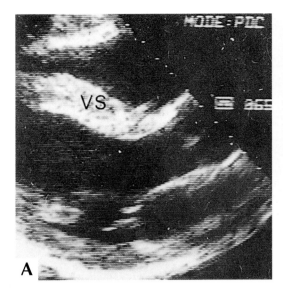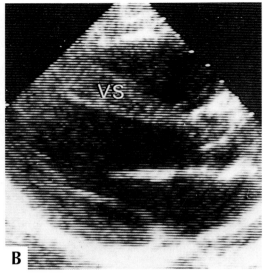

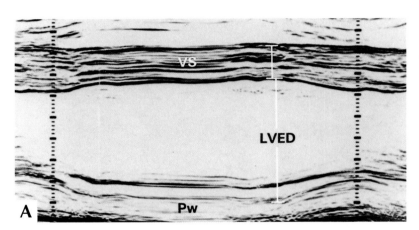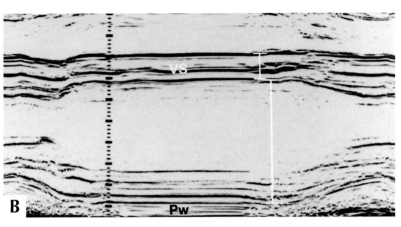

FIGURE 9-25. Dynamic change in left ventricular wall thickness associated with athletic deconditioning, constituting evidence for "physiologic" hypertrophy (*ie*, athlete's heart). Shown are serial M-mode echocardiograms recorded just below the mitral valve level in a 26-year-old Olympic rower at peak training (**A**) and after more than 8 months of complete deconditioning (**B**).

The ventricular septal (VS) thickness decreased from an abnormally increased value of 15 mm to within the normal range (*ie*, 10 mm). In addition, there was a small decrease in the left ventricular end-diastolic cavity dimension (LVED). The large calibration marks are 1 cm apart. Pw—posterior wall. (*Adapted from* Maron and coworkers [16]; with permission.)

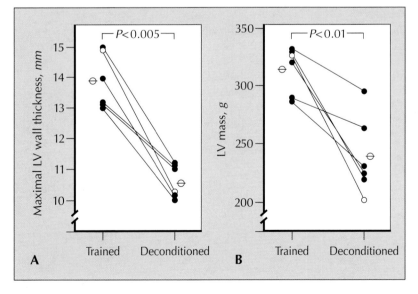

FIGURE 9-26. Changes in left ventricular (LV) wall thickness (**A**) and mass (**B**) associated with deconditioning in six Olympic athletes after the Seoul Games in 1988 show the dynamic regression of "physiologic" hypertrophy with deconditioning. Such alterations in LV dimensions argue strongly against the presence of primary cardiac hypertrophy (*ie*, hypertrophic cardiomyopathy). *Open circles* represent one athlete who retired from training and competition after the Olympic Games and had been deconditioned for 34 weeks at the time of the most recent echocardiographic study (*see* Fig. 9-25.) *Split circles* indicate mean values. (*Adapted from* Maron and coworkers [16]; with permission.)

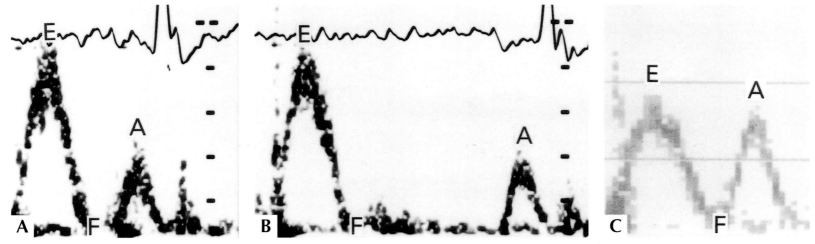

FIGURE 9-27. Clinical method for potentially distinguishing athlete's heart from hypertrophic cardiomyopathy (HCM) using pulsed Doppler echocardiography to assess transmitral flow velocity (as a reflection of left ventricular [LV] filling). Waveforms of transmitral flow velocity are shown for a sedentary 20-year-old man without cardiovascular disease (**A**), an 18-year-old highly trained football player (**B**), and a sedentary 19-year-old asymptomatic patient with HCM (**C**). The magnitude of LV wall thickening was similar in the athlete and in the patient with HCM, falling in the intermediate or "gray zone" of 13 to 15 mm. In the normal nonathlete (*panel A*), the diastolic waveform is normal; deceleration of flow velocity in early diastole (E-F slope) is rapid, and the height of the early diastolic peak of flow velocity (E) is more than twice that of the late diastolic peak (A). In the trained athlete (*panel B*), the pattern of the transmitral flow velocity waveform is similar to that of the nonathlete in *panel A*. In contrast, in the patient with HCM (*panel C*), the pattern of transmitral flow velocity is abnormal; deceleration of flow velocity in early diastole (the E-F slope) is decreased, and the ratio of the early (E) to late (A) peak of flow velocity is reduced. Each vertical division represents a 20 cm/s increment in flow velocity. Horizontal time divisions are 40 ms apart. (*Adapted from* Lewis and coworkers [17]; with permission.)

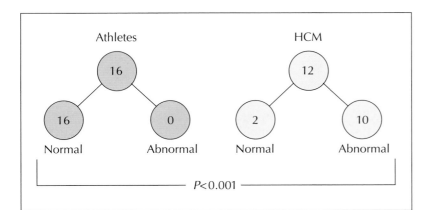

FIGURE 9-28. Distinguishing athlete's heart, in which left ventricular wall (LV) thickening is in the "gray zone," from nonobstructive hypertrophic cardiomyopathy (HCM) can be accomplished using the Doppler transmitral waveform as a reflection of LV filling. None of the 16 trained athletes studied showed abnormalities in the Doppler waveform, while 10 of the 12 asymptomatic patients with nonobstructive HCM and relatively mild hypertrophy had abnormalities in the peak E/A ratio or in the slope (descent) of the early (rapid) filling peak. Therefore, an abnormal transmitral waveform substantiates the diagnosis of HCM, while a normal waveform is consistent with both conditions (since 20% of patients with HCM have normal diastolic waveforms).

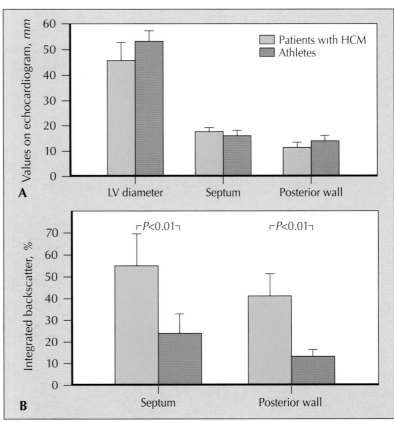

FIGURE 9-29. Role of ultrasonic myocardial reflectivity in differentiating hypertrophic cardiomyopathy (HCM) from athlete's heart. Bar graphs of histograms represent conventional echocardiographic measurements (left ventricular end-diastolic dimension [LVED] and wall thickness) (**A**) and quantitative ultrasound data (percent integrated backscatter, indicative of myocardial tissue reflectivity) (**B**) in 10 patients with HCM and 10 trained athletes with similar LV wall thicknesses, showing differentiation of the two conditions. (*Adapted from* Lattanzi and coworkers [18]; with permission from the American Heart Association, Inc.)

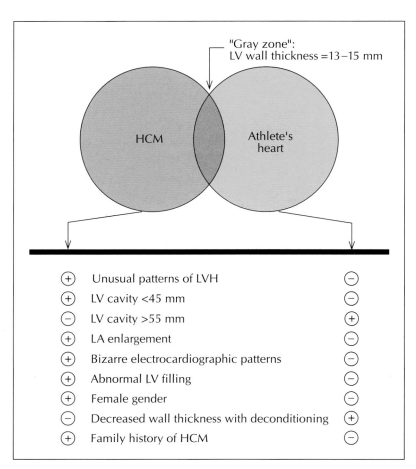

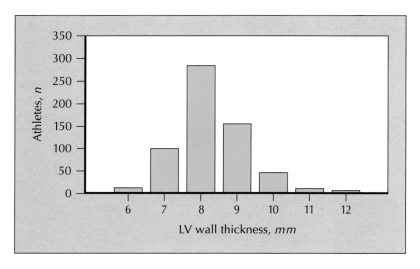

FIGURE 9-30. Summary of parameters for distinguishing hypertrophic cardiomyopathy (HCM) from athlete's heart when morphologic findings are within the "gray zone" of overlap consistent with both diagnoses (*ie*, left ventricular [LV] wall thickness of 13 to 15 mm). HCM is assumed to be of the nonobstructive type, since the presence of mitral valve systolic anterior motion per se would confirm the diagnosis of obstructive HCM in a competitive athlete. LV hypertrophy (LVH) may involve a variety of morphologic abnormalities, including a heterogeneous distribution of LVH in which asymmetry is prominent and adjacent regions may be of much different thickness, with sharp transitions evident between segments. Also evident are patterns in which the anterior ventricular septum is spared from the hypertrophic process and the region of predominant thickening is in the posterior portion of the septum or the anterolateral or posterior free wall, or apex. LA—left atrium. (*Adapted from* Maron and coworkers [19]; with permission from the American Heart Association, Inc.)

FIGURE 9-31. Athlete's heart in women. The distribution of maximal left ventricular (LV) wall thicknesses in 607 highly trained elite Italian female athletes shows that these values did not exceed 11 mm. Thus, compared with their male counterparts, female athletes exposed to similar training appear to have lesser wall thicknesses and do not often project into the borderline "gray zone" (13 to 15 mm) between physiologic and pathologic hypertrophy. Therefore, in female athletes suspected of having cardiac disease, wall thicknesses of 13 mm or are more much more consistent with hypertrophic cardiomyopathy than with athlete's heart.

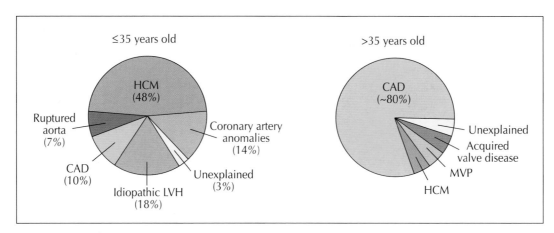

FIGURE 9-32. Pathologic substrate underlying sudden cardiac death in competitive athletes [20–22]. Estimated prevalences of those diseases responsible for death are compared in the youthful (age 35 years or less) and older (than age 35 years) athlete. Young athletes die from a variety of congenital cardiac malformations, with hypertrophic cardiomyopathy (HCM) being the most common. These catastrophes usually occurred on the athletic field (during practice or a game), most commonly in high school but also in college or even at the professional level. The vast majority of older athletes died of coronary artery disease (CAD). These data were collated from available studies in the literature. LVH—left ventricular hypertrophy; MVP—mitral valve prolapse. (*Adapted from* Maron and coworkers [20]; with permission from the American College of Cardiology.)

CAUSES OF UNEXPECTED DEATHS IN ATHLETES

CARDIOVASCULAR CONDITION/DISEASE	PATIENTS, n(%)
Hypertrophic cardiomyopathy	
Probable/definite	30 ⎫
Possible	10 ⎬ (45)
Coronary artery anomalies	13(15)
Normal*	11(12)
Myocarditis	7(8)
Ruptured aorta (including Marfan syndrome)	5(6)
Dilated cardiomyopathy	3(4)
Sarcoid	2(2)
Mitral valve prolapse	2(2)
Right ventricular dysplasia	2(2)
Coronary artery disease	2(2)
Aortic valvular stenosis	1(1)

COMPETITIVE SPORTS RELATED TO SUDDEN CARDIAC DEATH

TYPE OF SPORT	ATHLETES, n(%)
Football	37(41)
Basketball	29(31)
Track	15(17)
Baseball	3(4)
Swimming	2(2)
Soccer	2(2)
Tennis	1(1)
Volleyball	1(1)
Wrestling	1(1)
Boxing	1(1)
Lacrosse	1(1)
Golf	1(1)

FIGURE 9-33. Spectrum of cardiovascular causes of sudden, unexpected "athletic field deaths" in a series of 88 young competitive athletes, 13 to 40 years of age, assembled nationally (primarily from newsmedia accounts); 55% were white and 45% were black. A variety of 10 separate disease entities are represented on this list, the most common being hypertrophic cardiomyopathy. A sizable subset of athletes (12%) were classified as having structurally normal hearts (*asterisk*); however, it is possible that known causes of sudden death in youthful individuals, such as Q-T interval prolongation syndrome, occult conduction system abnormalities, or certain undetected forms of drug abuse, were responsible for such deaths.

FIGURE 9-34. Spectrum of 12 sports engaged in by 88 young competitive athletes with underlying cardiovascular disease who died suddenly, usually on the athletic field. The sports involved most commonly were football and basketball by a substantial margin, probably reflecting a high level of participation. (Percentages add up to more than 100% because several individual athletes competed in more than one sport.)

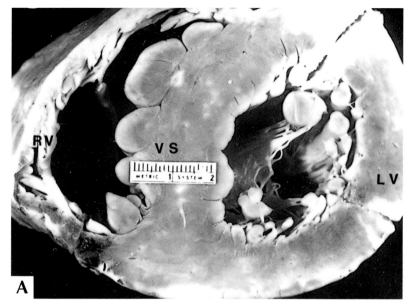

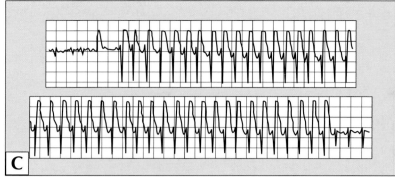

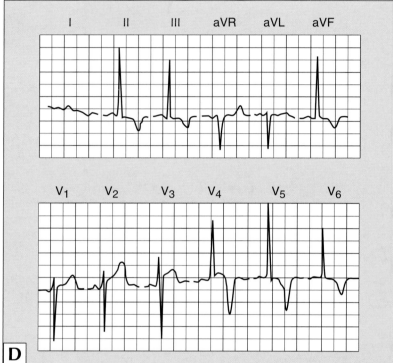

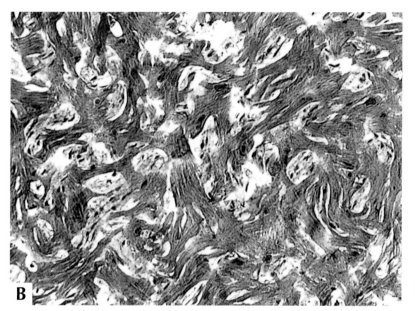

FIGURE 9-35. Clinical and morphologic features of athletes with hypertrophic cardiomyopathy (HCM), the most common cause of sudden cardiac death in young competitive athletes. **A,** Heart of a 13-year-old male football and baseball player showing disproportionate hypertrophy of the ventricular septum (VS) with respect to the left ventricular (LV) free wall. **B,** Marked disorganization of cardiac muscle cells in the thickened septum, with adjacent myocardial cells arranged at oblique and perpendicular angles rather than aligned in the normal, monotonous parallel orientation. **C,** Sustained

ventricular tachycardia that occurred in the second minute of recovery after a routine treadmill exercise test and terminated spontaneously; from a 23-year-old college basketball player with HCM who died suddenly some time later during a workout. **D,** Standard 12-lead electrocardiogram obtained under basal conditions showing marked symmetric T-wave inversions (up to 15 mm in depth) as well as LV hypertrophy in the same athlete shown in *panel C.* RV—right ventricular wall. (*Adapted from* Maron and coworkers [20]; with permission from the American College of Cardiology.)

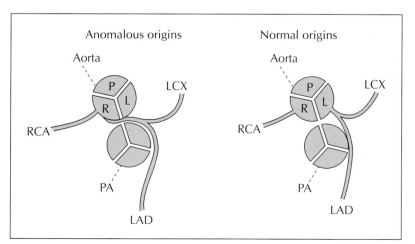

FIGURE 9-36. Congenital coronary anomalies are a relatively infrequent cause of sudden death in young athletes. Anomalous origin of the left anterior descending coronary artery (LAD) from the right (anterior) sinus of Valsalva is the most common of those coronary anomalies implicated in sudden cardiac death. The LAD may have a common (or separate) ostium with the right coronary artery (RCA), since both vessels arise from the right sinus of Valsalva. Note the acute leftward and posterior course of the LAD between the aorta and pulmonary artery (PA). (The normal origins—*ie,* LAD from the left sinus of Valsalva and RCA from the right sinus of Valsalva—are shown for comparison.) R—right (anterior) coronary cusp; L—left coronary cusp; P—posterior (noncoronary) cusp; LCX—left circumflex coronary artery.

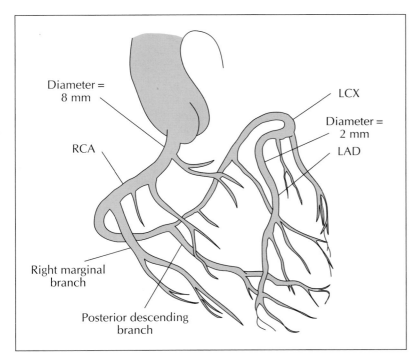

FIGURE 9-37. Sketch of a single, enlarged right coronary artery (RCA) noted on postmortem examination of Pete Maravich, a long-time elite professional basketball player. The left main coronary artery and its ostium are absent. Arteriosclerotic narrowing was minimal. The greatly dilated RCA circled the heart, gave off marginal and posterior descending branches, and anastomosed posteriorly with the circumflex branch of the left coronary artery (LCX). Although the left anterior descending (LAD) branch was diminutive (2 mm in diameter), it followed its normal course. Heart weight was 560 g, and the cardiac chambers were dilated, with widespread but patchy scarring. (*Adapted from* Choi and Kornblum [23]; with permission.)

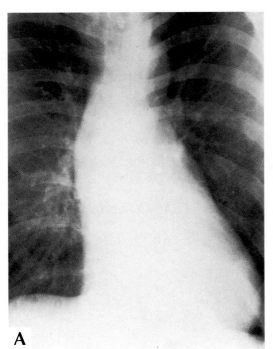

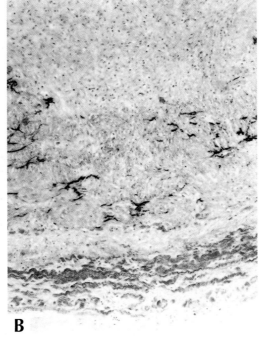

FIGURE 9-38. Sudden death in a young athlete due to Marfan syndrome. **A,** Chest radiograph from an 18-year-old male collegiate swimmer who died 2 months later of a ruptured aorta. Note prominent dilatation of the ascending aorta. **B,** Histologic section of the ascending aorta. Note that the elastic fibers in the aortic media (which stain darkly) are greatly reduced in number. Intima is at the top and adventitia is at the bottom. Elastic van Gieson stain, ×80. (*Adapted from* Maron and coworkers [19]; with permission from the American Heart Association, Inc.)

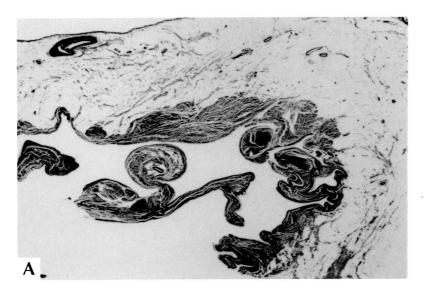

FIGURE 9-39. Sudden death in a young athlete due to right ventricular cardiomyopathy (dysplasia) of the lipomatous type. **A,** Lower-power view of the anterior right ventricular wall showing massive lipomatous infiltration (azan, ×5). (*continued*)

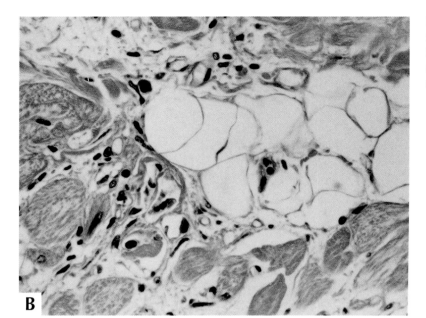

FIGURE 9-39. (*continued*) **B,** High-power view of right ventricular myocardium showing myocardial degeneration and lipomatous infiltration (hematoxylin and eosin, ×300). (*Adapted from* Thiene and coworkers [24]; with permission from the *New England Journal of Medicine*.)

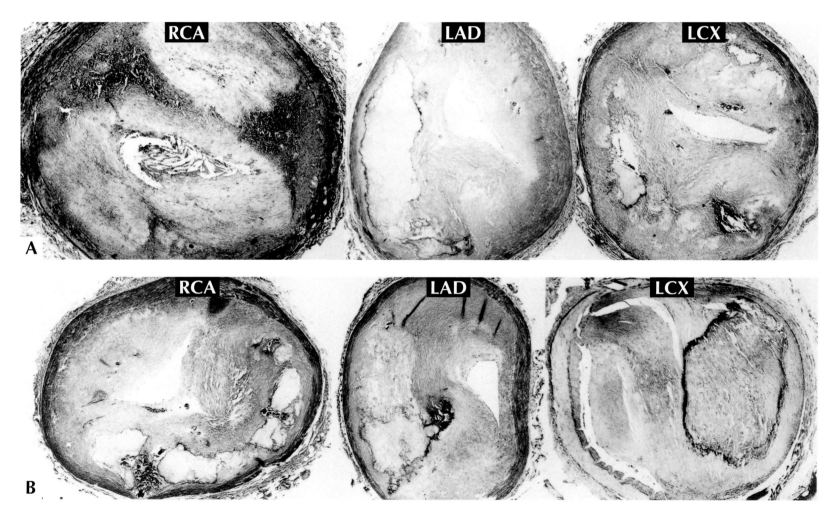

FIGURE 9-40. Sections of coronary arteries from a 49-year-old man who ran an average of about 170 km per week and successfully completed six marathons and seven 8-km races but subsequently died suddenly of coronary heart disease. The right (RCA), left anterior descending (LAD), and left circumflex (LCX) coronary arteries are shown at the sites of maximal atherosclerotic narrowing in both the proximal (**A**) and the distal (**B**) halves of the respective arteries. (*Adapted from* Maron and coworkers [19]; with permission from the American College of Cardiology.)

References

1. Rost R, Hollman W: Athlete's heart: a review of its historical assessment and new aspects. *Int J Sports Med* 1983, 4:147–165.

2. Maron BJ: Structural features of the athlete heart as defined by echocardiography. *J Am Coll Cardiol* 1986, 7:190–203.

3. Allen HD, Goldberg SJ, Sahn DJ, *et al.*: A quantitative echocardiographic study of champion childhood swimmers. *Circulation* 1977, 55:142–145.

4. Hauser AM, Dressendorfer RH, Vos M, *et al.*: Symmetric cardiac enlargement in highly trained endurance athletes: a two-dimensional echocardiographic study. *Am Heart J* 1985, 109:1038–1044.

5. Morganroth J, Maron BJ, Henry WL, *et al.*: Comparative left ventricular dimensions in trained athletes. *Ann Intern Med* 1975, 82:521–524.

6. Pelliccia A, Maron BJ, Spataro A, *et al.*: The upper limit of physiologic cardiac hypertrophy in highly trained elite athletes. *N Engl J Med* 1991, 324:295–301.

7. Longhurst JC, Kelly AR, Gonyea WJ, *et al.*: Chronic training with static and dynamic exercise: cardiovascular adaptation and response to exercise. *Circ Res* 1981, 48(suppl I):171–178.

8. Pelliccia A, Maron BJ, Spataro A, *et al.*: Absence of left ventricular hypertrophy in athletes engaged in intense power training. *Am J Cardiol* 1993, 72:1048–1054.

9. Ehsani AA, Hagberg JM, Hickson RC: Rapid changes in left ventricular dimensions and mass in response to physical conditioning and deconditioning. *Am J Cardiol* 1978, 42:52–56.

10. Fagard R, Aubert A, Lysens R, *et al.*: Noninvasive assessment of seasonal variations in cardiac structure and function in cyclists. *Circulation* 1983, 67:896–901.

11. DeMaria AN, Neumann A, Lee G, *et al.*: Alterations in ventricular mass and performance induced by exercise training in man evaluated by echocardiography. *Circulation* 1978, 57:237–244.

12. Nishimura T, Yamada Y, Kawai C: Echocardiographic evaluation of long-term effects of exercise on left ventricular hypertrophy and function in professional bicyclists. *Circulation* 1980, 61:832–840.

13. Douglas PS, O'Toole ML, Hiller DB, *et al.*: Left ventricular structure and function by echocardiography in ultraendurance athletes. *Am J Cardiol* 1986, 58:805–809.

14. Granger CB, Karuimeddini MK, Smith VE, *et al.*: Rapid ventricular filling in left ventricular hypertrophy. I. Physiologic hypertrophy. *J Am Coll Cardiol* 1985, 5:862–868.

15. Talan DA, Bauernfeind RA, Ashley WW, *et al.*: Twenty-four hour continuous ECG recordings in long-distance runners. *Chest* 1982, 82:19–24.

16. Maron BJ, Pelliccia A, Spataro A, *et al.*: Reduction in left ventricular wall thickness after deconditioning in highly trained Olympic athletes. *Br Heart J* 1993, 69:125–128.

17. Lewis JA, Spirito P, Pelliccia A, *et al.*: Usefulness of Doppler echocardiographic assessment of diastolic filling in distinguishing "athlete's heart" from hypertrophic cardiomyopathy. *Br Heart J* 1992, 68:296–300.

18. Lattanzi F, Di Bello V, Picano E, *et al.*: Normal ultrasonic myocardial reflectivity in athletes with increased left ventricular mass. A tissue characterization study. *Circulation* 1992, 85:1828–1834.

19. Maron BJ, Pelliccia A, Spirito P: Cardiac disease in young trained athletes: insights into methods for distinguishing athlete's heart from structural heart disease, with particular emphasis on hypertrophic cardiomyopathy. *Circulation*, 1995, 91:1596–1601.

20. Maron BJ, Epstein SE, Roberts WC: Causes of sudden death in the competitive athlete. *J Am Coll Cardiol* 1986, 7:204–214.

21. Maron BJ, Shirani J, Mueller FO, *et al.*: Cardiovascular causes of "athletic field" deaths: analysis of sudden death in 84 competitive athletes [abstract]. *Circulation* 1993, 88(suppl I):I-50.

22. Maron BJ, Roberts WC, McAllister, *et al.*: Sudden death in young athletes. *Circulation* 1980, 62:218–229.

23. Choi JH, Kornblum RN: Peter Maravich's incredible heart. *J Forensic Sci* 1990, 35:981–986.

24. Thiene G, Nava A, Corrado D, *et al.*: Right ventricular cardiomyopathy and sudden death in young people. *N Engl J Med* 1988, 318:129–133.

Evaluating Cardiac Patients at Special Risk: Noncardiac Surgery and Occupational, Environmental, and Recreational Considerations

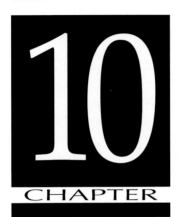

10

CHAPTER

David R. Ferry, James D. Anholm, C. Gunnar Blomqvist, Benjamin D. Levine, Lynda D. Lane, Jay C. Buckey, and Chris Wachholz

A variety of conditions and circumstances—namely, surgical procedures, aviation, high-altitude environments, space flight, and diving—can affect the cardiovascular system in unique ways. All may pose a threat to a person's safety, especially if that person has heart disease or is at risk for cardiovascular problems. In the case of recreational or professional endeavors, such as deep-sea exploration or aircraft piloting, such risk can extend to others.

Cardiac morbidity and mortality are the commonest perioperative complications in several types of surgical procedures, and the preoperative assessment of these patients is a common, difficult, complex, and expensive problem. A variety of methods for preoperative assessment—from clinical scoring systems to noninvasive and invasive techniques—have been devised, but all have various difficulties with sensitivity and specificity. Another difficult issue is how to use the information provided by preoperative evaluation. These issues are discussed in this chapter and an algorithm for preoperative evaluation is presented.

Aircrew fitness is an important consideration in commercial, military, and recreational flying. Guidelines for determining whether or not pilot certification can be conferred take into account a candidate's cardiac status and potential risk for disability during flight. For this purpose, certain diagnostic tests are recommended and described, including specific examples in patients with and without heart disease. The effects of high altitude on the cardiovascular system can be significant. For example, acute mountain sickness can progress to cerebral and/or pulmonary edema, which—despite descent—can lead to permanent neurologic damage or death. Lifesaving measures are discussed, as are the results of studies carried out in decompression chambers to simulate the effects of high altitude on the cardiovascular system.

The increased popularity of underwater recreation has led to strategies for evaluating diving fitness. Although the military and certain industrial organizations have strict standards regarding qualification for diving, no other regulatory agencies exist to ensure that recreational divers be fit to participate in this sport, which can be responsible for barotrauma and decompression sickness. For this reason, all potential divers with health problems, including the disabled, should be examined prior to entering the underwater environment.

SPACE FLIGHT

Despite the predictions of prominent physicians and physiologists that the microgravity (μG) of space would produce incapacitating and even lethal derangements of human cardiovascular physiology [1,2], the United States and the Soviet Union proceeded to develop manned space programs during the 1950s. During the 1950s, Yuri Gagarin, a 27-year-old Soviet Air Force officer, became the first human to circle the earth on April 12, 1962 [3]. As of October 1994, 322 men and women have flown in space, 221 on US and 101 on Soviet space craft. Although deaths attributable to space craft failure have occurred, no fatalities or known cases of permanent disability have resulted specifically from exposure to μG. Nevertheless, major μG-induced physiologic changes that affect multiple organ systems have been well documented. Early studies within the US and Soviet space programs demonstrated that μG produces vestibular dysfunction; hypovolemia, with rapid loss of plasma volume and red cell volume during flights that last more than a few days; and postflight orthostatic intolerance, skeletal muscle atrophy, and progressive loss of calcium, with consequent decreases in bone density [3,4].

Following the Apollo series of flights that took Americans to the moon in 1969 [4], the Skylab flights in 1973 carried three US crews to a well-equipped laboratory for detailed physiologic studies during progressively longer flights, reaching 84 days with Skylab 4 [5]. At this time, the Soviet space program had developed the technology required to accomplish flights of even longer duration, initially based on their experience with the Salyut orbital station, which was later replaced by an advanced modular space-station complex, Mir ("Peace"), in 1986. A Russian cardiologist, Dr. Oleg Atkov, spent 237 days in space in 1984, and in 1987 Mir supported flights of 365 days for two crew members, Titov and Manarov [3].

As has been well documented, the earth's gravitational field defines important aspects of the operating conditions for the human cardiovascular system. During the 1960s, Gauer established the concept that the distribution of intravascular pressures and volumes in the upright body position, rather than the conventional clinical supine baseline values, represents the physiologic norm [6]. This view explains why human cardiovascular dysfunction is invariably induced by prolonged exposure to conditions that minimize hydrostatic gradients (*eg*, bed rest and space flight) [7,8]. Physical inactivity is a contributing factor, but even prolonged and heavy exercise during exposure to μG and its analogs cannot prevent postexposure dysfunction, primarily manifest as orthostatic intolerance. The most likely sequence of cardiovascular events at μG is as follows:

1. Left ventricular (LV) end-diastolic volumes (as determined by echocardiography) and stroke volume (as determined by foreign-gas rebreathing) initially remain at or above supine preflight levels [9,10].

2. The initial hemodynamic state while the individual is in orbit reflects a central (or headward) fluid shift that produces high LV end-diastolic and stroke volumes. This activates a cascade of neurohumoral control mechanisms, including cardiopulmonary and arterial baroreflexes and the multiple mechanisms that regulate body fluid volumes. Early on, there is a loss of intravascular volume into the subcutaneous space, manifest as facial swelling. Ground-based simulations usually produce an early diuresis [8]. A more common early pattern during actual space flight is decreased fluid intake, resulting in a negative fluid balance. In either case, plasma volume decreases by about 500 to 600 mL, and total body mass is reduced by 1 to 2 kg [3,5]. LV end-diastolic and stroke volumes decrease and reach 1 G upright levels within a few days [11]. The hemodynamic state after adaptation to μG approaches that documented during preflight studies in the standing position [10]. Maximal oxygen uptake (as measured during bicycle exercise) is maintained at preflight levels on orbit after a week in space [12]—a strong indication that cardiac pump capacity and major regulatory mechanisms remain intact at μG.

3. Early after return from space, orthostatic intolerance is manifest in a large fraction of the crew members, with the incidence and severity tending to increase the longer the space flight. More than half the crew is unable to complete a 10-minute stand test after a flight of 10 to 14 days [11,13].

Postflight orthostatic intolerance was first reported after a 9-hour Mercury space flight in 1962 [3] and has remained a significant problem, with major operational and clinical implications. Conventional countermeasures, including in-flight exercise regimens and oral fluid loading immediately before return to 1 G, have had only limited impact, as is evident from physiologic data recently obtained from 14 crew members [11,13].

An important portion of the human studies carried out during the Mir flights has been devoted to developing countermeasures to prevent both cardiovascular and musculoskeletal deconditioning.

Although there has been no formal evaluation of the procedures, which included exercise and lower-body negative pressure, the program is considered an essential component of all prolonged Russian flights [14]. The most serious health problems during future interplanetary flight, however, will be caused by the various forms of ionizing radiation, including galactic cosmic rays, trapped belt radiation, and solar particle events. For example, heavy particles in galactic cosmic radiation can penetrate thick shielding, and at present no known practical measures can be taken to eliminate the risk of harmful exposure [15].

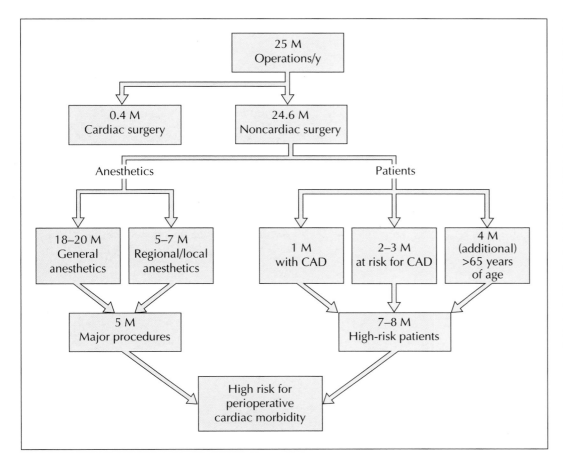

Figure 10-1. Estimates of the number of operations performed in the United States in 1988 [16]. Of the 25 million procedures, 400,000 were cardiac. Of the remaining group, 5 million (M) patients underwent major intra-abdominal, thoracic, vascular, neurologic, or orthopedic procedures, which are potentially more stressful to the cardiovascular system. In patients referred for peripheral vascular surgery, for instance, the incidence of coronary artery disease (CAD) is 40% to 70% [17]. In addition, one million patients referred for surgery had documented CAD, another 2 to 3 million had two or more risk factors for CAD, and 4 million were over age 65 and at increased risk for CAD. Patients who are about to undergo a major surgical procedure or who have known or suspected CAD are therefore at increased risk for perioperative cardiac morbidity. (*Adapted from* Mangano [16]; with permission.)

Figure 10-2. Estimated incidence of perioperative cardiac morbidity based on data drawn from multiple studies [16]. Although the incidence of the different outcomes varies widely because of the heterogeneity among study populations, in definitions of events, and in the methodologies used to identify events, the risk for perioperative cardiac complications is apparently substantial. CAD—coronary artery disease; MI—myocardial infarction. (*Adapted from* Mangano [16]; with permission.)

ESTIMATED INCIDENCE OF PERIOPERATIVE CARDIAC MORBIDITY

OUTCOMES	INCIDENCE, %
Myocardial ischemia	
Preoperative	24
Intraoperative	18–74
Postoperative	27–38
MI	
General population	0.1–0.7
Prior MI	1.9–7.7
Vascular surgery	1–15
Recent MI	0–37
Unstable angina	Unknown
Congestive heart failure	
Intraoperative	4.8
Postoperative	3.6
Serious dysrhythmias	
Intraoperative	0.9–36.0
Postoperative	14.0–40.5
Cardiac death	
Without CAD	0.5
With CAD	2.4
With perioperative MI	36–70

PREOPERATIVE CARDIAC RISK SCORING SYSTEM OF GOLDMAN

GOLDMAN CRITERIA	POINTS
History	
Age >70 y	5
MI in previous 6 mo	10
Physical examination	
S_3 gallop or jugular venous distention	11
Important aortic valve stenosis	3
Electrocardiogram	
Rhythm other than sinus or APBs on last preoperative ECG	7
> 5 VPBs/min documented at any time before operation	7
General status	
PO_2 < 60 or PCO_2 > 50 mm Hg, K < 3.0	3
or HCO_3 < 20 mEq/L, BUN > 50	
or CR > 3.0 mg/dL, abnormal SGOT, signs of chronic liver disease, or patient bedridden from noncardiac causes	
Operation	
Intraperitoneal, intrathoracic, or aortic	3
Emergency	4
Total number of points possible	**53**

FIGURE 10-3. Goldman's classic 1977 preoperative cardiac risk scoring system [18]. The Goldman index was prospectively derived from a detailed analysis of the history, physical examination, and basic laboratory studies of 1001 patients referred for surgery. By multivariate analysis, these components were found to be associated with an increased risk for a perioperative cardiac event. A point score was assigned to each criterion according to the groups based on their total scores (*see* Fig. 10-4). APBs—atrial premature beats; BUN—blood urea nitrogen; CR—creatinine; HCO_3—bicarbonate; MI—myocardial infarction; PO_2—partial pressure of oxygen; PCO_2—partial pressure of carbon dioxide; SGOT—serum glutamic oxalacetic transaminase; VPBs—ventricular premature beats. (*Adapted from* Goldman and coworkers [18]; with permission.)

PERIOPERATIVE COMPLICATIONS IN 1001 PATIENTS

CLASS	POINT TOTAL	NO OR ONLY MINOR COMPLICATIONS (n=943) n(%)	LIFE-THREATENING COMPLICATION (n=39) n(%)	CARDIAC DEATHS (n=19) n(%)
I (n=537)	0–5	532(99)	4(0.7)	1(0.2)
II (n=316)	6–12	295(93)	16(5)	5(2)
III (n=130)	13–25	112(86)	15(11)	3(2)
IV (n=18)	≥26	4(22)	4(22)	10(56)

FIGURE 10-4. Perioperative complications in the 1001 patients described in Fig. 10-3 [18]. Note that the likelihood of complication was substantial in those in classes III and IV but was extremely low in those in class I. (*Adapted from* Goldman and coworkers [18]; with permission.)

CARDIAC RISK SCORING SYSTEM OF DETSKY

PREOPERATIVE VARIABLES	POINTS
CAD	
MI within 6 mo	10
MI more than 6 mo previously	5
Canadian Cardiovascular Society angina	
Class 3	10
Class 4	20
Unstable angina within 3 mo	10
Alveolar pulmonary edema	
Within 1 week	10
Ever	5
Valvular disease	
Suspected critical aortic valve stenosis	20
Arrhythmias	
Sinus rhythm plus APBs or rhythm other than sinus on last preoperative ECG	5
More than 5 VPBs at any time prior to surgery	5
Poor general medical status	5
Age > 70 y	5
Emergency operation	10

FIGURE 10-5 Detsky's 1986 preoperative cardiac risk scoring system [19,20]. These and other cardiac risk indices have been applied to various noncardiac surgical populations with reasonably good reproducibility [21–23]. However, in an extensive review in 1990, Mangano [16] pointed out that the only uncontested indicators of increased perioperative risk were recent myocardial infarction (MI), the presence of preoperative congestive heart failure, and factors such as advanced age or diabetes that increase the risk for coronary artery disease (CAD). More recent studies have questioned the reliability of these indices in delineating a low-risk group, particularly in populations in which CAD is prevalent, such as those patients referred for peripheral vascular surgery [24,25]. The recognition of these limitations provided the impetus for the use of various noninvasive tests to evaluate risk for perioperative complications. APBs—atrial premature beats; ECG—electrocardiogram; VPBs—ventricular premature beats. (*Adapted from* Detsky and coworkers [19]; with permission.)

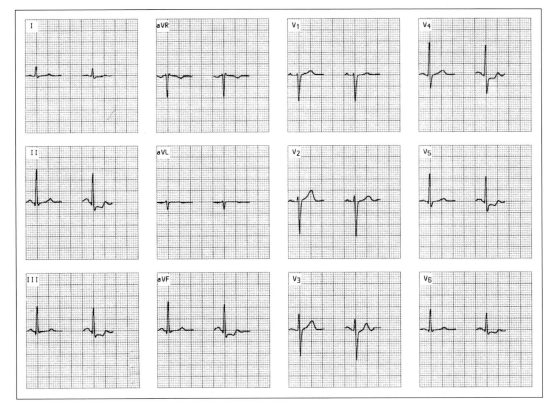

FIGURE 10-6. Rest and peak exercise electrocardiograms (ECGs) from a 53-year-old man being considered for semiurgent cholecystectomy. The patient had a history of single-vessel right coronary artery (RCA) disease and had undergone successful angioplasty for that lesion 2 years earlier. For the past several months, he had experienced moderate, stable angina on exertion. After exercising for 9 minutes using a modified Bruce protocol to a maximal heart rate of 116 bpm and a peak systolic blood pressure of 158 mm Hg, the patient experienced chest pain, evident on the ECG as 2-mm ST-segment depression. Subsequent cardiac catheterization demonstrated a recanalized occlusion of the mid-RCA and moderate hypokinesis of the inferior left ventricular wall. He was treated medically with β-blockers and nitrates, and the gallbladder surgery was uneventful.

The use of exercise stress test results as a preoperative indicator of risk has been evaluated extensively [26–30]. Several studies have concluded that (1) only about 30% of patients being considered for peripheral vascular surgery were able to achieve 85% of their maximal predicted heart rate, (2) the relatively few patients who achieved 85% of their maximal heart rate and had a negative stress test were at low risk for a preoperative cardiac event, and (3) the sensitivity and specificity of the test in this population was low.

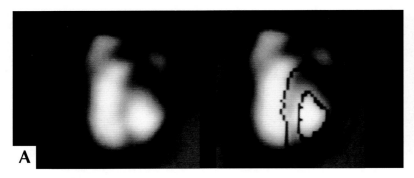

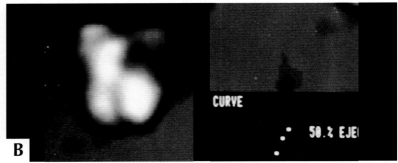

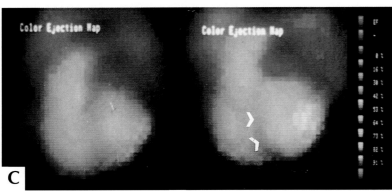

FIGURE 10-7. Rest (**A**) and stress (**B**) radionuclide ventriculograms from a patient suspected of having coronary disease [31]. Between the rest and the stress images there is no increase in ejection fraction (EF). **C** and **D**, Color-enhanced versions of the images shown in *A* and *B*. The images in *C* are coded for regional function and show a fall in the septal EF with stress (*arrowheads*). The phase images in *D* demonstrate more clearly a fall in septal intensity with stress, consistent with a decrease in regional stroke volume (*arrowhead*). These findings are consistent with stress-induced regional ischemia, which obviously implicates coronary artery disease.

Since patients with depressed left ventricular (LV) systolic function have been considered to be at increased risk, the usefulness of resting radionuclide ventriculography as a predictor of periop-erative cardiac morbidity has been evaluated by several investiga-tors [26,33–38]. Initial studies in patients referred for peripheral vascular surgery found that a resting LVEF below 35% was associ-ated with a 75% risk for a perioperative complication, whereas complications did not develop in patients with an EF above 56%. In later studies, however, resting EF was not predictive of outcome in patients undergoing vascular surgery. (*Adapted from* Botvinick and coworkers [31]; with permission.)

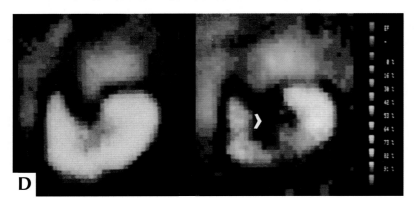

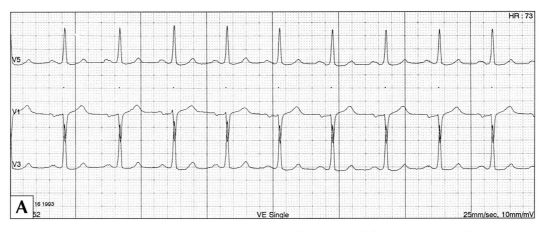

FIGURE 10-8. Ambulatory electrocardiograms (ECGs) obtained from a 73-year-old man 5 days before scheduled repair of a 7-cm aneurysm of the abdominal aorta. The tracings show minimal (**A**) and maximal (**B**) ST-segment depression. He had no history of coronary disease and was asymptomatic during ambulatory monitoring, although the ECG showed three episodes of sustained (15 to 23 minutes) ST-segment depression of at least 2 mm. These findings prompted cardiac catheterization, which demonstrated moderate two-vessel disease. The patient was treated with β-blockers and calcium antagonists and underwent aneurysm repair. (*continued*)

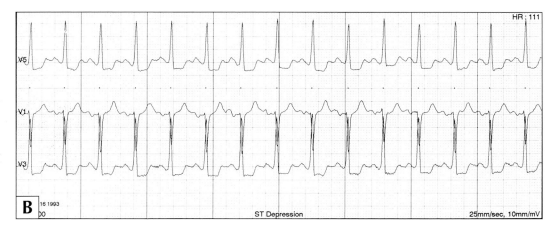

FIGURE 10-8. (*continued*) On the second postoperative day atrial fibrillation occurred. The ECG showed ischemic ST-segment changes, and the serum creatine kinase-MB fraction rose to twice the upper limit of normal. After intravenous diltiazem was given to control the ventricular rate, his heart rhythm converted to sinus within 24 hours.

As a screening technique ambulatory ECG monitoring has the advantages of being noninvasive, easy to perform, and relatively inexpensive. In several studies of patients referred for vascular surgery, risk for perioperative complications increased significantly if there were episodes of ischemia on the preoperative ambulatory ECG [38–41]. Often, these episodes were asymptomatic. Patients without such evidence of ischemia were at low risk for complications. In a more recent study by Mangano *et al.* [42], preoperative and intraoperative ischemic events in patients undergoing major surgery were associated with an increased risk for postoperative complications, but absence of ischemia on monitoring did not identify those at low risk, particularly in the subset undergoing vascular surgery.

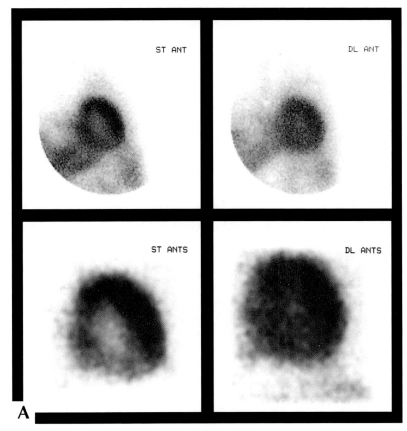

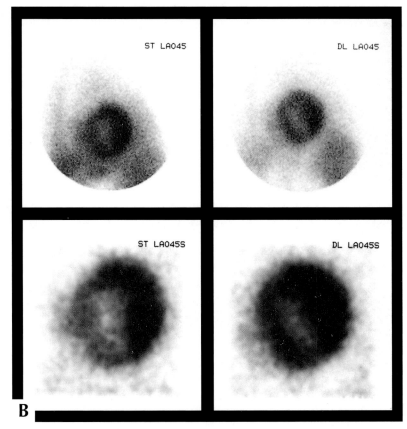

FIGURE 10-9. Unsubtracted (*top*) and background-subtracted (*bottom*) dipyridamole thallium scans in the anterior (**A**), 45° left anterior oblique (**B**), and 70° left anterior oblique (**C**) views in a 68-year-old man scheduled for iliofemoral bypass. Immediate post-infusion images are on the *left*, while corresponding 4-hour delayed images are on the *right* in each panel. Note that the perfusion defects in the inferoposterior, anteroseptal, and septal walls evident in the initial scans have filled in substantially in the delayed images.

Because previously described scoring systems have been unable to identify adequately those patients at low risk for perioperative complications after major surgery, particularly among those undergoing peripheral vascular procedures, myocardial perfusion studies have been evaluated extensively in this setting [24,30,43–45]. Initial reports were encouraging, with dipyridamole thallium imaging having a remarkable ability to identify groups at both high and low risk [30,45,46]. (*continued*)

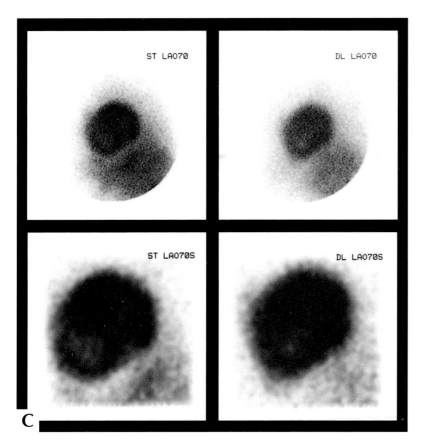

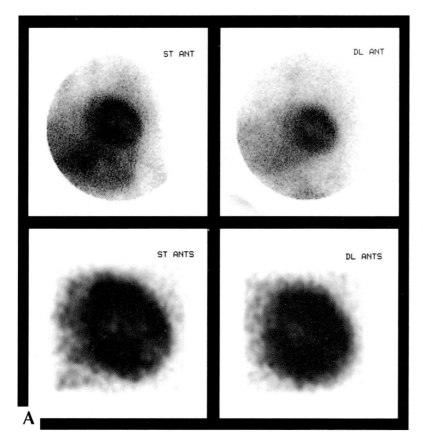

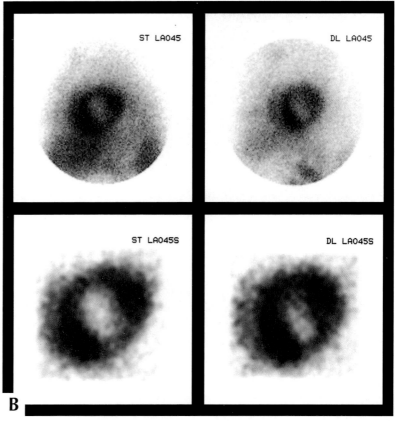

FIGURE 10-9. (*continued*) Recently, however, several investigators have questioned the accuracy of such testing in this setting [47–50]. Most of these studies evaluated consecutive patients referred for preoperative consultation because they were considered to be at high risk. Furthermore, nearly all the previous studies had found reversible thallium defects to be associated with a higher perioperative risk, while McFalls *et al.* found that *fixed*, irreversible defects were predictive of increased risk [51].

In response to these conflicting reports, Massie and Mangano [52] concluded that preoperative risk assessment is an imperfect art. Because the annual cost of dipyridamole thallium screening in high-risk populations referred for noncardiac surgery would exceed $10 billion, these authors recommended the approaches described by Eagle *et al.* [45] and Wong and Detsky [26] (*see* Fig. 10-12).

FIGURE 10-10. Unsubtracted (*top*) and background subtracted (*bottom*) dipyridamole thallium images in the anterior (**A**), 45° left anterior oblique (**B**), and 70° left anterior oblique (**C**) views in a 63-year-old man referred for carotid artery surgery. (*continued*)

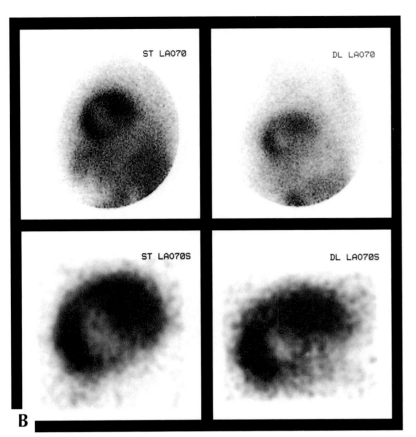

FIGURE 10-10. *(continued)* Immediate postinfusion images are on the *left*, while the corresponding 4-hour delayed images are on the *right*. The perfusion defects evident in the inferobasilar and posterolateral walls in the postinfusion scans have minimally recovered in the delayed images, indicating a fixed defect (*see* Fig. 10-9 for a complete discussion).

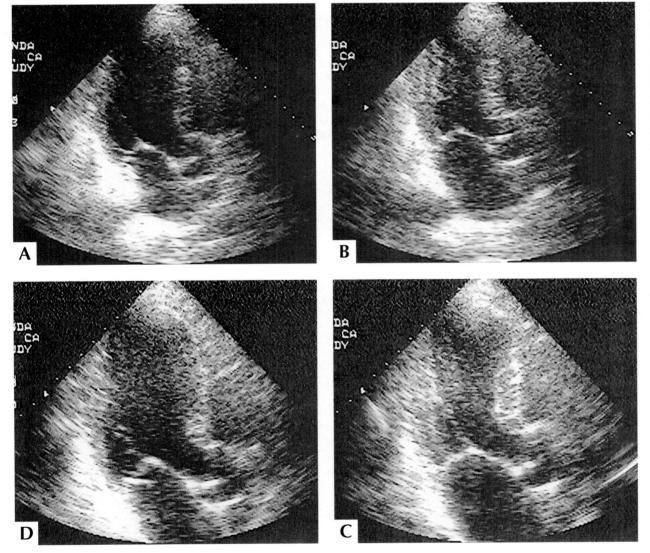

FIGURE 10-11. Two-dimensional echocardiograms in the apical long-axis view during diastole (**A** and **C**) and systole (**B** and **D**) in a 76-year-old man referred for peripheral vascular surgery. The images in *A* and *C* were obtained at rest, while those in *B* and *D* were obtained after the intravenous infusion of 20 µg/kg/min of dobutamine. Left ventricular wall motion was normal at rest, but with dobutamine distal septal and apical dyskinesis has appeared. Although the patient was asymptomatic, ischemic ST-segment depression was noted in leads V_4 to V_6 on the electrocardiogram. The usefulness of dobutamine stress echocardiography was recently evaluated in patients referred for vascular surgery and proved accurate in predicting both high-risk and low-risk groups [53–54a]. However, more studies are needed to validate these findings.

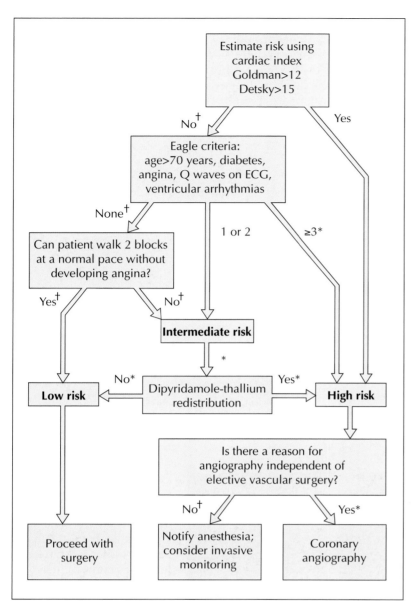

FIGURE 10-12. Wong and Detsky's approach to preoperative cardiac risk assessment for patients referred for vascular surgery [26]. *Asterisks* indicate strategies that (according to the authors) require validation; *daggers* indicate strategies based on untested hypotheses. Although most patients who are at high risk can be identified successfully, those at intermediate or low risk are much more difficult to detect.

An even more vexing question concerns the usefulness of risk stratification in patients referred for noncardiac surgery. Once a patient is identified preoperatively as being at high risk for a cardiac complication, there are only three situations in which a preoperative risk evaluation should be performed: (1) if the results would cause the surgery to be cancelled or would dictate a different operative procedure, (2) if the results would suggest that coronary revascularization precede noncardiac surgery, and (3) if the results would alter perioperative management [52]. Preoperative revascularization is expensive and adds its own substantial morbidity and mortality to that of the subsequent surgery.

In addition, the impact of perioperative complications and long-term survival has not been studied prospectively, and the need for more aggressive medical management of patients at high risk remains controversial. Whether preoperative β-blockade or other medical therapy or intraoperative monitoring with continuous electrocardiography, right heart catheterization, or transesophageal echocardiography are of benefit remains to be determined. (*Adapted from* Wong and Detsky [26]; with permission.)

AIRCREW SAFETY AND CARDIOVASCULAR RISK

AIRCREW FITNESS—THE "1% RULE"

1% = Annual cardiovascular mortality for persons 65 to 69 years of age

1% = Risk of second pilot not responding in an emergency if the first becomes completely disabled (based on flight simulator data)

Risk for sudden collapse causing an accident is greatest during 10% of the flight

Projected risk for accident from cardiovascular incapacity if pilot has annual catastrophic risk of 1% (10^{-6}):

$$10^{-6} \times 10^{-2} \times 10^{-1} = 10^{-9}$$

FIGURE 10-13. Origin of the "1% rule" with regard to aircrew fitness. In general, an annual rate of 10^{-9} for a commercial aircraft accident due to catastrophic cardiac dysfunction has been considered acceptable [55]. This could be accomplished (calculated as shown) in a multicrew aircraft as long as the annual cardiac mortality of any crew member did not exceed 1% [56]. Although mortality is lower for younger pilots and women, older pilots should not be excluded arbitrarily, since their greater experience and judgment may offset their higher cardiac risk. The chance that *two* pilots would simultaneously become disabled from cardiovascular causes has been estimated to be 10^{-14}. Any cardiac condition or combination of conditions that is likely to result in an annual cardiac mortality exceeding 1% is considered justification for decertification of a commercial pilot. This strategy appears to be effective, since there has been no commercial air accident from a cardiovascular cause in 20 years [57,58].

MANAGEMENT OF HYPERTENSION IN AN AIRCREW

UNACCEPTABLE AGENTS			ACCEPTABLE AGENTS
Centrally acting drugs	α-Adrenoceptor blockers	Direct vasodilators	ACE inhibitors
Clonidine	Doxazosin	Hydralazine	Calcium antagonists
Guanabenz	Phenoxybenzamine	Minoxidil	Diuretics
Guanficine	Phentolamine		Hydrophilic β-blockers
Lipophilic β-blockers (possibly)	Prazosin		
	Terazosin		
Methyldopa	Trimazosin		
Reserpine	Urapidil		

FIGURE 10-14. Management of hypertension in aircrew members [59]. Agents deemed "unacceptable" may have significant side effects that would interfere with task performance. Although evidence that centrally acting agents could impair performance is difficult to find, other agents are better tolerated. The α-adrenoceptor blockers and direct vasodilators may cause unacceptable orthostatic hypotension. In contrast, the side effect profiles for diuretics, hydrophilic β-blockers (*eg*, atenolol, metoprolol), calcium antagonists, and angiotensin-converting enzyme (ACE) inhibitors are considered acceptable for an aircrew. To avoid additive side effects, successive monotherapy with these agents is recommended.

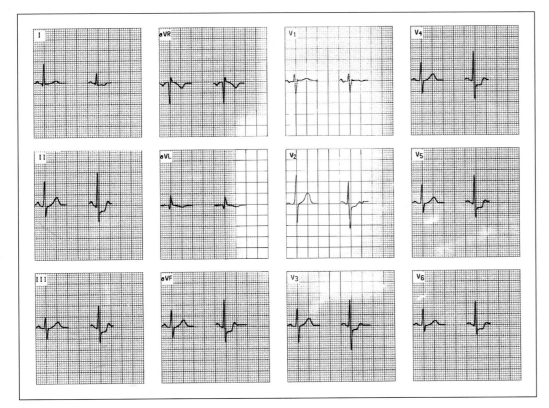

FIGURE 10-15. Computerized summary of resting (*left tracings*) and maximal exercise (*right tracings*) electrocardiograms (ECGs) in a 48-year-old asymptomatic aircrew member showing 2 mm of ST-segment depression at peak exertion (*ie*, 10 minutes using a Bruce protocol at a heart rate of 157 bpm). The implications of exercise tolerance testing (ETT) in aircrew have been studied extensively [60]. In the *asymptomatic* aircrew population, ETT is sufficiently sensitive to exclude this low-risk group from further investigation, if (1) exercise time is adequate—the subject reaches stage III using a Bruce protocol, exerts 10 metabolic equivalents (METs), or has a VO_2 of 35 mL/kg or more—and (2) there are few or no ST-segment changes. False-positive tests in this population are uncommon, but in equivocal cases must be evaluated further with thallium scintigraphy or coronary angiography.

Although prognosis can be predicted reasonably for a group with ischemic ST-segment changes, individual risk cannot be predicted accurately and requires coronary angiography in an aircrew member whose stress test is unequivocally positive. Several recommendations about testing have been made for aircrew members who have had a myocardial infarction: (1) anti-arrhythmic or anti-anginal medications should be discontinued prior to testing; (2) a period of 3 months of exercise training should precede the test, so results will be sufficiently stable; (3) the test must be symptom-limited; (4) systolic blood pressure should increase at least 50 mm Hg from the resting state; (5) the ECG should show no more than 1 mm of ST-segment change; (6) there should be no significant ectopy; and (7) the subject must achieve the exercise capacity previously described. Under these circumstances, and if coronary angiography shows no more than a 30% narrowing of all but the infarct-related artery (*see* Fig. 10-16), the aircrew member could be certified to fly. Follow-up testing at least annually is advised.

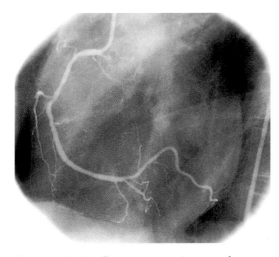

FIGURE 10-16. Coronary angiogram from a 56-year-old male commercial aviator with atypical chest pain and an equivocal tolerance test. The proximal and midportions of the right coronary artery show several areas of minimal irregularity, while the left

coronary artery and left ventricle were normal. Coronary angiography is frequently necessary in aircrew members with known or suspected cardiac disease because the results have prognostic significance and because the predictive value of noninvasive testing is not adequate. A completely normal coronary angiogram and normal left ventricular (LV) function is consistent with an extremely favorable 5- to 7-year survival rate of 96% to 99% [61,62]. These and other studies have demonstrated that prognosis in patients with coronary disease is directly related to the severity of the lesions on angiography [63], and that the outlook for patients with less than 50% diameter narrowing is reasonably good. Clearly, however, even minimal disease indicates that the atherosclerotic process is established and these lesions can serve as a nidus for plaque rupture, thrombus formation, and a sudden cardiac event.

In keeping with the "1% rule" (*see* Fig. 10-13), the following recommendations have been made [64]: (1) if the coronary angiogram shows less than 30% narrowings, certification to fly with a copilot may be considered if both the left ventricle and the results of a maximal exercise tolerance test are normal; (2) if the exercise test results are equivocal or coronary stenoses are greater than 30% but less than 50%, certification can be considered only if LV function is normal; (3) if coronary narrowing is greater than 50%, certification should be denied. In view of the progressive nature of coronary disease, careful follow-up of aircrew members whose angiograms are abnormal is mandatory and should include yearly exercise tests and repeat angiography at regular intervals (*eg*, every 5 years). Coronary angiography may also be useful in preventing unnecessary disqualification of pilots in whom symptoms or noninvasive tests suggest the possibility of coronary artery disease.

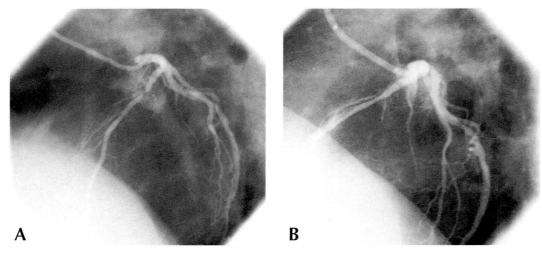

A **B**

FIGURE 10-17. Two cranially angulated left anterior oblique frames from a coronary angiogram of a 52-year-old pilot with a strongly positive exercise tolerance test. **A,** A 90% stenosis of the midportion of the left anterior descending coronary artery, with severe disease in a small diagonal branch. **B,** The same vessel immediately after percutaneous transluminal coronary angioplasty (PTCA) showing mild residual stenosis and occlusion of the small diagonal branch. This patient subsequently had an uncomplicated clinical course and a negative exercise test.

The emergence of PTCA as a therapy for coronary artery disease has offered a form of treatment with a significant chance for symptomatic relief without the associated morbidity of a cardiothoracic surgical procedure. Nevertheless, several problems with this technique have been identified. First, there is a small but significant risk of acute myocardial infarction and death, and 1% to 3% of angioplasties require urgent coronary bypass surgery owing to a complication of the procedure. Second, the rate of restenosis is 25% to 50% within 6 months, and the angiographic restenosis rate is higher than that suggested by symptoms alone. The role of PTCA in multivessel coronary disease in patients who would otherwise be considered surgical candidates is being investigated in at least five major trials in the United States and Europe. In addition, the ultimate contribution of a multitude of newer devices and techniques (including atherectomy, laser-assisted angioplasty, plaque extraction devices, and stents) remains to be determined. It is currently recommended that aircrew members who have undergone single-vessel angioplasty should have follow-up coronary angiography at 6 months; if the lesion has not recurred [65] and results of a concomitant maximal exercise test are normal, certification for flight status could be considered. Because of the poor predictive value of exercise testing in identifying restenosis, coronary angiography at regular intervals (*eg*, every 2 to 3 years) may be required in this group.

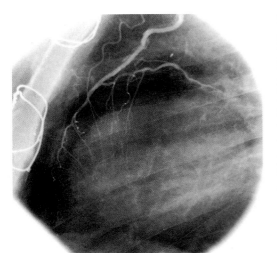

FIGURE 10-18. Coronary angiogram showing a patent internal mammary artery bypass graft to the left anterior descending coronary artery 4 years after uncomplicated single-vessel coronary artery bypass surgery (CABG). The role of CABG in aircrew members has been evaluated extensively [66]. In keeping with the "1% rule" (*see* Fig. 10-13), it has been recommended that a pilot could be considered for restricted flight certification if he or she has had uncomplicated bypass surgery (preferably including one or both internal mammary arteries) with normal left ventricular function postoperatively, remains asymptomatic, takes meaningful steps toward reducing cardiac risk, and has a normal maximal exercise tolerance test. A period of at least 9 months after CABG should be anticipated to allow physical and mental recovery, risk modification, and recurrence of symptoms (if any). Coronary angiography 5 years postoperatively and at least every 2 years thereafter to ensure graft patency is also recommended.

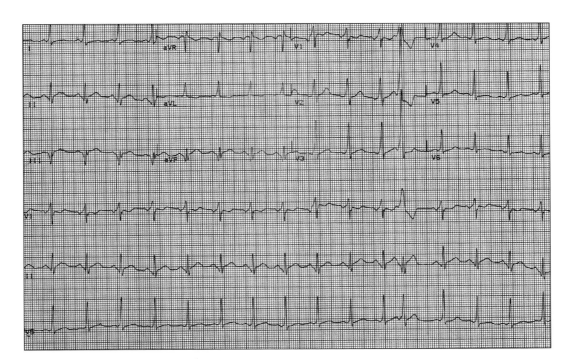

FIGURE 10-19. An electrocardiogram (ECG) from a 34-year-old asymptomatic aircrew member showing typical features of the Wolff-Parkinson-White (WPW) syndrome—*ie*, a short P-R interval and delta waves in multiple leads. Pre-excitation is relatively common, having a prevalence of 0.1% to 0.2% [67]. In long-term studies, the percentage of patients with WPW syndrome who eventually experience arrhythmias has varied widely. Guize *et al*. [68] found the frequency increased with age from 10% in patients 20 to 39 years of age to 36% in those over age 60. WPW syndrome may produce symptoms by virtue of various re-entrant tachycardias, atrial fibrillation (AF), or (uncommonly) AF with a rapid ventricular response degenerating into ventricular fibrillation.

A WPW population at sufficiently low risk to consider flight certification can be identified by both noninvasive and invasive means [69]. Subjects are deemed to be at low risk if they are asymptomatic and have no documented sustained arrhythmia, no documented episodes of spontaneous AF, no sick sinus syndrome, no arrhythmia on ambulatory or exercise ECG, and an electrophysiologic study that shows an accessory pathway antegrade refractory period greater than 300 ms, no inducible re-entrant tachyarrhythmia, no multiple pathways, and either no inducible AF or the shortest delta-delta interval during AF greater than 300 ms. Surgical and, more recently, catheter ablation techniques have been shown to be highly effective in abolishing the accessory pathway in the majority of patients [70]. Flight recertification may be considered 6 months after successful surgical ablation and 3 months after catheter ablation as long as results of noninvasive and electrophysiologic studies are normal. An annual cardiologic review is also recommended.

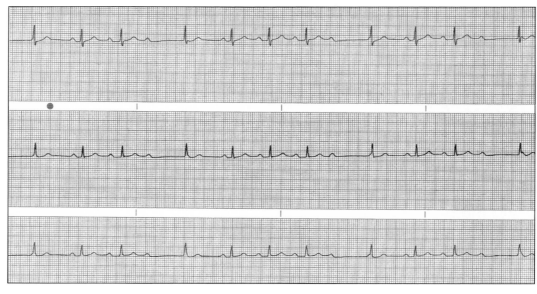

FIGURE 10-20. A rhythm strip from a 39-year-old male veteran who complained of intermittent syncope showing an extreme case of Mobitz type I second-degree atrioventricular (AV) block. Progressive lengthening of the P-R interval from 800 to 1000 ms is present until there is failure of AV nodal conduction. The topic of varying degrees of sinoatrial nodal, AV nodal, and intraventricular conduction disturbances as they relate to aircrew certification has been reviewed extensively [71]. Disturbances determined to be sufficiently benign to allow consideration for flight status include sinus pauses of up to 2.2 seconds in duration, first-degree AV block, Mobitz type I second-degree AV block (as long as the episodes are intermittent and of short duration and higher degrees of AV block are never present), isolated bundle branch block, and left anterior and left posterior fascicular blocks. Aircrew members with sinus pauses of 2.2 to 2.5 seconds who are not well-conditioned athletes should undergo exercise stress testing and ambulatory monitoring prior to certification; it is not clear what course should be taken with athletic individuals with sinus pauses exceeding 2.5 seconds. Persons with left bundle branch block require exercise thallium scintigraphy and perhaps coronary angiography before they can be certified. Conduction abnormalities associated with symptoms as well as Mobitz type II second-degree AV block and third-degree AV block are indications for decertification.

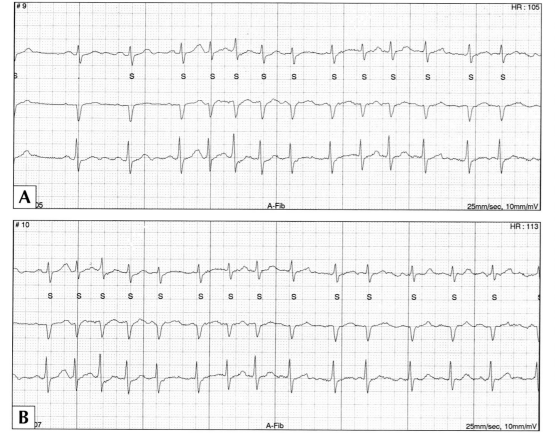

FIGURE 10-21. A three-lead rhythm strip from a 44-year-old hypertensive man showing an episode of paroxysmal atrial fibrillation (AF) (**A**); the ventricular rate becomes more rapid (**B**) and then slows down (**C**), and the entire episode lasted 35 minutes. Arrhythmias in aircrew members are obviously grounds for extreme concern and have been reviewed extensively in this context [72,73]. A pilot who has a single episode of AF should be grounded for 6 months. If exercise tolerance testing, echocardiography, and at least four 24-hour ambulatory electrocardiograms are normal, unlimited certification should be considered. Paroxysmal AF is a more difficult problem. If there is no indication of coronary disease and the pilot is asymptomatic during the episodes, and if the ventricular rate is controlled by an approved medication (*see* Fig. 10-22), restricted certification may be considered after 6 months of grounding. Chronic AF (and to a lesser extent paroxysmal AF) is associated with an increased risk of stroke [74]. (*continued*)

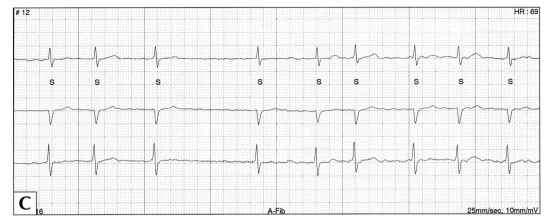

FIGURE 10-21. (*continued*) The risk of stroke or disabling symptoms from the arrhythmia itself is enough to disqualify for a single crew certification. Pilots without hypertension or evidence of coronary disease who are on an acceptable medication and have achieved good control of the ventricular response at rest and during flight simulation testing may be considered for multicrew certification. Currently, warfarin therapy precludes flying status, although low-dose warfarin prophylaxis has not been considered. Paroxysmal AF is sufficiently unstable to deny flight certification.

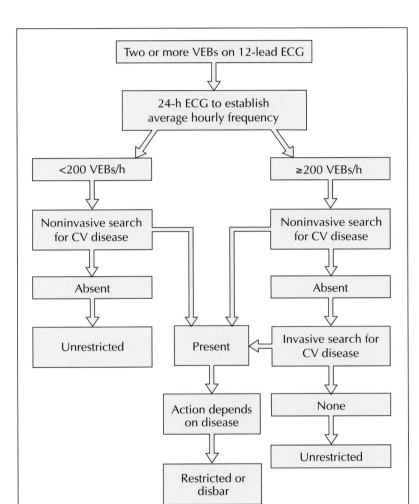

FIGURE 10-22. Algorithm for investigation and management of aircrew who present with two or more ventricular ectopic beats (VEBs) on electrocardiography (ECG) [75]. In the absence of identifiable heart disease, fewer than 200 VEBs/h on ambulatory monitoring is associated with less than the annual mortality allowed by the 1% rule. When VEBs complicate heart disease, mortality may exceed 1%/y, and flight certification should be considered only after extensive evaluation. Almost all individuals with nonsustained ventricular tachycardia (VT) (more than three successive VEBs at a rate of 120 bpm) have an unacceptable yearly mortality and should not be licensed. Another algorithm has been designed for the vigorous evaluation of potential aircrew with VT, which recommends restricted certification for a few selected cases [75]. CV—cardiovascular. (*Adapted from* Campbell [75]; with permission.)

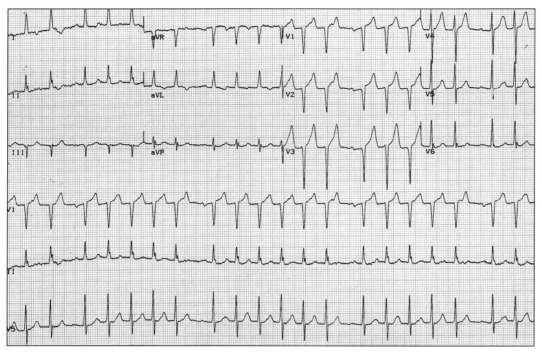

FIGURE 10-23. Electrocardiogram (ECG) from a 37-year-old male aviator with occasional palpitations. The intermittent narrow-complex tachycardia is consistent with atrioventricular (AV) nodal re-entry. A 24-hour ECG recording showed several such episodes, the longest lasting 11 minutes. The patient's exercise tolerance test was normal, and echocardiography showed no structural heart disease. Oral verapamil completely ameliorated the arrhythmia.

Gorgels *et al.* [76] have considered the implications of arrhythmias and anti-arrhythmia medication in the context of aviation. They suggest that arrhythmias that may be accept-

able in aircrew include infrequent supraventricular ectopic beats (< 2% of total), infrequent ventricular ectopic beats (< 2% of total; *see* Fig. 10-22), chronic atrial fibrillation with controlled ventricular response (*see* Fig. 10-21), AV nodal tachycardia when completely controlled by permissible anti-arrhythmic drugs, and AV re-entrant tachycardia via an accessory pathway following demonstrably complete catheter ablation (*see* Fig. 10-19). Class IA agents (by the Vaughan Williams classification [77]) such as quinidine and procainamide have pro-arrhythmic effects, class IB agents have unacceptable neurologic side effects, and class IC agents such as flecainide are also pro-arrhythmic; none of these agents is acceptable for flight certification. Class II agents, the β-blockers, have an acceptable profile for aircrew if they are of the hydrophilic type. Class III drugs such as amiodarone and sotalol have a variety of side effects that disqualify their use by aircrew; however, class IV agents such as verapamil and diltiazem are permissible. Digitalis is acceptable if levels are monitored and toxicity is avoided. When any of these agents is prescribed, grounding for 3 months, 24-hour ambulatory ECG, and flight simulator testing are necessary.

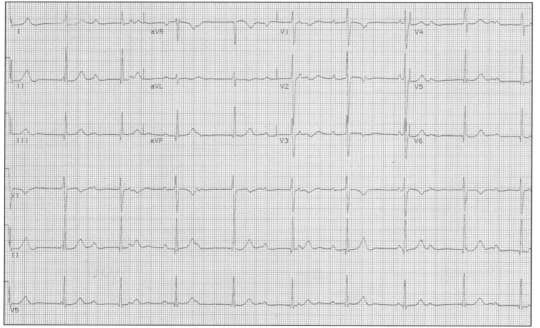

FIGURE 10-24. Electrocardiogram (ECG) from an asymptomatic 23-year-old flight attendant candidate who had been told as a child that she had an irregular heartbeat. The findings are consistent with third-degree atrioventricular (AV) block. On exercise testing, neither her sinus rate nor her ventricular rate increased more than 20% from baseline. A diagnosis of complete heart block with chronotropic incompetence was made, and an AV sequential pacemaker with rate responsiveness was implanted. The use of permanent pacemakers has

increased dramatically over the past decade as devices have become more sophisticated and reliable and the benefits of AV synchrony have become obvious. Indications for permanent pacemaker implantation have been published [78].

Application of these devices to aviation has been reviewed, and the following recommendations were made [79]: Pilots with pacemakers should have only restricted licenses because of the remote possibility of device failure or electromagnetic interference. If restricted certification is contemplated, it should be delayed for 3 months, the person should have no other cardiac conditions, devices known to be at higher risk for failure should be excluded, subjects dependent on atrial sensing should be excluded, bipolar pacing leads are preferred, the pacing mode and programming should be appropriate to the clinical setting, and follow-up should be done every 6 months by a cardiologist and with routine ambulatory ECG recordings. The implant date and serial numbers of the pacemaker and leads should be on file with the licensing agency. Persons with implanted antitachycardia and defibrillator devices must not be certified.

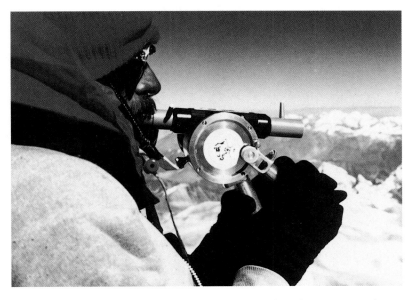

FIGURE 10-25. Dr. Christopher Pizzo taking alveolar gas samples on the summit of Mt. Everest (October 24, 1981) during the American Medical Research Expedition. It has been estimated that

in the United States more than 40 million people travel to high altitude annually [80]. For most purposes, high altitude begins above 2440 m (8000 ft), the height at which oxygen saturation usually falls below 90% [81]. High-altitude illness occurs when the rate of ascent exceeds the rate of acclimatization and the body's ability to adapt to an acute lowering of arterial oxygen content [82].

At extreme elevations, such as at the summit of Everest at 8872 m (29,107 ft, barometric pressure 253 torr), maximal oxygen uptake is reduced to 20% to 25% of that at sea level, and only extraordinary measures allow a person to function [83].

Investigations carried out at the summit of Everest during this expedition and in simulated ascents in decompression chambers (Operation Everest I and II) have shown that an alveolar PO_2 of about 35 torr can be maintained only by vigorous hyperventilation, which produces an alveolar PCO_2 of 7.5 to 11.0 torr [84,85]! Under these conditions, it has been estimated that arterial PO_2 is less than 30 torr at rest and may be lower on exercise. This degree of hyperventilation was associated with an estimated pH of over 7.7 on the summit [84,86]. Given these conditions, it is extraordinary that Everest has been climbed by more than 50 people without supplemental oxygen. (*Adapted from* West and Lahiri [86a]; with permission.)

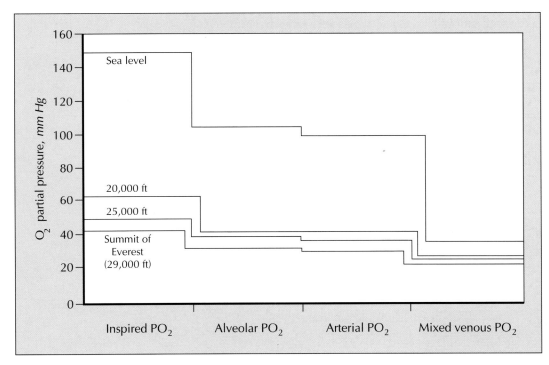

FIGURE 10-26. Oxygen tensions at various elevations. At very high altitudes, oxygen availability falls substantially. A variety of illnesses occur at increasing altitudes, and Tso [87] has provided an excellent review of these conditions. The most common is acute mountain sickness (AMS), which has been reported in 1.4% to 25.0% of persons visiting elevations of

2060 to 2440 m (6754 to 8000 ft) [88,89], and most persons will experience some symptoms of AMS above 3050 m (10,000 ft) [90].

The classic symptoms of AMS are headache, insomnia, anorexia, nausea, and dizziness. Other findings include vomiting, weakness, fatigue, oliguria, irregular respirations during sleep, thirst, cough, chest discomfort, peripheral edema, rales, and retinal hemorrhages. AMS can usually (but not always) be avoided by gradual ascent and is cured by descent. Most episodes are benign and transient, but 5% to 10% of cases progress to a more serious condition: high-altitude cerebral edema (HACE) and high-altitude pulmonary edema (HAPE) [91]. Although much less common than HAPE, HACE may affect up to 1.8% of travelers to high altitude, usually above 3660 m (12,000 ft) [92,93]. Neurologic symptoms include severe headache, marked ataxia, altered mental status, focal neurologic deficits, seizures, emotional lability, and frank psychosis [93]. There is a significant risk for death or permanent neurologic deficit, sometimes in spite of descent. (*See* Fig. 10-27 for a more complete discussion of HAPE.)

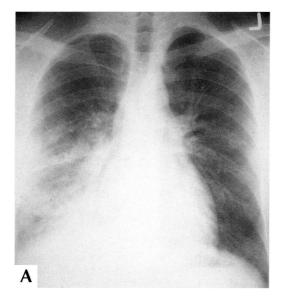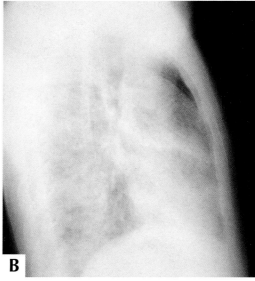

FIGURE 10-27. **A** and **B,** Chest roentgenograms of a 25-year-old medical student who drove and climbed from sea level to 2743 m (9000 ft) where he spent the night. He spent the next night in a snow cave at 3780 m (12,400 ft). When attempting to climb still higher on the following day, he developed extreme fatigue, dyspnea, headache, and a cough productive of yellowish sputum. He was able to descend with assistance and later improved slowly. These radiographs, obtained 18 hours later, show patchy edema in the right lung.

High-altitude noncardiogenic pulmonary edema (HAPE) develops in 0.5% to 15.0% of persons who ascend rapidly to high altitudes [94]. These persons as well as younger persons and those with a previous episode of HAPE are more susceptible. Signs and symptoms include persistent cough, weakness, fever, cyanosis, tachycardia, tachypnea, orthopnea, and rales. Pink frothy sputum and hemoptysis may develop [95]. Without descent or supplemental oxygen, mortality was as high as 44% in early studies [96].

Prior to 1960, HAPE was thought to represent congestive heart failure [97]. Hultgren [98] proposed unevenly distributed hypoxic pulmonary vasoconstriction as the underlying mechanism in HAPE. Schoene *et al.* [99] showed that the protein content of bronchoalveolar lavage specimens obtained from victims of HAPE on Denali was increased, consistent with a noncardiogenic etiology. Recently, West *et al.* [100] have suggested that HAPE is due to stress failure of pulmonary capillaries caused by hypoxia-induced acute pulmonary hypertension. Treatment would include descent, supplemental oxygen, and nifedipine [101]. In addition, nifedipine has been useful in preventing HAPE [102]. In cases of severe high-altitude cerebral or pulmonary edema, a Gamow hyperbaric bag may be lifesaving (*see* Fig. 10-28).

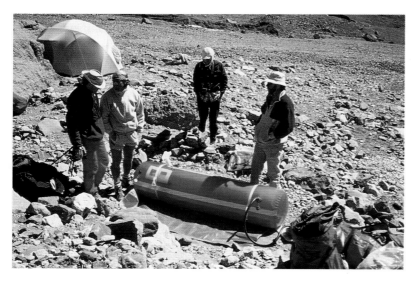

FIGURE 10-28. Mountaineers at base camp (elevation, 4200 m [13,800 ft]) on Aconcagua in Argentina, with a Gamow bag, a portable emergency recompression device (*see* Fig. 10-27). By means of a manual pumping system, the pressure inside the bag can be raised about 100 mm Hg above ambient pressure. The Gamow bag has proved effective in treating numerous cases of high-altitude illness [103–105].

ALTITUDE LIMITS (WITHOUT SUPPLEMENTAL OXYGEN) FOR PATIENTS WITH MEDICAL CONDITIONS

MAXIMUM ALTITUDE, ft	PROBLEM
2000	Cardiac patients in CHF
	MI within last 8 weeks
	Cyanosis, cor pulmonale, *and* respiratory acidosis
4000	Severe cardiac disease with cyanosis or recent decompensation
	Patients with any two of the following: cyanosis, cor pulmonale, *or* respiratory acidosis
6000	Recent MI (within 8 to 24 wk)
	Angina pectoris
	Sickle cell disease
	Alveolar block with cyanosis
	Any one the following: cyanosis, cor pulmonale, *or* respiratory acidosis
8000	Mildly symptomatic cardiopulmonary disease without failure or marked ventilatory restriction
10,000	Suspected or symptomatic cardiopulmonary disease

FIGURE 10-29. Recommendations regarding the limits on high-altitude travel (without supplemental oxygen) for patients with various cardiac conditions [87]. During commercial air travel, the cabin is pressurized to altitudes that usually range from 1675 to 2440 m (5500 to 8000 ft) [106]. Much higher altitudes may be experienced in small airplanes and helicopters. About 5% of all air travelers have some chronic illness, and 0.2% (of these approximately 686,000 who fly annually in the United States) may be adversely affected by altitude [107]. In studies from the Seattle-Tacoma and Los Angeles International Airports, about one person in 39,000 experienced an in-flight emergency [107–109]. The most common complaints were abdominal pain, chest pain, dyspnea, hyperventilation, headache, and nausea. About 50 altitude-related deaths occur annually in the United States (*ie*, about 1/6.4 to 7.0 million passengers), mainly owing to myocardial infarction (MI), other cardiac-related processes, or stroke. Many investigators disagree as to which patients with various cardiac disorders should not be allowed to travel by commercial airplane or to ascend to high altitudes. In reality, many patients with cardiopulmonary disease have tolerated travel to altitudes of 2300 m (about 7500 ft) or higher without difficulty [110]. CHF—congestive heart failure. (*Adapted from* Tso [87]; with permission.)

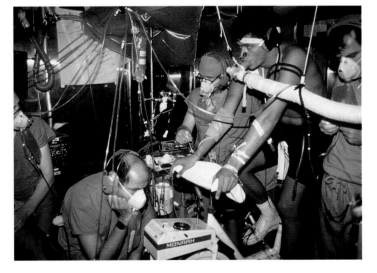

FIGURE 10-30. Subject performing an exercise test in a decompression chamber. Pulmonary and radial arterial lines are in place, and exhaled gas is being collected. The researchers are using supplemental oxygen. During Operation Everest II (1985), subjects lived continuously in a decompression chamber in which the pressure was decreased gradually over 35 days to simulate an ascent of Mt. Everest [111]. Right heart catheterizations were performed at various simulated altitudes, the highest being equivalent to Everest's summit. Right heart pressures, oxygen consumption, and arterial and mixed venous oxygen tensions were measured, and cardiac output and pulmonary vascular resistances were calculated. These data were collected at rest and during upright bicycle ergometry. Mean pulmonary arterial pressures increased from 15 mm Hg at rest to 33 mm Hg with exercise at sea level and from 34 to 54 mm Hg during exercise at 7620 m (25,000 ft) [112]. Heart rate for any given oxygen uptake and stroke volume for a given right atrial or pulmonary capillary wedge pressure were well preserved, and cardiac contractile function was maintained at extreme altitudes [113].

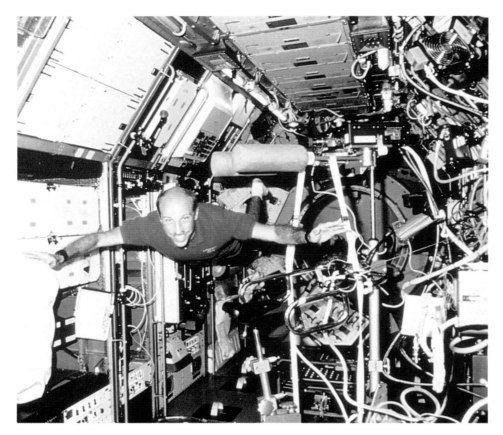

FIGURE 10-31. Interior of the Spacelab module as it appeared during the 1991 US Space Shuttle flight Spacelab Life Sciences-1 (SLS-1). The Spacelab, developed and built by the European Space Agency [114], is a multipurpose laboratory unit carried in the payload bay of the Space Shuttle. It was first flown in 1983 and has since supported a long series of US and international scientific flights. SLS-1 was dedicated to the life sciences and was designed to carry out 18 human and animal (rodent and jellyfish) experiments that addressed a wide range of questions concerning cardiovascular and pulmonary physiology, body fluid metabolism, disuse atrophy of the musculoskeletal systems, and neurovestibular physiology. The SLS-1 crew of seven included three physicians: Dr. James Bagian, an anesthesiologist (shown here floating in the module); Dr. Andrew Gaffney, a cardiologist; and Dr. Rhea Seddon, a surgeon. Facilities included a mass spectrometer, an echocardiograph, a bicycle ergometer, and a rotating chair for vestibular testing, as well as computers for prompting and digital recording of experimental results, modules for tissue culture, freezers and refrigerators, and a mass measuring device. In addition, there were holding facilities and an enclosed workstation for rodent experiments. This laboratory truly represented the state of the art with respect to biomedical research in space. (Courtesy of NASA Photo, Lyndon B. Johnson Space Center, Houston, TX.)

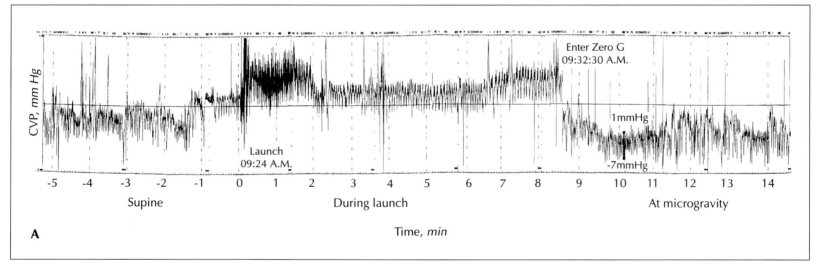

FIGURE 10-32. Central venous pressure (CVP) has recently been monitored during Space Shuttle launches and during the initial adaptation to microgravity (μG). **A,** The first record obtained was this continuous tracing of CVP from a crew member of Spacelab Life Sciences-1 (SLS-1) in 1991 [115]. (*continued*)

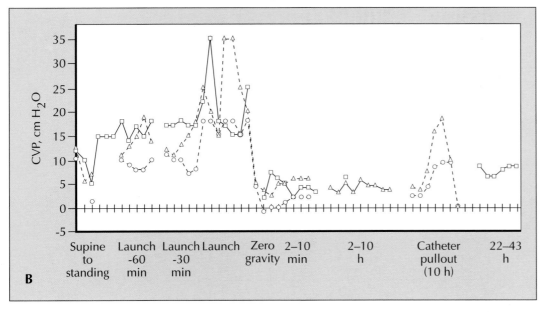

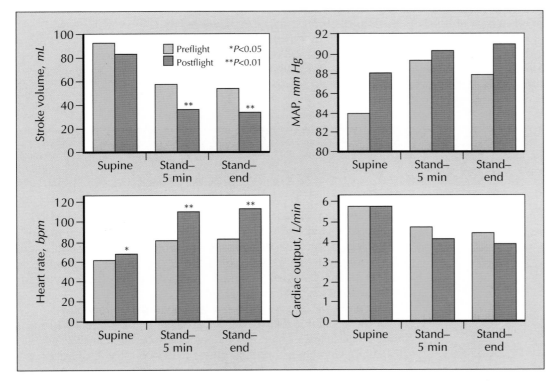

designed safe, stable, and accurate fluid-filled system in which a catheter was inserted in an arm vein with its tip positioned in the superior vena cava immediately peripheral to the right atrium [115]. The continuous recording (*A*) shows that CVP rises well above normal supine levels during launch, when acceleration forces compress the chest from front to back. On arrival in µG, CVP falls precipitously to levels approximating preflight upright measurements. These data can be reconciled with the high left ventricular end-diastolic volume at µG only by assuming a change in the normal relation between measured and effective cardiac filling pressures, which most likely reflects altered mechanical properties of the chest at µG. These findings were unexpected and inconsistent with prevailing concepts, yet the response of the three subjects was uniform (*B*). Catheter pullout pressure data document the integrity of the measurement system, *ie*, an initial increase as the tip moved peripherally and a return to a zero baseline upon complete pullout. (Part A *adapted from* Buckey and coworkers [116]; with permission from *New England Journal of Medicine*; part B *adapted from* Buckey and coworkers [11]; with permisson.)

FIGURE 10-32. (*continued*) **B,** Summary of CVP data from two US flights, including information from *panel A* and the results from two additional crew members instrumented during the launch of SLS-2 in 1993. Similar information was also recorded in one crew member by Foldager and Norsk during the launch of another Spacelab flight (D-2), also in 1993 (Foldager N, Norsk P, personal communication). The µG condition leads to a major redistribution of body fluids, including intravascular volume. Measurement of CVP is currently the only practical means of obtaining a continuous, quantitative measure of cardiac filling pressure during launch. These data were collected from a subject instrumented with a specially

FIGURE 10-33. Orthostatic intolerance is a common finding early on return after prolonged space flight [9,11]. Summary of pre- and postflight hemodynamic responses of 14 crew members (11 men and 3 women, 31 to 50 years of age) studied before and after three Space Shuttle flights between 1991 and 1993: two US Spacelab

Life Sciences flights (SLS-1 and SLS-2) and an international flight (D-2), which carried a mixed science payload and was managed by the German Space Agency. All crew members completed a 10-minute preflight stand test, but after the flight, only five of the 14 were asymptomatic and able to finish the test. All but three participants (two finishers and one nonfinisher) had used NASA's oral fluid-loading procedure designed to prevent orthostatic intolerance. The preflight data illustrate the typical normal orthostatic hemodynamic response: supine stroke volume decreased 43%, from 94 to 54 mL, on standing, and mean arterial pressure (MAP) (and thus cerebral perfusion) was maintained by mean increases of 21 bpm in heart rate and 45% in total peripheral resistance (*see* Fig. 10-34). After the flight, stroke volume was insignificantly reduced at supine baseline (84 vs 94 mL preflight), with no change in MAP. During standing, the final stroke volume was significantly lower than preflight levels (35 vs 54 mL, $P<0.001$), and heart rate was increased (113 vs 82 bpm, $P<0.001$).

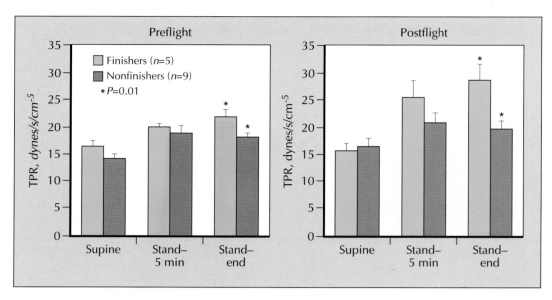

FIGURE 10-34. Principal hemodynamic difference in postflight responses between stand-test finishers and nonfinishers [9,11,13]. Most striking was the marked relative attenuation of the systemic vasoconstrictor response in the nonfinishers, measured as a change in total peripheral resistance (TPR). (TPR is measured as the ratio of mean arterial pressure (mm Hg) to cardial output [L/min].) The specific underlying mechanism(s) remain to be defined. An apparent limitation in the dynamic range of systemic vasoconstrictor response may reflect functional defect(s) at one or more of multiple regulatory levels (eg, differences in afferent reflex mechanisms, central integration, neural efferent activity, and/or end-organ responsiveness). Paradoxical vasodepressor drive, produced by systolic stimulation of ventricular mechanoreceptors under conditions that include markedly reduced ventricular filling, may also contribute. However, the orthostatic heart rate response was (as might have been expected) significantly larger in the nonfinishers (see Fig. 10-33, lower left). On the other hand, a μG-induced blunting of the heart rate response, as mediated by the carotid baroreflex, has been described by Eckberg et al. [116,117]. Perhaps these apparent contradictions can be reconciled during future flights by studies testing the hypothesis that the adaptation to μG alters the central integration of cardiovascular neurohumoral regulatory mechanisms. (Adapted from Blomqvist and coworkers [9]; with permission.)

DIVING AND CARDIOLOGY

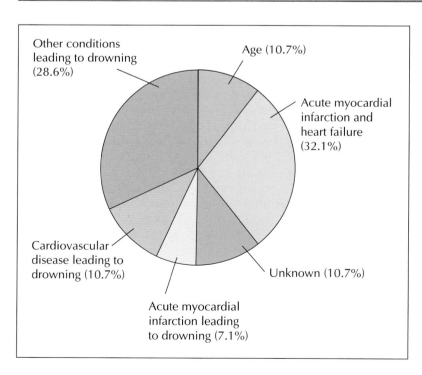

FIGURE 10-35. Estimates of causes of death among divers in 1991 provided by Divers Alert Network [118]. Although the number of deaths is accurate, this organization emphasizes that the causes are often presumptive and based on indirect evidence. Nevertheless, these data are obviously of concern to medical personnel involved in the evaluation and care of divers.

The number of divers who use a self-contained underwater breathing apparatus (SCUBA) has increased over the last 20 years in the United States. Over 50,000 divers were certified in 1987; as of 1992, there were up to 4 million divers in this country. As diving has become more popular, so has the number of medical complications of this activity. Physicians and other health care providers have had to evaluate the diving fitness of persons with various underlying medical conditions and have had to develop strategies for assessing and managing diving emergencies. As shown here, coronary artery disease and other cardiovascular diseases are responsible for a significant proportion of diving deaths in divers over age 40 [119]. Therefore, it is essential that, before entering the underwater environment, all potential divers who have significant health problems undergo a thorough medical history and a physical examination performed by a clinician familiar with the problems associated with this activity. (Adapted from Divers Alert Network [118]; with permission.)

CARDIAC CONTRAINDICATIONS TO DIVING CLEARANCE

MI in the previous 12 months
Symptomatic CAD or demonstrable inducible ischemia
Symptomatic valvular heart disease
Heart failure
High-grade or symptomatic arrhythmias
Unexplained syncope
Intracardiac shunting

FIGURE 10-36. Cardiac contraindications to clearance for diving [119,120]. Most authors recommend disqualification of anyone with known coronary artery disease (CAD). Under special circumstances some divers have been certified despite a history of CAD, a previous myocardial infarction (MI), percutaneous transluminal coronary angioplasty, or coronary artery bypass graft surgery. In these cases, a year should have elapsed since the MI or intervention, and they should be asymptomatic and should be able to reach at least 13 metabolic equivalents (METs) on an exercise test (equivalent to stage 4 of a Bruce protocol) without arrhythmias or evidence

of ischemia. They should be evaluated yearly, and their diving leaders and companions should be made aware of their situation.

There are no regulatory agencies in the United States charged with setting medical standards for recreational diving fitness. Furthermore, there are no legal requirements for a recreational diver to have a medical evaluation or even formal training before purchasing equipment and entering the water. However, most diving instructors, outfitters, and expedition leaders do require evidence of medical fitness, although a certifying physician may not be familiar with the particular problems associated with the underwater environment. Finally, a diver may never be required to undergo a medical re-evaluation for diving fitness. On the other hand, military and industrial organizations usually have strict regimens for determining continuing fitness for diving.

Guidelines that represent the consensus opinion of diving physicians have been published with regard to the medical evaluation of the recreational diver as well as criteria for disqualification from diving [119,120]. According to these authors, diving is a strenuous activity that requires considerable physical fitness, and recreational diving is a voluntary effort that is not necessary for the diver's livelihood. Furthermore, although it is laudable to include persons with physical disabilities in recreational activities, disabled recreational divers may endanger not only themselves but other divers who attempt rescue, and disabled divers cannot render assistance to others. Thus, the authors recommend a conservative approach to certification in such cases.

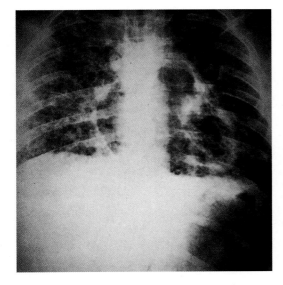

FIGURE 10-37. Chest roentgenogram in a fatal case of *pulmonary barotrauma* [121]. The cardiac cavities are filled with air, as are the splenic vessels. Two medical conditions are specific to the underwater environment: barotrauma and decompression sickness (*see* Fig. 10-38). Barotrauma refers

to tissue injury resulting from the failure of a gas-filled body (*eg*, the lungs, middle ear, sinuses) to equalize its internal pressure to correspond to changes in ambient pressure [121–123]. Pulmonary barotrauma, which occurs during ascent, is the most severe and life-threatening form of this condition. During ascent, gases in the lungs expand; if they are not properly equalized by exhalation, the lungs will become distended. Stretching and tearing of the alveolar basement membranes result in numerous small air leaks, which may lead to pneumothorax, pneumomediastinum, or subcutaneous emphysema. The diver may experience voice changes, chest fullness, dyspnea, dysphagia, and pleuritic pain. A large pneumothorax can compromise cardiovascular function and, rarely, lead to shock and death.

The most serious complication of pulmonary barotrauma is arterial air embolism, owing to passage of gas into the pulmonary veins and hence to the systemic circulation. Gas bubbles may lodge in cerebral, coronary, or other vascular beds and lead to central nervous system symptoms, myocardial infarction or arrhythmias, skin marbling, or retinal hemorrhages. Unconsciousness or other neurologic manifestations in a diver suggest decompression sickness (*see* Fig. 10-38). Treatment of pulmonary barotrauma includes maintaining respiration and an adequate oxygen tension. High concentrations of oxygen should be delivered to treat the hypoxia that may occur as a result of intrapulmonary hemorrhage, aspiration, or pneumothorax. The high oxygen concentration will lower the concentration of nitrogen in the blood, and hence in the tissues, thus facilitating the diffusion *out* of tissue bubbles. Mechanical ventilation may be necessary, and tube thoracostomy may be required to alleviate a pneumothorax. Patients with severe symptoms unresponsive to these measures as well as those with air embolism should be transported immediately to the nearest medical facility for stabilization and then to a hyperbaric oxygen facility for emergency recompression (*see* Fig. 10-38). (*Adapted from* Elliott and Moon [121]; with permission.)

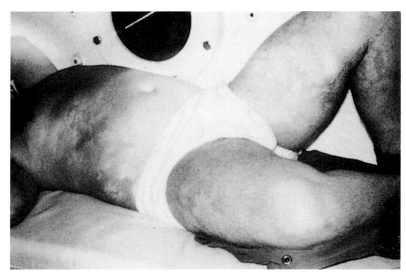

Decompression sickness traditionally has been divided into types I and II based on the clinical manifestations [121,123,124]. Type I included localized joint pain ("the bends") caused by the liberation of gas bubbles into the poorly perfused tight connective tissues during decompression. The pain may be mild or severe, generally develops within 1 hour, and may gradually worsen over 24 to 36 hours. Type II symptoms usually occur within 10 to 30 minutes after surfacing but may develop insidiously over several days. Central nervous system (CNS) involvement is often characterized by spinal cord damage and may lead to paraparesis and paraplegia. Loss of bowel and bladder control and referred abdominal pain are common with spinal cord involvement. Other symptoms include severe headache, visual disturbances, dysarthria, dizziness, and changes in mental status. CNS symptoms may also represent gas embolism from pulmonary barotrauma (*see* Fig. 10-37). Skin marbling is considered a type II manifestation.

Several authorities in the diving community consider the previous classification to be outdated, and they emphasize that *any* manifestation of decompression sickness should be considered serious and should be treated aggressively. Contrary to what was believed previously, type II manifestations are now understood to be as common as type I.

The US Navy has published recommendations for the treatment of diving accidents [125]. These guidelines are representative of those developed to deal with diving emergencies [126,127]. Divers Alert Network at Duke University Medical Center is an excellent source of information about all aspects of diving and medicine and maintains a 24-hour hotline for consultation and diving emergencies: (919) 684-8111. (*Adapted from* Elliott and Moon [121]; with permission.)

FIGURE 10-38. Appearance of a patient with *decompression sickness*. When a diver breathes air under increased pressure, the tissues are loaded with increased quantities of oxygen and nitrogen. Although oxygen is used in metabolism, nitrogen (which is physiologically inert) is not. When the diver returns to the surface, the excess nitrogen may lead to liberation of free gas from the tissues and produce the features of decompression sickness. Gas bubbles may block capillaries, rupture cell membranes, activate clotting sequences, and compress various structures. Decompression sickness can usually be avoided by controlled ascent with stops at appropriate depths, as specified in decompression tables provided by the US Navy. Still, even meticulous adherence to these schedules may not prevent this problem.

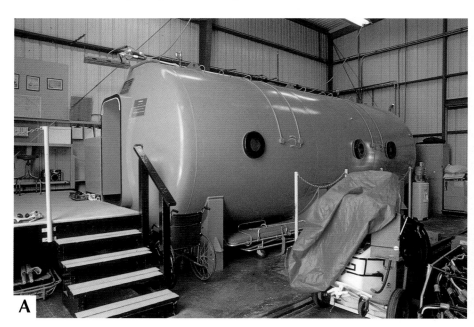

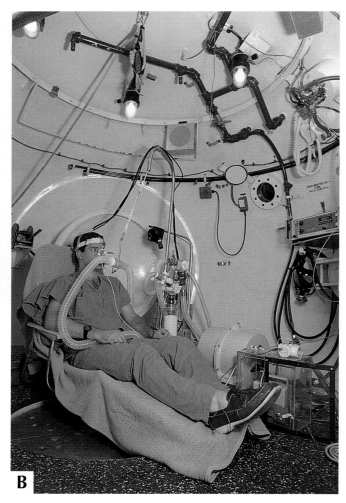

FIGURE 10-39. External (**A**) and internal (**B**) views of a hyperbaric chamber. The modern chamber is large enough to accommodate the patient, a considerable amount of medical equipment, and one or more physicians or other personnel. Every effort should be made to transport a patient with pulmonary barotrauma or decompression sickness as rapidly as possible to a facility with appropriate equipment and expertise to treat these conditions. (Courtesy of F. G. Hall Hyperbaric Center, Duke University Medical Center, Durham, NC.)

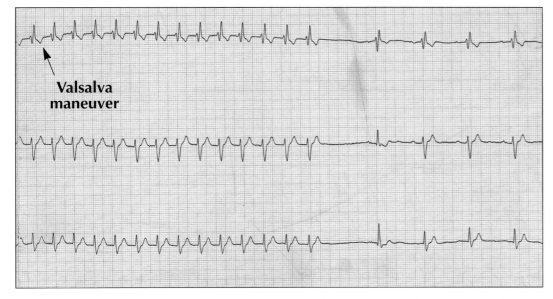

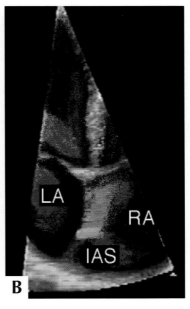

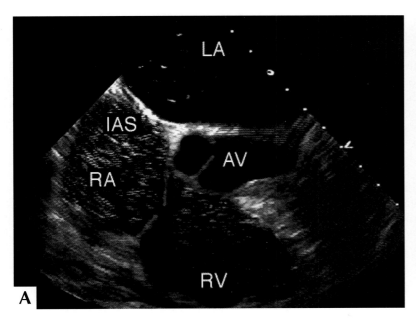

Valsalva maneuver

FIGURE 10-40. Electrocardiogram showing conversion from paroxysmal supraventricular tachycardia (PSVT) to sinus rhythm using a vagal maneuver. Over a century ago, Paul Bert of France observed pronounced bradycardia in ducks during diving, and this phenomenon has been noted in all diving animals [128]. Human breath-hold divers also show distinct brady-cardia during diving; the heart rate begins to decrease with the onset of the dive and reaches a minimal level in 20 to 30 seconds. Usually the lowest heart rate is 60% to 70% of the pre-dive level. Although diving bradycardia is usually associated with intense peripheral vasocon-striction, the latter is not considered to cause the decrease in heart rate. The intensity of the bradycardia is related to the temperature of the water and is more profound in colder temperatures. Moreover, diving bradycardia can be induced by immersing only the face in cold water. Therefore, the trigger of the reflex must be multifactorial and probably includes intrathoracic volume receptors, facial cold receptors, baroreceptors in various locations within the body, and PO_2 and PCO_2 chemoreceptors.

Breath-hold face immersion in cold water has been shown to be effective in termi-nating PSVT in many patients and may be a useful adjunct to carotid sinus massage [129]. Observations in pearl divers have demonstrated frequent abnormal P waves, junctional and idioventricular rhythms, and premature supraventricular and ventricular beats [130]. To what extent these abnormalities contribute to fatal diving accidents is not known.

FIGURE 10-41. Evidence of patent foramen ovale by microbubble contrast echocardiography (**A**) and color Doppler study (**B**). In *panel A*, sonicated saline was injected in a peripheral arm vein during echocardiography. As expected, microbubbles appeared in the right atrium (RA), although there were only a few bubbles in the left atrium (LA) and adjacent to the interatrial septum (IAS). *Panel B* shows flow away from the patent foramen ovale. Moon *et al.* [131] suggested that sports divers with this defect have a higher incidence of decompression sickness. A patent foramen ovale might allow asymptomatic bubbles to enter the arterial circulation and be responsible for some features of decompression sickness. Preliminary studies suggest a fivefold risk for neurologic disorders related to decompression sickness in divers with a patent foramen; however, these authors empha-size that although venous bubbles are relatively common in recently surfaced divers, the overall risk for neurologic decompression sickness is very low (probably less than one in 10,000). The depth of the dive and the age and gender of the diver also appear to be impor-tant factors. Investigators at Divers Alert Network are continuing to evaluate the applicability of this technique as part of a larger study to observe recreational divers for decompression sickness and to compare these observations with in-depth profiles retrieved from dive computers (Moon RE, personal communication). AV—aortic valve; RV—right ventricle. (Courtesy of Ramdas G. Pai, MD, Loma Linda University School of Medicine, Loma Linda, CA.)

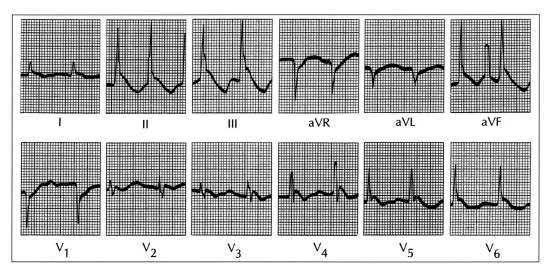

FIGURE 10-42. Electrocardiogram (ECG) showing Osborne or "J" waves in a person with hypothermia. Intentional or unintentional exposure to the aquatic environment poses a significant potential risk for hypothermia, since water has 1000 times the heat capacity and 26 times the thermal conductivity of air. The use of standard foamed neoprene wet suits retards heat loss moderately, but such protection may not be adequate in colder temperatures, during prolonged immersion, or at depths greater than 15 m, when the air cells in the material become compressed, reducing its insulating effectiveness.

With mild hypothermia (core temperature, 35°C to 37°C) the person is awake, complains of cold, and is able to answer questions appropriately. Moderate hypothermia (32°C to 35°C) is characterized by apathy, mild confusion, slurred speech, and poor cooperation, while severe hypothermia (less than 32°C) may cause coma and possibly cardiac arrest and the victim may appear clinically dead. All three stages of hypothermia are emergencies requiring prompt attention; however, since rough handling, chest compressions, airway manipulations, and attempts at rewarming in the field may increase mortality, rescue and medical personnel should be thoroughly trained and follow established treatment guidelines [132,133].

From a cardiopulmonary standpoint, severe hypothermia may produce profound bradycardia, supraventricular and ventricular ectopy, ventricular fibrillation, or asystole. Hypotension may be severe even without fibrillation or asystole. The respiratory rate may be profoundly depressed or absent, and there may be pulmonary edema. The ECG may show the characteristic J-point elevation, the so-called Osborne wave. (*Adapted from* Fisch [134]; with permission.)

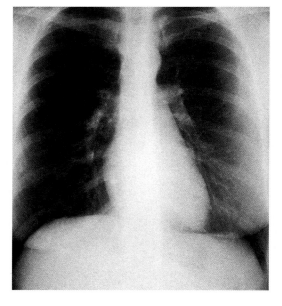

FIGURE 10-43. Chest roentgenogram of a 35-year old female diver who experienced severe dyspnea 25 minutes into a dive to a depth of 20 m. Slight pulmonary vascular redistribution, peribronchial cuffing, and minimal hazy infiltration of the hila can been seen. She responded rapidly to oxygen and diuretic therapy. Pulmonary edema occurring in otherwise healthy persons has been described during scuba diving in cold water [135]. Dyspnea, cough, hemoptysis, and expectoration of frothy sputum may occur while one is swimming or diving in shallow water or during the descent to or after attaining greater depths. These features are distinct from dyspnea from decompression sickness, which occurs during or after surfacing from a time-depth exposure extensive enough to cause inert gas loading. The mechanism in the pulmonary edema of immersion is probably cardiogenic and may involve increased cardiac preload due to water immersion, high inspiratory breathing resistance, and increased afterload due to cold water vasoconstriction. (Courtesy of F. G. Hall Hyperbaric Center, Duke University Medical Center, Durham, NC.)

REFERENCES

1. Engle L, Lott AS: *Man in Flight. Biomedical Achievements in Aerospace.* Annapolis, MD: Leeward Publications; 1979.

2. Dietlein LF: Skylab: a beginning. In *Biomedical Results from Skylab* (NASA SP-377). Edited by Johnston RS, Dietlein LF. Washington, DC: National Aeronautics and Space Administration, Scientific and Technical Information Office; 1977:408–420.

3. Nicogossian AE, Leach Huntoon C, Pool SL, eds: *Space Physiology and Medicine*, ed 3. Philadelphia: Lea & Febiger; 1994.

4. Johnston RS, Dietlein LF, Berry CA, eds: *Biomedical Results of Apollo* (NASA SP-368). Washington, DC: National Aeronautics and Space Administration, Scientific and Technical Information Office; 1975.

5. Johnston RS, Dietlein LF, eds: *Biomedical Results from Skylab* (NASA SP3-77). Washington, DC: National Aeronautics and Space Administration, Scientific and Technical Information Office; 1977.

6. Thron HL, Gauer OH: Postural changes in the circulation. In *Handbook of Physiology: Circulation*, Section 2, Volume III. Edited by Hamilton WE. Washington, DC: American Physiological Society; 1965:2408–2439.

7. Blomqvist CG, Stone HL: Cardiovascular adjustment to gravitational stress. In *Handbook of Physiology: The Cardiovascular System, Part 2: Peripheral Circulation and Organ Blood Flow*, Section 2, Volume III. Edited by Shepherd JT, Abboud FM. Washington, DC: American Physiological Society; 1983:1025–1063.

8. Baisch F, Beck L, Blomqvist CG, *et al.*: Head-down tilt bed test. HDT '88—an international collaborative effort in integrated systems physiology. *Acta Physiol Scand* 1992, 144:1–141.

9. Blomqvist CG, Buckey JC, Gaffney FA, *et al.*: Cardiovascular adaptation to zero gravity. In *Spacelab Life Sciences-2 180-Day Report.* Houston: National Aeronautics and Space Administration, Lyndon B. Johnson Space Center; 1994:31–41

10. Prisk GK, Guy HJB, Elliott AR, *et al.*: Pulmonary diffusing capacity, capillary blood volume, and cardiac output during sustained microgravity. *J Appl Physiol* 1993, 75:15–26.

11. Buckey JC, Lane LD, Levine BD, *et al.*: Orthostatic intolerance after space flight. *J Appl Physiol,* in press.

12. Levine BD, Lane LD, Gaffney FA, *et al.*: Maximal exercise performance after adaptation to microgravity [abstract]. *Med Sci Sports Exer* 1994, 26:S112.

13. Blomqvist CG, Buckey JC, Gaffney FA, *et al.*: Mechanisms of postflight orthostatic intolerance. *J Gravit Physiol* 1994, 1:P122–P124.

14. Atkov OE, Bednenko VS: *Hypokinesia and Weightlessness. Clinical and Physiological Aspects.* Madison, CT: International Universities Press; 1992.

15. Robbins DE, Yang TC: Radiation and radiobiology. In *Space Physiology and Medicine*, ed 3. Edited by Nicogossian AE, Leach Huntoon C, Pool SL. Philadelphia: Lea & Febiger; 1994:167–210.

16. Mangano DT: Perioperative cardiac morbidity. *Anesthesiology* 1990, 72:153–184.

17. Hertzer NR, Beven EG, Young JR, *et al.*: Coronary-artery disease in peripheral vascular patients. A classification of 1,000 coronary angiograms and results of surgical management. *Ann Surg* 1984,199:223–233.

18. Goldman L, Caldera DL, Nussbaum SR, *et al.*: Multifactorial index of cardiac risk in noncardiac surgical procedures. *N Engl J Med* 1977, 297:845–850.

19. Detsky AS, Abrams HB, Forbath N, *et al.*: Cardiac assessment for patients undergoing noncardiac surgery. A multifactorial clinical risk index. *Arch Intern Med* 1986, 146:2131–2135.

20. Detsky AS, Abrams HB, Mclaughlin JR, *et al.*: Predicting cardiac complications in patients undergoing non-cardiac surgery. *J Gen Intern Med* 1986, 1:211–219.

21. Zeldon RA, Math B: Assessing cardiac risk in patients who undergo noncardiac surgical procedures. *Can J Surg* 1984, 27:402–404.

22. Jeffrey CC, Kunsman J, Cullen DJ, *et al.*: A prospective evaluation of cardiac risk index. *Anesthesiology* 1983, 58:462–464.

23. Goldman L: Multifactorial index of cardiac risk in noncardiac surgery: Ten-year status report. *J Cardiothorac Anesth* 1987, 1:237–244.

24. Lette J, Waters D, Lassonde J, *et al.*: Multivariate clinical models and quantitative dipyridamole-thallium imaging to predict cardiac morbidity and death after vascular reconstruction. *J Vasc Surg* 1991, 14:160–169.

25. Lette J, Waters D, Bernier H, *et al.*: Preoperative and long-term cardiac risk assessment. *Ann Surg* 1992, 216: 192–204.

26. Wong T, Detsky AS: Perioperative cardiac risk assessment for patients having peripheral vascular surgery. *Ann Intern Med* 1992, 116:743–753.

27. Cutler BS, Wheeler HB, Paraskos JA, *et al.*: Assessment of operative risk with electrocardiographic exercise testing in patients with peripheral vascular disease. *Am J Surg* 1979, 137:484–490.

28. Cutler BS, Wheeler HB, Paraskos JA, *et al.*: Applicability and interpretation of electrocardiographic stress testing in patients with peripheral vascular disease. *Am J Surg* 1981, 141:501–506.

29. McPhail N, Calvin JE, Shariatmadar A, *et al.*: The use of preoperative exercise testing to predict cardiac complications after arterial reconstruction. *J Vasc Surg* 1988, 7:60–68.

30. McPhail NV, Ruddy TD, Calvin JE, *et al.*: A comparison of dipyridamole-thallium imaging and exercise testing in the prediction of postoperative cardiac complications in patients requiring arterial reconstruction. *J Vasc Surg* 1989, 10:51–56.

31. Botvinick EH, Dae M, Barron H, *et al.*: Nuclear cardiology: the scintigraphic evaluation of the cardiovascular system. In *Cardiology*, Vol I. Edited by Parmley W, Chatterjee K. Philadelphia: JB Lippincott; 1995:1–65.

32. Pasternack PF, Imparato AM, Bear G, *et al.*: The value of radionuclide angiography as a predictor of perioperative myocardial infarction in patients undergoing abdominal aortic aneurysm resection. *J Vasc Surg* 1984, 1:320–325.

33. Pasternack PF, Imparato AM, Riles TS, *et al.*: The value of the radionuclide angiogram in the prediction of perioperative myocardial infarction in patients undergoing lower extremity revascularization procedures. *Circulation* 1985, 72(suppl II):1113–1117.

34. Mosley JG, Clarke JMF, Marston A: Assessment of myocardial function before aortic surgery by radionuclide angiocardiography. *Br J Surg* 1985, 72:886–887.

35. Kazmers A, Cerqueira MD, Zierler RE: The role of preoperative radionuclide ejection fraction in direct abdominal aortic aneurysm repair. *J Vasc Surg* 1988, 8:128–136.

36. Franco CD, Goldsmith J, Veith FJ, *et al.*: Resting gated pool ejection fraction: a poor predictor of perioperative myocardial infarction in patients undergoing vascular surgery for infrainguinal bypass grafting. *J Vasc Surg* 1989, 10:656–661.

37. McPhail NV, Ruddy TD, Calvin JE, *et al.*: Comparison of left ventricular function and myocardial perfusion for evaluating perioperative cardiac risk of abdominal aortic surgery. *Can J Surg* 1990, 33:224–228.

38. McCann RL, Wolfe WG: Resection of abdominal aortic aneurysm in patients with low ejection fractions. *J Vasc Surg* 1989, 10:240–244.

39. Ouyang P, Gerstenblith G, Furman WR, *et al.*: Frequency and significance of early postoperative silent myocardial ischemia in patients having peripheral vascular surgery. *Am J Cardiol* 1989, 64:1113–1116.

40. Raby KE, Goldman L, Creager MA, *et al.*: Correlation between preoperative ischemia and major cardiac events after peripheral vascular surgery. *N Engl J Med* 1989, 321:1296–1300.

41. Pasternack PF, Grossi EA, Baumann FG, *et al.*: The value of silent myocardial ischemia monitoring in the prediction of perioperative myocardial infarction in patients undergoing peripheral vascular surgery. *J Vasc Surg* 1989, 10:617–625.

42. Mangano DT, Browner WS, Hollenberg M, *et al.*: Association of perioperative myocardial ischemia with cardiac morbidity and mortality in men undergoing noncardiac surgery. *N Engl J Med* 1990, 323:1781–1788.

43. Boucher CA, Brewster DC, Darling RC, *et al.*: Determination of cardiac risk by dipyridamole-thallium imaging before peripheral vascular surgery. *N Engl J Med* 1985, 312:389–394.

44. Leppo J, Plaja J, Gionet M, *et al.*: Noninvasive evaluation of cardiac risk before elective vascular surgery. *J Am Coll Cardiol* 1987, 9:269–276.

45. Eagle KA, Coley CM, Newell JB, *et al.*: Combining clinical and thallium data optimizes preoperative assessment of cardiac risk before major vascular surgery. *Ann Intern Med* 1989, 110:859–866.

46. Levinson JR, Boucher CA, Coley CM, *et al.*: Usefulness of semiquantitative analysis of dipyridamole thallium 201 redistribution for improving risk stratification before vascular surgery. *Am J Cardiol* 1990, 66:406–410.

47. Marwick TH, Underwood DA: Dipyridamole-thallium imaging may not be a reliable screening test for coronary artery disease in patients undergoing vascular surgery. *Clin Cardiol* 1990, 13:14–18.

48. Fliesher LA, Hawes AD, Rosenbaum SH: The limited predictive value of dipyridamole thallium imaging in noncardiac surgery patients [abstract]. *Anesthesiology* 1990, 73:A75.

49. Bertrand M, Coriat P, Baron JF, *et al.*: Dipyridamole thallium scan is not accurate in detecting coronary stenoses in patients undergoing abdominal aortic surgery [abstract]. *Anesthesiology* 1990, 73:A86.

50. Mangano DT, London MJ, Tubau JF, *et al.*: Dipyridamole thallium-201 scintigraphy as a preoperative screening test. A reexamination of its predictive potential. *Circulation* 1991, 84:493–502.

51. McFalls EO, Doliszny KM, Grund F, *et al.*: Angina and persistent exercise thallium defects: independent risk factors in elective vascular surgery. *J Am Coll Cardiol* 1993, 21:1347–1352.

52. Massie BM, Mangano DT: Assessment of perioperative risk: have we put the cart before the horse? *J Am Coll Cardiol* 1993, 21:1353–1356.

53. Lalka SG, Sawada SG, Dalsing MC, *et al.*: Dobutamine stress echocardiography as a predictor of cardiac events associated with aortic surgery. *J Vasc Surg* 1992, 15:831–842.

54. Poldermans D, Fiorette PM, Forster T, *et al.*: Dobutamine stress echocardiography for assessment of perioperative cardiac risk in patients undergoing major vascular surgery. *Circulation* 1993, 87:1506–1512.

54a. Dávila-Romá VG, Waggonar AD, Sicard GA, *et al.*: Dobutamine stress echocardiography predicts surgical outcome in patients with an aortic aneurysm and peripheral vascular disease. *J Am Coll Cardiol* 1993, 21:957–963.

55. Chaplin JC: In perspective: the safety of aircraft, pilots, and their hearts. *Eur Heart J* 1988, 9(suppl G):17–20.

56. Tunstall-Pedoe H: Cardiovascular risk and risk factors in the context of aircrew certification. *Eur Heart J* 1992, 13(suppl H):16–20.

57. Joy M: Introduction and summary of principal conclusions to the first European workshop in aviation cardiology. *Eur Heart J* 1992, 13(suppl H):1–9.

58. Bennet G: Medical cause accidents in commercial aviation. *Eur Heart J* 1992, 13(suppl H):13–15.

59. Brunner HR, Waeber B, Nussberger J: Strategies for the management of hypertension in aircrew. *Eur Heart J* 1992, 13(suppl H):45–49.

60. Broustet JP, Douard H, Oysel N, *et al.*: What is predictive of exercise electrocardiography in the investigation of male aircrew aged 40-60 years old? *Eur Heart J* 1992, 13(suppl H):59–69.

61. Papanicolaou MN, Califf RM, Hlatky MA, *et al.*: Prognostic implications of angiographically normal and insignificantly narrowed coronary arteries. *Am J Cardiol* 1986, 58:1181–1187.

62. Kemp HG, Kronmal RA, Vlietstra RE, and Coronary Artery Surgery Study Investigators: Seven year survival of patients with normal or near normal coronary arteriograms: A CASS registry study. *J Am Coll Cardiol* 1986, 7:479–483.

63. Proudfit WL, Bruschke AVG, Sones FM Jr: Clinical course of patients with normal or slightly or moderately abnormal coronary arteriograms: 10 year follow-up of 521 patients. *Circulation* 1980, 62:712–717.

64. Bruschke AVG, Van der Wall EE, Manger Cats V: The natural history of angiographically demonstrated coronary artery disease. *Eur Heart J* 1992, 13(suppl H):70–75.

65. Serruys PW, Breeman A: Coronary angioplasty: long term follow-up results and detection of restenosis: guidelines for aviation cardiology. *Eur Heart J* 1992, 13(suppl H):76–88.

66. Dargie HJ: Late results following coronary artery bypass grafting. *Eur Heart J* 1992, 13(suppl H):89–95.

67. Ferrer MI: *Pre-excitation Including the Wolff-Parkinson-White Syndrome and Other Related Syndromes*. Mt Kisco, NY: Futura; 1976.

68. Guize L, Soria R, Chaouat JC, *et al.*: Prevalence et evolution du syndrome de Wolff-Parkinson-White dans une population de 138,048 subjects. *Ann Med Interne* 1985, 136:474–478.

69. Toff WD, Camm AJ: Ventricular pre-excitation and professional aircrew licensing. *Eur Heart J* 1992, 13(suppl H):149–161.

70. Jackman W, Wang X, Fiday KJ, *et al.*: Catheter ablation of accessory atrioventricular pathways (Wolff-Parkinson-White syndrome) by radiofrequency current. *N Engl J Med* 1991, 324:1605–1611.

71. Rowland E, Morgado F: Sino-atrial node dysfunction, atrioventricular block and intraventricular conduction disturbances. *Eur Heart J* 1992, 13(suppl H):130–135.

72. Kulbertus HE: Implications of lone atrial fibrillation/flutter in the context of cardiovascular fitness to fly. *Eur Heart J* 1992, 13(suppl H):136–138.

73. Brand FN, Abbot RD, Kannel WB, *et al.*: Characteristics and prognosis of lone atrial fibrillation. 30-year follow-up in the Framingham study. *JAMA* 1985, 254:3449–3453.

74. Petersen P, Boysen G, Godtfudsen J, *et al.*: Placebo controlled randomised trial of warfarin and aspirin for prevention of thromboembolic complications in chronic atrial fibrillation. The Copenhagen AFASAK Study. *Lancet* 1989, 1:175–179.

75. Campbell RWF: Ventricular rhythm disturbances in the normal heart. *Eur Heart J* 1992, 13(suppl H):139–143.

76. Gorgels APM, Wellens HJJ, Vos MA: Aviation and antiarrhythmic medication. *Eur Heart J* 1992, 13(suppl H):144–148.

77. Cobb SM: Clinical usefulness of the Vaughan Williams classification system. *Eur Heart J* 1987, 8(suppl A):65–69.

78. Dreifus LS, Fisch C, Griffin JC, *et al.*: Guidelines for implantation of cardiac pacemakers and anti-arrhythmia devices. A report of the American College of Cardiology/American Heart Association Task Force on assessment of diagnostic and therapeutic cardiovascular procedures (committee on pacemaker implantation). *J Am Coll Cardiol* 1991, 18:1–13.

79. Toff WD, Edhag OK, Camm AJ: Cardiac pacing and aviation. *Eur Heart J* 1992, 13(suppl H):162–175.

80. Moore LG: Altitude-aggravated illness: examples from pregnancy and prenatal life. *Ann Emerg Med* 1987, 16:965–973.

81. Auerbach PS, Kizer KW: High-altitude illnesses. In *Emergency Medicine: A Comprehensive Study Guide*, ed 2. Edited by Tintinalli JE, Krome RL, Ruiz E. New York: McGraw-Hill; 1988:776–780.

82. Hackett PH, Hornbein TF: Disorders of high altitude. In *Textbook of Respiratory Medicine*. Edited by Nadel J, Murray J. Philadelphia: WB Saunders; 1989:1646–1663.

83. West JB: Limiting factors for exercise at extreme altitudes. *Clin Physiol* 1990, 10:265–272.

84. West JB, Hackett PH, Maret KH, *et al.*: Pulmonary gas exchange on the summit of Mt. Everest. *J Appl Physiol* 1983, 55:678–687.

85. Sutton JR, Reeves JT, Wagner PD, *et al.*: Operation Everest II: Oxygen transport during exercise at extreme simulated altitude. *J Appl Physiol* 1988, 64:1309–1321.

86. Winslow RM, Samaja M, West JB: Red cell function at extreme altitude on Mount Everest. *J Appl Physiol* 1984, 56:109–116.

86a. West JB, Lahiri E, eds: *High Altitude and Man*. American Physiological Society Clinical Physiology Series. Baltimore: Williams and Wilkins; 1984.

87. Tso E: High altitude illness. *Env Emerg* 1992, 10:231–247.

88. Montgomery AB, Mills J, Luce JM: Incidence of acute mountain sickness at intermediate altitude. *JAMA* 1989, 261:732–734.

89. Pigman EC, Karakla DW: Acute mountain sickness at intermediate altitude: military mountainous training. *Am J Emerg Med* 1990, 8:7–10.

90. Hultgren HN: High altitude medical problems. *West J Med* 1979, 131:82–83.

91. Hackett PH, Rennie D: The incidence, importance, and prophylaxis of acute mountain sickness. *Lancet* 1976, 2:1149–1154.

92. Meehan RT, Zavala DC: The pathophysiology of acute high-altitude illness. *Am J Med* 1982, 73:395–403.

93. Houston CS, Dickinson J: Cerebral forms of high-altitude illness. *Lancet* 1975, 2:758–761.

94. Schoene RB: High-altitude pulmonary edema: pathophysiology and clinical review. *Ann Emerg Med* 1987, 16:987–992.

95. Schoene RB: Pulmonary edema at high altitude. Review, pathophysiology and update. *Clin Chest Med* 1985, 6:491–507.

96. Lobenhoffer HP, Zink RA, Brendel W: High altitude pulmonary edema: analysis of 166 cases. In *High Altitude Physiology and Medicine*. Edited by Brendel W, Zink RA. New York: Springer; 1982.

97. Houston CS: Acute pulmonary edema of high altitude. *N Engl J Med* 1960, 263:478–480.

98. Hultgren HN: High altitude pulmonary edema. In *Lung Water and Solute Exchange*. Edited by Staub NC. New York: Marcel Dekker; 1978:437–469.

99. Schoene RB, Hackett PH, Henderson WR, *et al.*: High altitude pulmonary edema: characteristics of lung lavage fluid. *JAMA* 1986 256:63–69.

100. West JB, Tsukinoto K, Mathieu-Cortello O, *et al.*: Stress failure in pulmonary capillaries. *J Appl Physiol* 1991, 70:1731–1742.

101. Oelz O, Maggiorini M, Ritter M, *et al.*: Nifedipine for high altitude pulmonary edema. *Lancet* 1989, 2:1241–1244.

102. Bärtsch P, Maggiorini M, Ritter M, *et al.*: Prevention of high-altitude pulmonary edema by nifedipine. *N Engl J Med* 1991, 321:1248–1289.

103. Gamow RI, Geer GS, Kasic JF, *et al.*: Methods of gas-balance control to be used with a portable hyperbaric chamber in the treatment of high altitude illness. *J Wilderness Med* 1990, 1:165–180.

104. Taber RL: Protocols for the use of a portable hyperbaric chamber for the treatment of high altitude disorders. *J Wilderness Med* 1990, 1:181–192.

105. King SJ, Greenlee RR: Successful use of the Gamow Hyperbaric Bag in the treatment of altitude illness at Mount Everest. *J Wilderness Med* 1990, 1:193–202.

106. Cottrell JJ: Altitude exposures during aircraft flight. *Chest* 1988, 92:81–84.

107. Rodenberg H: Medical emergencies aboard commercial aircraft. *Ann Emerg Med* 1987, 16:1373–1377.

108. Cummins RO: High-altitude flights and risk of cardiac stress. *JAMA* 1988, 260:3669.

109. Cummins RO Schubach JA: Frequency and types of medical emergencies among commercial air travelers. *JAMA* 1989, 261:1295–1299.

110. Gong HL: Air travel and patients with chronic obstructive pulmonary disease. *Ann Intern Med* 1984, 100:595–597.

111. Houston CS, Sutton JR, Cymerman A, *et al.*: Operation Everest II: man at extreme altitude. *J Appl Physiol* 1987, 63:877–882.

112. Groves BM, Reeves JT, Sutton JR, *et al.*: Operation Everest II: elevated high-altitude pulmonary resistance unresponsive to oxygen. *J Appl Physiol* 1987, 63:521–530.

113. Reeves JT, Groves BM, Sutton JR, *et al.*: Operation Everest II: preservation of cardiac function at extreme altitude. *J Appl Physiol* 1987, 63:531–539.

114. Lord DR: *Spacelab: An International Success Story* (NASA SP-487). Washington, DC: National Aeronautics and Space Administration, Scientific and Technical Information Division; 1987.

115. Buckey JC, Gaffney FA, Lane LD, *et al.*: Central venous pressure in space. *N Engl J Med* 1993, 328:1853–1854.

116. Fritsch JM, Charles JB, Bennett MM, *et al.*: Short-duration space flight impairs human carotid baroreflex responses. *J Appl Physiol* 73:664–671, 1992.

117. Eckberg DL, Fritsch JM: Influence of ten day head-down bedrest on human carotid-cardiac reflex function. *Acta Physiol Scand* 1992; Suppl 604:69–76.

118. Divers Alert Network: Report on 1991 diving accidents. Durham, NC: Duke University Medical Center; 1992.

119. Bove AA: Cardiovascular disorders in diving. In *Diving Medicine*, ed 2. Edited by Bove AA, Davis JC. Philadelphia: WB Saunders, 1990:239–248.

120. Mebane GY, McIver NKI: Fitness to dive. In *The Physiology and Medicine of Diving*, ed 4. Edited by Bennett PB, Elliott DH. Philadelphia: WB Saunders; 1993:53–76.

121. Elliott DH, Moon RE: Manifestations of the decompression disorders. In *The Physiology and Medicine of Diving*, ed 4. Edited by Bennett PB, Elliott DH. Philadelphia: WB Saunders; 1993:481–505.

122. Bradley ME: Pulmonary barotrauma. In *Diving Medicine*, ed 2. Edited by Bove AA, Davis JC. Philadelphia: WB Saunders; 1990:188–191.

123. Melamed Y, Shupak A, Bitterman H: Medical problems associated with underwater diving. *N Engl J Med* 1992, 32:630–635.

124. Francis TRJ, Dutka AJ, Hallenback JM: Pathophysiology of decompression sickness. In *Diving Medicine*, ed 2. Edited by Bove AA, Davis JC. Philadelphia: WB Saunders; 1990:170–187.

125. United States Navy: *Diving Manual*, Vol I (Air Diving). Revision 3. Washington, DC: US Government Printing Office. February 13, 1993:8-41–8-44.

126. Davis JC: Treatment of decompression sickness and arterial gas embolism. In *Diving Medicine*, ed 2. Edited by Bove AA, Davis JC. Philadelphia: WB Saunders; 1990:249–260.

127. Moon RE, Gorman DF: Treatment of the decompression disorders. In *The Physiology and Medicine of Diving*, ed 4. Edited by Bennett PB, Elliott DH. Philadelphia: WB Saunders; 1993:506–541.

128. Hong SK: Breath-hold diving. In *Diving Medicine*, ed 2. Edited by Bove AA, Davis JC. Philadelphia: WB Saunders; 1990:65–67.

129. Gooden BA: The diving response in clinical medicine. *Aviat Environ Med* 1982, 53:273–276.

130. Scholander PF, Hammel HT, LeMessurier H, *et al.*: Circulatory adjustment in pearl divers. *J Appl Physiol* 1967, 23:18–22.

131. Moon RE, Camporesi EM, Kisslo JA: Patent foramen ovale and decompression sickness in divers. *Lancet* 1989, 1:513–514.

132. Mebane GY: Hypothermia. In *Diving Medicine*, ed 2. Edited by Bove AA, Davis JC. Philadelphia: WB Saunders; 1990:95–104.

133. Sterba JA: Thermal problems: prevention and treatment. In *The Physiology and Medicine of Diving*, ed 4. Edited by Bennett PB, Elliott DH. Philadelphia: WB Saunders; 1993:301–341.

134. Fisch C: Electrocardiography and vectorcardiography. In *Heart Disease*, 4th ed. Edited by Braunwald E. Philadelphia: WB Saunders; 1992:116–160.

135. Wilmshurst PT, Byrne JC, Webb-Peploe MM: Relation between interatrial shunts and decompression sickness in divers. *Lancet* 1989, 2:1302–1306.

INDEX